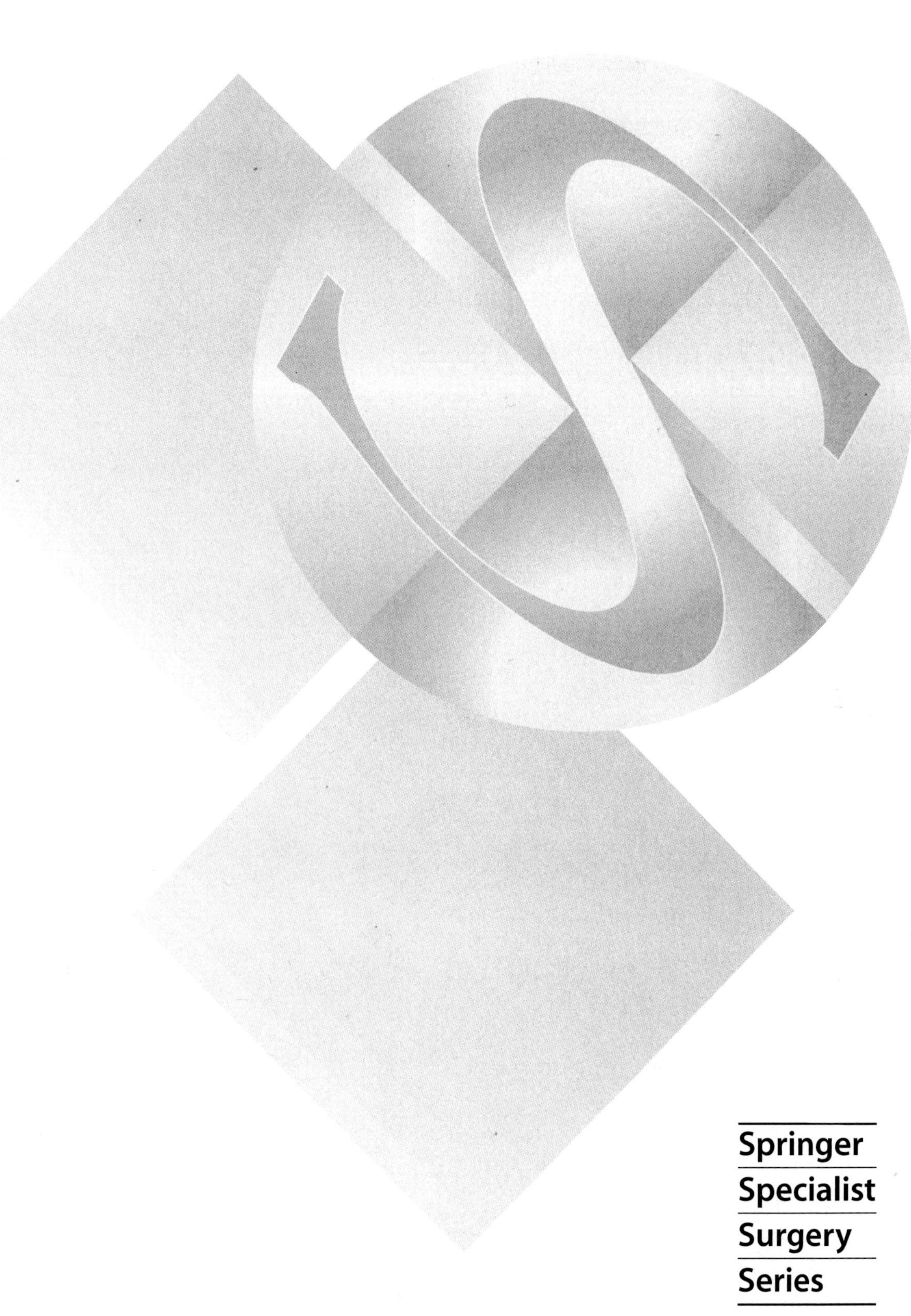

Springer
Specialist
Surgery
Series

Other titles in this series include:

Upper Gastrointestinal Surgery, edited by Fielding & Hallissey, 2005
Neurosurgery: Principles and Practice, edited by Moore & Newell, 2004
Transplantation Surgery, Edited by Hakim & Danovitch, 2001

Alun H. Davies and Colleen M. Brophy (Eds)

Vascular Surgery

With 46 Illustrations

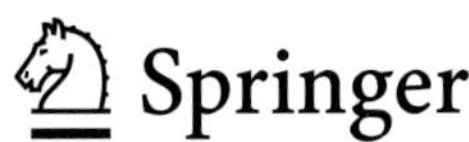 Springer

Alun H. Davies, MA, DM, FRCS
Department of Vascular Surgery
Reader and Honorary Consultant in Surgery
Imperial College London
Charing Cross Hospital
London, UK

Colleen M. Brophy, MD, FACS
Chief of Vascular Surgery
Carl T. Hayden VAMC
Research Professor Bioengineering
Arizona State University
Clinical Professor of Surgery
University of Arizona
Phoenix, AZ
USA

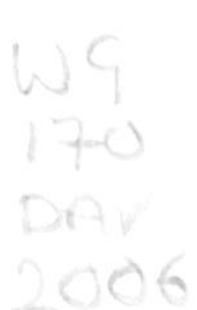

A catalogue record for this book is available from the British Libuary

Library of Congress Control Number: 2005923614

ISBN-10: 1-85233-288-3   Printed on acid-free paper.
ISBN-13: 978-1-85233-288-4

Printed in the United States of America.   (BS/MVY)

9 8 7 6 5 4 3 2 1

Springer Science+Business Media
springeronline.com

Preface

This book provides coverage of a broad range of topics in the field of vascular surgery to residents, registrars in training, and to recent graduates of training programs. The book is meant to be a practical rendition of the basic knowledge and clinical management required for optimal care of vascular surgical patients. Each chapter contains input from specialists in vascular surgery from the United States and Great Britain. There are up-to-date perspectives on common clinical conditions and emerging techniques encountered by vascular surgeons from both an American and British perspective. The chapters are organized under broad topics including medical management, noninvasive and invasive diagnostic approaches, perioperative care, indications and approaches for vascular procedures, and a discussion of newer endovascular techniques. The information contained in this text is not meant to be exhaustive, but rather a practical overview that will be useful in directing the management of patients with vascular diseases. The information in this text is also meant to be useful for certification examinations and recent graduates of vascular surgical training programs can utilize this text as an update of the most important vascular topics.

Alun H. Davies
Colleen M. Brophy

Contents

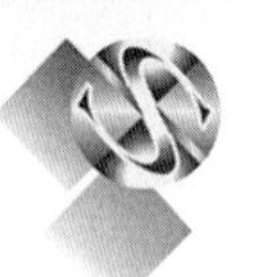

Contributors

Jill J.F. Belch, MB ChB, MD, FRCP
Peripheral Vascular Diseases Research Unit,
Department of Medicine, Ninewells Hospital
and Medical School, Dundee, UK

Andrew W. Bradbury, BSc, MB ChB, MD, FRCS
University Department of Vascular Surgery,
Research Institute, Birmingham Heartlands
Hospital, Birmingham, UK

Colleen M. Brophy, MD, FACS
Chief of Vascular Surgery, Carl T. Hayden
VAMC, Research Professor Bioengineering
Arizona State University, Clinical Professor of
Surgery, University of Arizona, Phoenix, AZ,
USA

Elliot L. Chaikof, MD, PhD, FACS
Division of Vascular Surgery, Brown
Whitehead Department of Surgery, Emory
University School of Medicine, Atlanta, GA,
USA

Nicholas J.W. Cheshire, MB ChB, MD, FRCS
Regional Vascular Unit, St Mary's Hospital,
London, UK

Jeremy S. Crane, MB ChB, MRCS
Regional Vascular Unit, St Mary's Hospital,
London, UK

R. Clement Darling III, MD
Institute for Vascular Health and Disease,
Albany Medical Center, Albany, NY, USA

Philip Davey, MB ChB
Newcastle upon Tyne, UK

Alun H. Davies, MA, DM, FRCS
Department of Vascular Surgery, Reader and
Honorary Consultant in Surgery, Imperial
College, Charing Cross Hospital, London, UK
London

Meryl Davis
Charing Cross Hospital, London, UK

Mark F. Fillinger, MD, FACS
Department of Vascular Surgery, Dartmouth
Medical School, Dartmouth-Hitchcock
Medical Center, Lebanon, NH, USA

F.G.R. Fowkes, MB ChB, PhD, FRCPE, FFPHM
Wolfson Unit for Prevention of Peripheral
Vascular Diseases, Public Health Sciences, The
University of Edinburgh, Edinburgh, UK

George Geroulakos, MD, FRCS, DIC, PhD
Vascular Unit, Ealing Hospital, London, UK

Vivienne J. Halpern, MD, FACS
Department of Surgery, Division of Vascular
Surgery, Long Island Jewish Medical Center,
New Hyde Park, NY, USA

Sacha Hamdani
Institute for Vascular Health and Disease,
Albany Medical Center, Albany, NY, USA

Jamal J. Hoballah, MD
Department of Surgery, Division of Vascular
Surgery, University of Iowa Hospitals and
Clinics, Iowa City, IA, USA

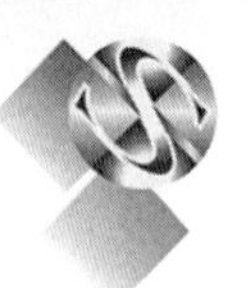

Jonathan R.B. Hutt, BA, MBBS
Department of Accident and Emergency,
Imperial College, Charing Cross Hospital,
London, UK

Paul B. Kreienberg, MD
Institute for Vascular Health and Disease,
Albany Medical Center, Albany, NY, USA

Christopher J. Kwolek, MD, FACS
Division of Vascular Surgery, Massachusetts
General Hospital, Boston, MA, USA

Peter H. Lin, MD, FACS
Division of Vascular Surgery and
Endovascular Therapy, Michael E. DeBakey
Department of Surgery, Baylor College of
Medicine, Houston, TX, USA

David C. Mitchell, MA, MS, FRCS
Department of Surgery, Southmead Hospital,
North Bristol NHS Trust, Bristol, UK

Farid Moulla, MD, MBA
Department of Anaesthetics, Charing Cross
Hospital, London, UK

Andrew H. Muir, MB ChB
Peripheral Vascular Diseases Research Unit,
Department of Medicine, Ninewells Hospital
and Medical School, Dundee, UK

A. Ross Naylor, MB ChB, MD, FRCS
Department of Vascular Surgery, Leicester
Royal Infirmary, Leicester, UK

C. Keith Ozaki, MD, FACS
Division of Vascular Surgery and
Endovascular Therapy, University of Florida
College of Medicine, Gainesville, FL, USA

Kathleen J. Ozsvath, MD
Institute for Vascular Health and Disease,
Albany Medical Center, Albany, NY, USA

Peter J. Pappas, MD
Department of Surgery, Section of Vascular
Surgery, University of Medicine and Dentistry
of New Jersey – New Jersey Medical School,
Newark, NJ, USA

Peter A. Robless, MB ChB, FRCS, MD, FEBVS
Department of Cardiac, Thoracic and Vascular
Surgery, National University Hospital,
Singapore, Republic of Singapore

Eva M. Rzucidlo, MD
Department of Vascular Surgery, Dartmouth-
Hitchcock Medical Center, Lebanon, NH,
USA

Rajabrata Sarkar, MD, PhD
Division of Vascular Surgery, University of
California, San Francisco, CA, USA

Sherry D. Scovell, MD
Division of Vascular Surgery, Beth Israel
Deaconess Medical Center, Boston, MA, USA

William L. Smead, MD
Division of General Vascular Surgery, Ohio
State University, Columbus, OH, USA

Frank C.T. Smith, BSc, MD, FRCS
University Department of Surgery, University
of Bristol, Bristol Royal Infirmary, Bristol, UK

Laila Tabatabai
Institute for Vascular Health and Disease,
Albany Medical Center, Albany, NY, USA

Kong T. Tan, MB ChB, BAO, FRCSI, FRCR
Sheffield Vascular Institute, Vascular Office,
Northern General Hospital, Sheffield, UK

William G. Tennant, BSc, MB ChB, MD, FRCS
Department of Vascular Surgery, Queens
Medical Centre, Nottingham, UK

Steven M. Thomas, MRCP, FRCR, MSc
Sheffield Vascular Institute, Vascular Office,
Northern General Hospital, Sheffield, UK

Gilbert R. Upchurch, Jr., MD
Surgery Department, Vascular Surgery
Section, University of Michigan Health
System, Ann Arbor, MI, USA

Michael G. Wyatt, MB BS, MSc, MD, FRCS
Department of Vascular Surgery, Freeman
Hospital, Newcastle upon Tyne, UK

1

The Epidemiology and Etiology of Atherosclerosis

Paul B. Kreienberg, R. Clement Darling III, and F.G.R. Fowkes

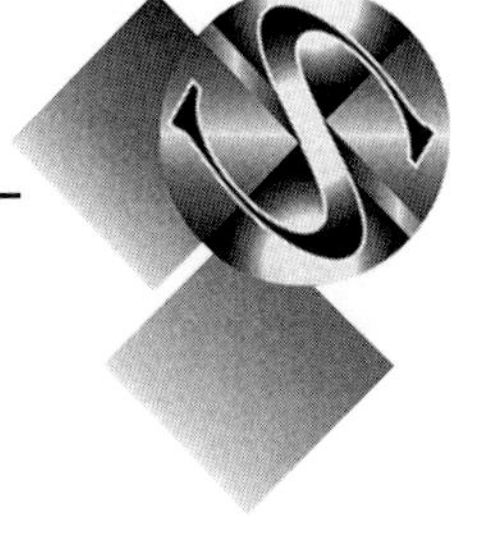

The underlying disorder in the vast majority of cases of cardiovascular disease is atherosclerosis, for which low-density lipoprotein (LDL) cholesterol is recognized as a major risk factor. Evidence from epidemiological and clinical studies continues to improve our understanding of the pathogenesis of atherosclerosis. Atherosclerosis contributes to myocardial infarction, stroke, and peripheral vascular disease. Despite major advances in the development of diagnostic methods and effective treatments, cardiovascular disease remains the leading cause of mortality in the Western world.

Vascular surgeons treat patients who have already developed end-stage cardiovascular disease. These surgeons have a unique opportunity to intervene not only in the arterial pathology itself, but also in the main factors that contribute to the development of atherosclerosis. Atherosclerosis is a systemic disorder and all aspects of the disease must be addressed in treating these patients.

Epidemiology

Cardiovascular disease is responsible for approximately 30% of all mortality worldwide, amounting to approximately 15 million deaths (Sueta et al., 1999). Furthermore, cardiovascular disease is the principal cause of mortality in all developed countries, responsible for 50% of all deaths, and is also emerging as a prominent public health problem in developing countries, representing approximately 16% of all deaths. In the United States cardiovascular disease is the most common cause of mortality in both men and women and accounts for almost 500,000 deaths/year. Additionally, 58,800,000 Americans have one or more types of cardiovascular disease according to current estimates (Table 1.1).

Coronary artery disease (CAD) has been recognized as the leading cause of death since the late 1940s. Hypertension, hypercholesterolemia, cigarette smoking, and diabetes mellitus were identified as key contributors to atherosclerosis and the development of cardiovascular risk. These risk factors are also related to cerebrovascular and peripheral vascular disease (Table 1.2).

The data support aggressive treatment of atherosclerosis in populations at risk. In patients with peripheral arterial disease (PAD), there is a high prevalence of myocardial infarction, stroke, and increased mortality. Lack of patient and physician awareness of peripheral vascular disease is associated with low atherosclerosis risk factor treatment intensity (Sueta et al., 1999). In this study of patients with known cardiovascular disease, only 35% had smoking behavior treated, 73% had lipid abnormalities treated, and 71% were on antiplatelet therapy. Recognition and treatment in patients with symptomatic or asymptomatic [ankle-brachial index (ABI) <0.9] PAD were significantly lower than the rates for patients with CAD.

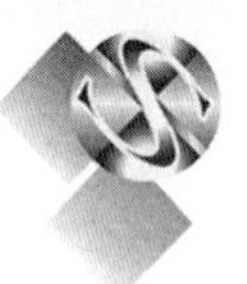

Table 1.1. Cardiovascular Disease in the United States: 58.8 million Americans have one or more types of cardiovascular disease

Type	Number (in millions)
Hypertension	50
Coronary artery disease	12
Stroke	4.4
Congestive heart failure	4.6
Peripheral arterial disease	8.4

Table 1.2. Selected risk factors for atherosclerosis

Age
Diabetes
Smoking
Hyperlipidemia
Hypertension
Hyperhomocystinemia
Hyperfibrinogenemia

Risk Factors

Smoking

Nearly 440,000 Americans die each year of smoking-related illness, at a cost of about $50 billion annually. In general, smoking is associated with a threefold increase in the risk for peripheral atherosclerosis (Hiatt et al., 1995). Two large follow-up studies of patients with intermittent claudication demonstrate the benefits of smoking cessation (Jonason and Bergstrom, 1987; Smith et al., 1996). In these studies, 11% to 27% of the patients complied with the advice to stop smoking. Within 3 years of stopping, there was no reduction in limb-threatening complications of the vascular disease. However, after 7 years, rest pain had developed in 16% of persistent smokers, but in none of those who had stopped smoking. After 10 years, 53% of persistent smokers suffered a myocardial infarction compared to only 11% of stopped smokers; 54% of persistent smokers died compared to 18% of stopped smokers. In a comprehensive review of the literature, abstinence from smoking was found to be associated consistently with better outcomes following revascularization, lower amputation rates, and improved survival (Hirsch et al., 1997). However, smoking cessation had probably only a minimal effect in improving walking distance in claudicants.

Hyperlipidemia

An estimated 50% of American adults have total blood cholesterol levels of 200 mg/dL and higher, and about 20% of American adults have levels of 240 mg/dL or higher. Levels of 240 mg/dL or higher are considered high risk and levels from 200 to 239 mg/dL are considered borderline high risk. Evidence linking lipids to atherosclerosis has grown, suggesting that lowering serum cholesterol, whether through diet and lifestyle modification alone or in combination with cholesterol-lowering pharmacotherapy, decreases the incidence of vascular events. For example a 1 mg/dL increase in high-density lipoprotein (HDL) cholesterol concentration is associated with a 2% to 3% decrease in CAD and a 4% to 5% decrease in cardiovascular mortality. Data from the Multiple Risk Factor Intervention Trial (MRFIT) demonstrate a strong, graded, positive correlation between serum cholesterol and cardiovascular mortality rate (Neaton and Wentworth, 1992). Elevations in lipoprotein (a) [Lp(a)] constitute a more recently recognized independent risk factor for cardiovascular disease. Elevations of LP(a) greater than 30 mg/dL increase the risk of CAD approximately twofold (Beckman et al., 2002).

Diabetes

Diabetes mellitus magnifies the risk of cardiovascular morbidity and mortality. Diabetics have a two- to fourfold increase in the risk of CAD. Diabetics, particularly those with non–insulin-dependent diabetes mellitus (NIDDM) are at high risk of vascular disease because of high levels of triglycerides, LDL, and very low-density lipoprotein (VLDL) particles. Patients with NIDDM tend to produce small, dense LDL particles that are more vulnerable to oxidation. Other mechanisms for the adverse effects of diabetes that promote vascular disease include glycation of arterial wall proteins, enhancement of LDL oxidation, microvascular disease of the vasa vasorum, change in cellular function, promotion of thrombogenesis, and the development of renal disease and hypertension (Beckman et al., 2002).

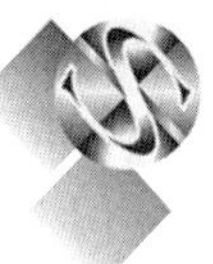

Hypertension

Hypertension is a well-recognized risk factor for atherosclerotic disease, particularly stroke and to a lesser extent ischemic heart disease and peripheral vascular disease. There are several possible mechanisms for the underlying potentiation of atherogenesis by hypertension, including direct mechanical disruptive effects, actions on vasoactive hormones, and changes in the response characteristics of the arterial wall. It is thought that, although hypertension may potentiate or enhance atherogenesis, hypertension alone is probably not sufficient for atherogenesis (Valentine et al., 1996).

Homocysteine

Alterations in homocysteine metabolism are an independent risk factor for the development of vascular disease. Elevations of plasma homocysteine levels are associated with increased risks of all forms of atherosclerotic vascular disease. Homocysteine can react with LDL cholesterol to form oxidized LDL, which is found in early atherosclerotic lesions. Through this mechanism homocysteine can promote endothelial dysfunction, lipid peroxidation, and oxidation of LDL cholesterol.

Atherogenesis and Lipid Metabolism

Central to the discussion of atherogenesis is the metabolism of the peripheral blood lipoproteins. These are a complex macromolecule of lipid and protein in which the nonpolar lipid core is surrounded by a polar monolayer of phospholipids and heads of free cholesterol and apolipoproteins. This structure allows for the transport of the relatively insoluble lipids through the liquid plasma. The lipoproteins differ in their proportions of lipid content and proteins found on their surface. Lipid disorders alter the composition and structure of the lipoprotein. For example, as mentioned earlier, patients with high triglycerides produce LDL with a higher protein-to-lipid ratio, yielding a small dense LDL.

Cholesterol

The body uses cholesterol for numerous functions including cell membrane biogenesis, steroid synthesis, and formation of bile acids. The human body can produce all the cholesterol it needs. The liver is the primary producer of endogenous cholesterol. Cholesterol is derived from the in vivo form acetate by a mechanism characterized by a rate-limiting step in which 3-hydroxy-3-methylglutaryl coenzyme A (HMG CoA) is converted into melavalonic acid by HMG CoA reductase. Statin-type drugs inhibits this step. This action decreases endogenous cholesterol production.

Lipoproteins

The major lipoproteins are chylomicrons, VLDL, intermediate-density lipoprotein (IDL), LDL, and HDL.

Chylomicrons are larger triglyceride carrying particles formed after ingestion of a meal. They result from the processing of ingested fat by intestinal mucosal cells. They are transported to the thoracic duct via the intestinal lymphatics to eventually end up in the peripheral circulation. At peripheral sites the chylomicrons are acted upon by lipoprotein lipase bound to capillary endothelium. Chylomicrons have the lowest density of any of the lipoproteins.

Very low-density lipoproteins are not as large as chylomicrons and are slightly more dense. They carry triglycerides and other fats synthesized in the liver. The IDLs are formed when some of the triglyceride is removed from VLDL. Under normal circumstances it is removed so rapidly from plasma that its concentration is quite low.

Low-density lipoprotein is normally produced from the catabolism of VLDL. It is the major carrier of cholesterol in the plasma. It is cleared by both receptor-mediated and non–receptor-mediated processes from the plasma. Low-density lipoprotein may be modified through acetylation, oxidation, or both. These modified forms are particularly important in the development of atherogenesis. First, these molecules are cytotoxic and may damage the vascular endothelium, initiating atherosclerosis. They may also aggregate in the intima of the vessel wall and are chemotactic for inflammatory cells such as monocytes. These modified LDL particles have a decreased affinity for the normal LDL receptor and thus require clearance through other scavenger pathways.

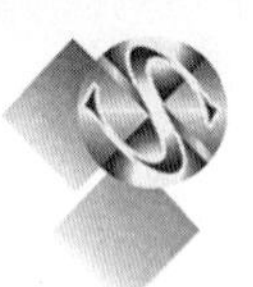

Lipoprotein (a)

Lipoprotein (a) [Lp(a)] is a particle comparable in size to LDL. It is assembled from LDL and a large glycoprotein called apolipoprotein (a). It has a decreased affinity for the LDL receptor compared with LDL itself. Evidence links elevated levels of Lp(a) with increased risk of vascular disease. Lipoprotein (a) may also be taken up by scavenger pathways and thus accumulates in foam cells in the early atherosclerotic lesion.

Small-Density LDL

Alterations of LDL metabolism may create species of LDL particles with higher protein-lipid concentrations. Increased levels of these types of particles (termed small, dense LDL) are associated with increased risk of atherosclerotic disease and with elevated triglycerides (TGs) and low levels of HDL cholesterol. The mechanism linking these particles and hypertriglyceridemia relates to the production of chylomicrons and VLDL that are particularly rich in TGs. Catabolism of these TG-saturated VLDL particles produce LDL particles that have higher than normal TG content. These TG-rich LDLs are susceptible to further lipolysis by hepatic lipase, producing a decrease in size and increase in the density of the particle. Small, dense LDLs are believed to be more susceptible to oxidative modification and hence are thought to be highly atherogenic. Metabolic disorders such as diabetes and insulin resistance syndrome often produce this lipid particle.

High-Density Lipoprotein

High-density lipoprotein is the lipoprotein responsible for the transport of cholesterol from cells to other lipoprotein or catabolic sites. High-density lipoprotein may be formed de novo in the liver and intestines, and intravascularly from the redundant surface material of chylomicrons and VLDL. Newly formed HDL consists of free cholesterol phospholipids and apoproteins. Free cholesterol from cells and perhaps from other lipoproteins reacts in the plasma with a complex containing the enzyme lecithin-cholesterol acetyltransferase (LCAT), apoprotein A-1, and an HDL-associated apoprotein D. This complex attaches to, and the cholesterol is esterified by, LCAT. As nonpolar esterified cholesterol migrates to the interior of the particle, a sphere with an outer coating of free cholesterol and an inner core of esterified cholesterol and small amounts of triglyceride is formed.

In epidemiological studies elevated HDL levels are associated with a reduced risk of atherosclerotic vascular disease. It is thought that HDL mediates this benefit through reverse cholesterol transport, which does not involve a direct route from peripheral tissues to the liver but rather depends on repeated transfer of cholesterol esters among lipoproteins before excretion through the liver.

Lipid Metabolism

Chylomicrons are formed in the intestine from ingested fat and taken by the intestinal lymphatics to peripheral blood and then to adipose and other tissues. There, most of the triglyceride is acted upon by the enzyme lipoprotein lipase, transported across the cell membrane as fatty acid and monoglyceride, resynthesized into triglyceride, and stored. When necessary, intracellular triglyceride can undergo lipolysis. The released fatty acid is then transported out of the cell and bound to albumin to be transported in the plasma. After lipolysis a remnant of the chylomicron is transported to the liver and catabolized as a portion of the particle apolipoprotein A [Apo(A)] free cholesterol, and phospholipid is transferred to HDL formed in the liver; HDL may also pick up free cholesterol from cells. The cholesterol from other cells is esterified under the influence of LCAT. This ester is then available for storage or transport.

Very low-density lipoprotein is synthesized in the liver from fatty acids obtained from the processing of chylomicrons or from endogenously produced triglyceride. These particles are smaller and more dense than chylomicrons. The apolipoproteins associated with VLDL are Apos B-100, C-1, C-II, C-III, and E.

Very low-density lipoprotein exchanges triglycerides for cholesterol esters from HDL. Like chylomicrons, lipoprotein lipase catalyzes the hydrolysis of triglyceride in VLDL to fatty acids that are used by muscle or stored as fat in adipose tissue. This hydrolysis step reduces VLDL to IDL. Intermediate-density lipoprotein can be taken up by the LDL receptor or be reduced to LDL by hepatic lipase. Intermediate-

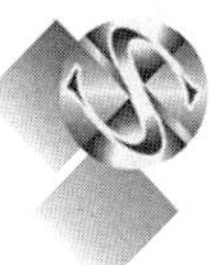

density lipoprotein clearance is mediated by Apo E, which has a higher affinity for the LDL receptor than Apo BB. Low-density lipoprotein contains only the apolipoprotein B-100. Two thirds of the LDL is cleared through the LDL receptor, 60% to 70% of which is located in the liver. Peripheral cells can also take up LDL for membrane biogenesis and steroid synthesis.

Low-density lipoprotein is removed from plasma by binding to these specific receptors located in many tissues, including the liver. After binding, LDL is internalized and metabolized to free cholesterol and other products. Cholesterol is stored in cells as the ester. Saturation of LDL receptors inhibits intracellular cholesterol synthesis by inhibiting HMG CoA reductase. This negative feedback system operates so that intracellular cholesterol synthesis varies inversely with the availability of intracellular LDL.

Theories of Atherogenesis

Numerous theories exist regarding the pathogenesis of atherosclerosis (Table 1.3). One unifying hypothesis linking the various theories is the "response to injury" model that in a broad context embraces many aspects of the theories (Ross, 1999).

The Atheroma

Whatever the initiating process, the first lesion of arteriosclerosis occurs with the entry of LDL through the intima and into the arterial wall. The lipids of human plasma are similar to what can be found in these early lesions. These early lesions, termed *fatty streaks*, are minimally raised yellow lesions found in the aorta of infants and children. The lipid deposits in these lesions are found within macrophages and smooth muscle cells. Foam cells, which are macrophages containing lipid particles, are

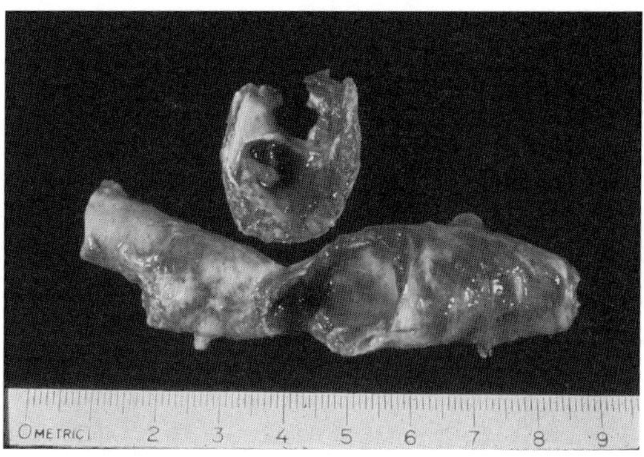

Figure 1.1. Atherosclerotic plaque. The appearance of complex atherosclerotic plaque removed during a carotid endarterectomy.

characteristic of these early lesions. It is believed that these lesions represent the precursor to more advanced atherosclerotic lesions. As these lesions grow they then intrude into the arterial lumen.

Fibrous plaques are composed of large numbers of smooth muscle cells and connective tissue forming a cap over an inner core containing mainly lipid cholesterol esters believed to be from disrupted foam cells. The fibrous cap may provide structural support or may function as a barrier to sequester thrombogenic debris in the underlying plaque from the arterial lumen. These plaques can show evidence of uneven and episodic growth. Intermittent ulceration and healing may occur, and there is evidence that thrombi formed on lesions are incorporated into them and resurfaced with a fibrocellular cap and an intact endothelial layer. Whether all fibrous plaques are characteristic of advanced atherosclerosis evolving from the fatty streak is uncertain. However, fibrous plaques often appear chronologically after fatty streaks in the same anatomical locations and characterize clinically apparent atherosclerosis.

Complicated plaques comprise the end stage of atherosclerosis and cause clinical symptoms (Fig. 1.1). These are fibrous plaques that have become calcified, ulcerated, or necrotic. The consensus, at least for coronary ischemic events, is that they are thrombotic in origin, resulting from the rupture of the complicated atherosclerotic lesions. In most patients myocardial infarction occurs as a result of erosion or

Table 1.3. Pathogenesis of atherogenesis

Response to injury
Monoclonal hypothesis
Lipid hypothesis
Inflammatory
Lesion regression
Unstable plaque

uneven thinning and rupture of the fibrous cap, often at the shoulders of the lesion where macrophages enter and accumulate. Degradation of the fibrous cap may occur by release of metalloproteinases, collagenases, and elastases by these cells.

Response to Injury

The response-to-injury hypothesis initially proposed that endothelial denudation was the first step in atherosclerosis. More recent data suggest that endothelial dysfunction rather denudation is the primary problem. According to this model, atherogenesis is a response to injury of the vascular endothelium. At its mildest, atherosclerosis may represent a reparative process that leads to thrombus formation and smooth muscle cell proliferation at the site of endothelial injury. The production of the endothelial injury may be from hypertension, cytotoxic molecules, or blood flow changes. Atherosclerosis develops at sites exposed to unusual shear stress, such as in the abdominal aortic bifurcation. Hypercholesterolemia, hyperhomocystinemia, and smoking may all contribute to endothelial injury.

Lipid Hypothesis

Cholesterol accumulation in atherosclerotic lesions was initially considered an incidental accompaniment of the degenerative changes in the arterial wall. Forty years ago the normal range of blood cholesterol encompassed everyone within two standard deviations from the mean. Cardiologists and cardiovascular surgeons concluded that serum cholesterol must be unimportant because most myocardial infarctions occurred in patients well below this arbitrary normal level. The notion that the mean cholesterol level in the average American was high enough to cause serious clinical illness seemed improbable, and thus the lipid hypothesis had few advocates.

However, the most important study to demonstrate that blood cholesterol is a risk factor for CAD is the Framingham study. The results of this study demonstrated the risk for developing clinically evident CAD was a continuous curvilinear function of blood cholesterol level. Larger trials would follow substantiating the link between cholesterol level and clinical

risk, so that eventually experts agreed on the causal link between blood cholesterol levels and CAD risk.

As mentioned previously, the endothelial injury hypothesis postulated the loss of endothelial cell integrity; however, in areas of atheroma often the endothelium remains intact. These results suggested that monocytes penetrate the intact endothelium, settle in the intima, and then take up cholesterol particles to become foam cells. The lesion is initiated by elevated blood cholesterol characterized by lipid accumulation in foam cells.

This process is accelerated in vivo under conditions in which the circulating LDL is modified to oxidized LDL. Many biological properties of oxidized LDL make it more atherogenic than native LDL including cytotoxicity. These facts are supported by data that demonstrate benefits of antioxidants in preventing oxidation of LDL on lesion progression.

Inflammatory Theory

This theory stems from the observations that atherosclerosis represents a different stage in chronic inflammatory process in the artery. Unchecked, this process may eventually result in the advanced complicated lesion.

The different forms of injury increase the adhesiveness of the endothelium to leukocytes and platelets. It also induces the endothelium to have procoagulant activities and to form vasoactive cytokines and growth factors. The response then triggers the migration and proliferation of smooth muscle cells that form the fibrous lesion. Macrophages and T lymphocytes regulate the majority of the inflammatory component of this process.

Macrophages have the ability to produce cytokines (such as tumor necrosis factor-α, interleukin-1, and transforming growth factor-β), proteolytic enzymes, and growth factors such as platelet-derived growth factor and insulin-like growth factor. In addition, they express class II histocompatibility antigens that allow them to present antigens to T lymphocytes.

Plaque Regression

Plaque regression refers to a discernible decrease in intimal plaque. Apparent regression

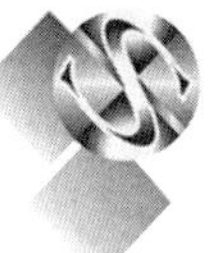

of atherosclerosis has been documented by serial contrast arteriography in both coronary and peripheral vascular beds. Although plaque regression is usually thought of as a decrease in plaque bulk, it may proceed by other means. This lessening of luminal intrusion on sequential angiography coincides experimentally with decreased plaque size and lipid content. However, as intimal plaques enlarge, a closely associated enlargement of the affected artery segment tends to limit the stenosing effect of the enlarging intimal plaque (Glagov et al., 1987). In the human left main coronary artery such enlargement keeps pace with increases in intimal plaque and is effective in preventing lumen stenosis until plaque area occupies on the average approximately 40% of the cross-sectional area. Continued plaque enlargement or complication apparently exceeds the ability of the artery to enlarge and stenosis may then develop. Thus the development of critical lumen stenosis, the maintenance of normal cross-sectional area, and the development of an increase in luminal diameter are dependent on the respective rates of plaque growth and arterial enlargement.

Unstable Plaque

Plaque rupture is the major cause of acute coronary syndromes (Table 1.4). Often, however, plaque rupture may be asymptomatic but contributes to the rapid growth of lesions as thrombus fibroses.

A number of characteristics distinguish stable plaque from the unstable plaque that might produce acute symptoms. The common underlying feature of the unstable plaque is thinning of the fibrous cap, which is composed mainly of vascular smooth muscle cells and matrix. In plaques that have ruptured, the fibrous cap at the shoulders of lesion where the cap meets the normal segment of the arterial wall is where this thinning occurs. Another typical feature of the unstable plaque is a large

necrotic core filled with lipid and cellular debris with intraplaque and intraluminal thrombosis. The final feature is that of intense macrophage infiltration. Proteases and elastases released form inflammatory cells may contribute to the thinning of the fibrous cap seen in these lesions. Additionally, they contribute to the thrombotic nature of the unstable plaque through the elaboration of tissue factor.

Prevention

Hypotheses of pathogenesis and etiology of atherosclerosis have been tested through the manipulation of risk factors associated with this disease process. Among the various strategies tried, only those strategies that promote a decrease in LDL or an increase in HDL have been associated with favorable changes in the plaque itself.

Additionally, large epidemiological studies have demonstrated that lower cholesterol levels are associated with a lower overall risk of morbidity and mortality due to CAD (Martin et al., 1986). Numerous clinical trials support these epidemiological data, and show that cholesterol lowering therapies lead to a significant reduction in morbidity and mortality associated with CAD. Additionally, these benefits extend to a population presenting with peripheral arterial disease as well. The benefits of statin therapy to decrease risk is seen as early as the first year of treatment and extend not only to prevention of cardiovascular disease but also to the quality of life. In this era of evidence-based medicine, it would be difficult not to treat patients identified at risk with statin therapy based on these data. Recommended treatment guidelines are given in Table 1.5.

However, one must understand that the treatment to prevent or stabilize atherosclerotic plaques extends not just to those patients with demonstrable severely stenotic lesions. In fact, it seems to be that most myocardial infarctions occur at sites that did not have prior angiographically recognized severe lesions. These facts are supported by the finding that thallium studies in stable CAD show that the site of stress-induced myocardial ischemia is frequently not the site of myocardial infarction. To extend this concept, it would seem reasonable to start statin therapy in patients at risk before the

Table 1.4. Characteristics of the unstable plaque

Thinning of fibrous cap
Lipid core
Intraplaque thrombosis
Macrophage infiltration

Table 1.5. Risk factors that modify low-density lipoprotein

Cigarette smoking
Hypertension (>140/90) or on antihypertensive
  medication
Low HDL cholesterol (<40 mg/dL)
Family history of premature coronary artery disease in
  male first-degree relative or female <65 years of
  age
Age (men >45 or women >55 years of age)

Risk categories that modify LDL cholesterol goals

Risk category	LDL goal
Coronary artery disease	<100 mg/dL
Multiple (2+) risk factors	<130 mg/dL
0–1 risk factors	<160 mg/dL

development of these unstable plaques or to stabilize the ones already present.

Controversy

The importance of treating patients to lower the cholesterol levels and to lessen the risk of developing atherosclerosis is well accepted. However, the question remains whether there is a threshold below which cholesterol reduction may translate into clinical benefit.

On average drug therapy with simvastatin loweres LDL cholesterol levels by 35% and reduces heart risk by 34% (Pedersen et al., 1998). The goal of this study was to reduce total cholesterol below 200. However, many patients achieved reductions greater than this and were associated with continuing but progressively smaller reductions in heart attack risk. This subgroup analysis estimated a 1% reduction in LDL, reducing the risk of major coronary events by 1.7%. However, at what point this benefit can be extrapolated to remains to be determined. Another active debate is whether the treatment for acute myocardial infarction in high-risk patients should be lipid-lowering therapy rather than revascularization (Forrester and Shah, 1997).

Additional therapeutic approaches that are receiving attention include antioxidant treatment such as vitamin E. In a situation where oxidation of LDL is a major target in atherogenesis, antioxidant therapy obviously might play a role. To what extent it may be of benefit is still under investigation.

Fundamental to the treatment of atherosclerosis is recognizing it as a systemic disease with the potential to affect a variety of end organs. Therefore, when patients are identified it appears advantageous to screen, counsel, and treat patients as soon as possible.

References

Beckman JA, Creager MA, Libby P. (2002) JAMA 287: 2570–81.
Forrester JS, Shah PK. (1997) Circulation 96:1360–2.
Glagov S, Weisenberg E, Zarins CK, Stankunavicius R, Kolettis GJ. (1987) N Engl J Med 316:1371–5.
Hiatt WR, Hoag S, Hamman RF. (1995) Circulation 91: 1472–9.
Hirsch AT, Treat-Jacobson D, Lando HA, Hatsukami DK. (1997) Vasc Med 2:243–51.
Jonason T, Bergstrom R. (1987) Acta Med Scand 221:253–60.
Martin MJ, Hulley SB, Browner WS, Kuller LH, Wentworth D. (1986) Lancet 2:933–6.
Neaton JD, Wentworth D. (1992) Arch Intern Med 152:56–64.
Pedersen TR, Olsson AG, Faergeman O, et al. (1998) Circulation 97:1453–60.
Ross R. (1999) N Engl J Med 340:115–26.
Smith I, Franks PJ, Greenhalgh RM, Poulter NR, Powell JT. (1996) Eur J Vasc Endovasc Surg 11:402–8.
Sueta CA, Chowdhury M, Boccuzzi SJ, et al. (1999) Am J Cardiol 83:1303–7.
Valentine RJ, Kaplan HS, Green R, Jacobsen DW, Myers SI, Clagett GP. (1996) J Vasc Surg 23:53–61, discussion 61–3.

2

Clinical Evaluation of Patients with Vascular Disease

William G. Tennant

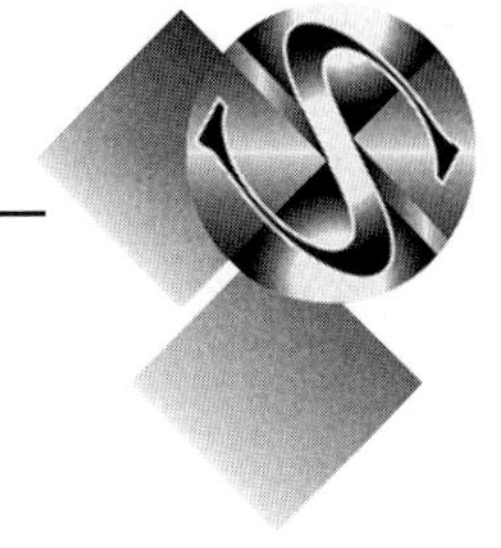

The primary goal of the clinical evaluation of patients with vascular disease is to decide which tests will help the surgeon treat the patients' problem while at the same time minimizing patient discomfort. Investigation of patients with vascular disease differs from that of other surgical patients and depends mainly on the underlying disease process. For instance, patients with lower extremity occlusive vascular disease suffer not only from their index problem (claudication, ischemic rest pain, gangrenous ulcers) but also from some of the conditions that have predisposed them to vascular disease in the first place (diabetes, hypercholesterolemia, etc.). In addition, they are likely to require a number of medications for these predisposing conditions, some of which require consideration in diagnosing and treating vascular disease. It is also important to keep in mind that the presence of occlusive vascular disease in the lower limbs indicates the likely involvement of other vessels (coronary, carotid, cerebral, renal, mesenteric, etc.). Because the underlying pathology is very different, the clinical evaluation of patients with aneurysmal disease is strikingly different. These patients are healthier overall and their clinical evaluation is less intense.

Patients' Characteristics

Vascular surgery patients suffer many of the fears and anxieties of other surgical patients. Added to this are fears of gangrene, amputa-tion, and aneurysm rupture. Many elderly patients suffer other severe illness or disability. They may, as a result, have limited aims and aspirations when seeking investigation and treatment. In contrast, younger patients' family life or career may be threatened by their disease, and very high expectations of investigation and treatment have to be realistically modified. It is these human characteristics that deserve our consideration when deciding on an investigative pathway. Although it is important to gain all the information required to execute an effective treatment plan, it is equally important to do this in as noninvasive and humane a way as possible. Fortunately, the technology is on our side in this regard, and the days of highly invasive investigations are probably numbered.

The History

The value of a good clinical history is increasingly overlooked as techno-diagnosis advances. One should remember that the history is usually the first interaction that takes place between the doctor and patient. It is at this time that the therapeutic relationship is forged. With skill and practice it is possible to elicit not only symptoms but also their significance to the patients, the patients' expectations and fears, and their attitudes toward treatment. It is possible to avoid unnecessary diagnostic tests and limit the investigative mill that the patient is put through.

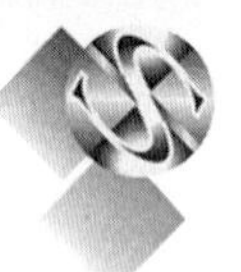

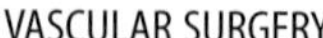

There are some general points in the clinical history that warrant mention:

1. Lifestyle. Risk factors that can lead to the progress of vascular disease such as smoking, diabetes, hypertension, and hyperlipidemia are ascertained in the history. Additionally, an adequate exercise history should be elicited. One question that elucidates the rate-limiting organ system is how far patients can walk, and what stops them (leg pain, shortness of breath, chest pain, etc.). It is also important to know if the patient is taking hormonal medications such as oral contraceptives or hormone replacement therapy. These medications can predispose to venous and occasionally arterial thrombosis. It is during the history taking that a physician can begin to address many of these risk factors. By recruiting antismoking clinics or eliciting the help of diabetes and cardiac specialist physicians, a surgeon can improve a patient's overall health both pre- and postoperatively.

2. Family history. It is especially important to question the patient about the prevalence of early cardiovascular disease or thrombosis (i.e., stroke, occlusive limb disease, or cardiac disease) that manifests before age 50. Aneurysm disease has a clear familial association, and an incidence approaching 20% in first-degree relatives.

3. Atherosclerosis. Atherosclerosis is a systemic disorder, so inclusion of a discussion of stroke/transient ischemic attacks and coronary artery disease/myocardial infarction/angina is important.

Although the points covered above may elicit factors predisposing the patient to vascular occlusive or aneurysm disease, they are non-specific and nondiagnostic. Because the symptoms of occlusive vascular, aneurysmal, and venous disease differ, they will be dealt with separately below. It should be remembered, however, that they may occur in combination.

Chronic Limb Ischemia

The principal symptom of chronic limb ischemia (CLI) is that of claudication (*claudicare*, to limp). This is effort-related muscular pain relieved by rest. In the lower limb, patients in the initial stages of disease complain of calf, thigh, or buttock pain brought on by walking, which is relieved after a few minutes of rest. This is commonly a condition that follows a variable course with periods of remission and relapse, often according to changes in lifestyle, medications, or the progress of a comorbid condition such as diabetes mellitus. With worsening ischemia, the patient begins to feel pain at night usually in the distal forefoot, toes, and instep (rest pain). As the patient becomes horizontal in bed (removing the effect of gravity on blood flow), and the blood pressure drops with the onset of sleep, perfusion of the lower limbs worsens. Patients often wake up in the middle of the night with pain that they can relieve only by getting out of bed and, paradoxically, walking around the bedroom. Some patients with rest pain learn to sleep with the affected leg hanging over the side of the bed to regain the assistance of gravity (Fig. 2.1). When patients sleep with ischemic limbs dependent, there is a gradual onset of edema and worsening tissue perfusion, which create a vicious circle of pathologies.

Acute Critical Limb Ischemia

Acute critical limb ischemia (ACLI) can be defined as sudden onset of severe limb ischaemia of less than 24 hours' duration. The principal causes are arterial embolism and thrombosis. A history should be taken to include the common sources of emboli (Table 2.1). A history suggestive of claudication in the affected limb makes thrombosis in situ of a chronic arterial stenosis more likely than embolus.

The symptoms of ACLI include paresthesia, pain in the limb at rest, numbness, coldness, and paralysis. Symptoms are likely to be more severe in cases of embolus than in cases of thrombosis because thrombosis usually occurs at the site of a chronic stenosis, completely occluding the vessel. Where a stenosis has existed, it is likely that a collateral circulation has developed that will continue to function even when the main vessel is occluded. In cases where an embolus has suddenly occluded a previously normal limb artery, there are no collaterals to support adequate perfusion.

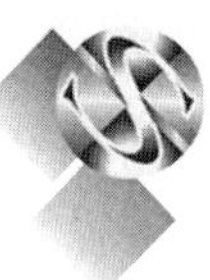

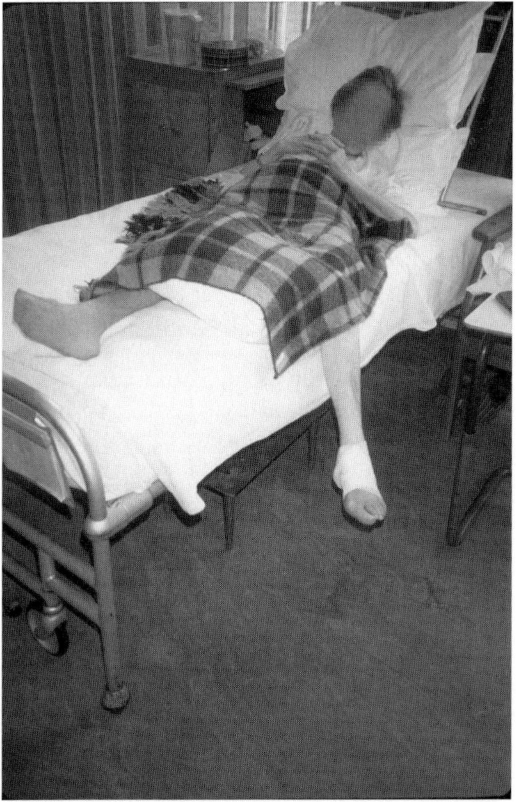

Figure 2.1. Rest pain. This elderly woman is adopting a classic posture, which gives gravity assistance to blood flow while she is recumbent.

Upper Limb Vascular Occlusive Disease

Chronic occlusive vascular disease in the arm is considerably less common than that in the leg.

Table 2.1. Common sources of emboli

Cardiac arrhythmias (commonly atrial fibrillation)
Cardiac mural thrombus from recent myocardial infarction
Diseased heart valves
Atheroma of aortic arch or more distal aorta
Areas of chronic arterial damage (cervical rib, thoracic outlet syndrome)
Aortic aneurysm (rare)
Broken catheter tips
Bullets and other materials introduced violently
Air
Amniotic fluid
Fat (long bone fractures)

Perhaps because of its rarity, the diagnosis is often made late and by exclusion. Arm claudication presents with effort-induced heaviness or tiredness that is relieved by rest. The patient may also complain of relative pallor and an impression of coldness of the affected limb, exacerbated by cold exposure.

Subclavian occlusive disease may also cause cerebrovascular symptoms because of the anatomical relationship between the vertebral arteries that arise off of the subclavian arteries. This is best exemplified by the subclavian steal syndrome. Tight stenosis or occlusion of the subclavian artery proximal to the origin of the vertebral artery leads to effort-induced reversal of flow in the vertebral artery that contributes to the arterial supply of the arm (Fig. 2.2). When the arm is exercised, increased (reversed) flow from the vertebral artery to the subclavian can lead to marked but transient symptoms of brainstem ischemia in addition to arm claudication. Although most patients with this condition have no symptoms of cerebrovascular steal at rest, symptoms can occur during exercise, including dizziness, ataxia, diplopia, and bilateral blurred vision.

Acute upper limb vascular disease is usually due to embolism. Trauma is a less common

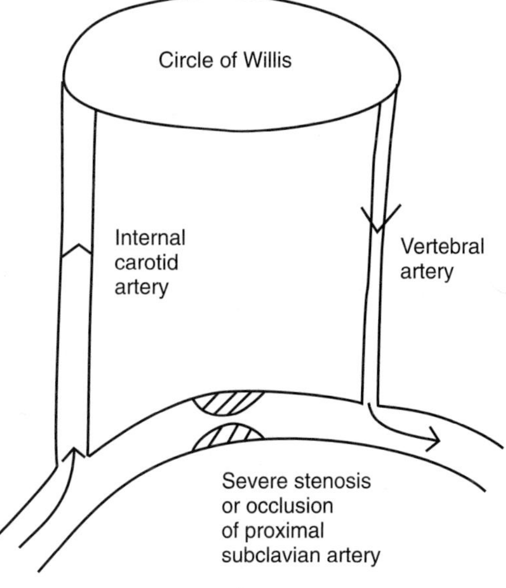

Figure 2.2. Subclavian stenosis can lead to reversal of flow in the vertebral artery and vertebrobasilar symptoms.

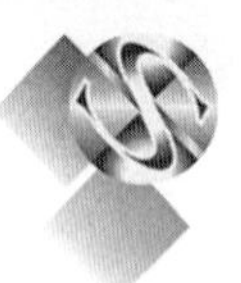

cause. The symptoms are the same as for acute lower limb disease: pain or numbness, paralysis, and pallor. A history of recent myocardial infarction or of known atrial fibrillation should be taken. Traumatic causes can range from a "simple" supracondylar humeral fracture to the massive bone and soft tissue disruption caused by motorcycle accidents. It is also important to find out how the symptoms have developed over time. For instance, many elderly patients with brachial emboli give a history of severe pain initially followed by gradual resolution over the succeeding hours. These patients then present to the vascular surgeon with viable limbs and minor symptoms. Other patients may complain of worsening symptoms, and the need for urgent intervention becomes obvious. Where an artery has been damaged by trauma, there may be a clear history of resolution of symptoms and restoration of pulses after, for instance, the reduction of a fracture.

Aortic Aneurysm

Whether the aneurysm affects the thoracic or abdominal aorta, there are usually very few symptoms. Chronic symptoms that do occur are usually due to pressure effects on the surrounding structures. Even in quite small abdominal aneurysms, erosion of adjacent vertebral bodies can occur, leading to back pain. One of the commonest symptoms of large thoracic aneurysms is dysphagia from direct pressure on the esophagus. Patients who notice abnormal abdominal pulsation (frequently while bathing, or in bed) often present with amusing self-diagnoses that belie the serious nature of the condition. This has been called "slipped-heart syndrome."

In the special case of inflammatory abdominal aortic aneurysm (vide infra), fibrosis can extend laterally in the retroperitoneum to include the ureters, which can result in ureteral stenosis. The presentation of such aneurysms is often via the urologist, the patient having presented with symptoms due to obstructive uropathy and hydronephrosis or even renal failure.

The acute presentation of abdominal aortic aneurysm is usually as a differential diagnosis of acute abdominal pain. Symptoms are not always due to rupture, and the aneurysm may be intact but acutely symptomatic. Symptoms in an intact aneurysm, though the etiology is unknown, are principally severe abdominal and back pain of sudden onset. The pain may radiate into the groin, flanks, or genitalia and can closely mimic renal colic. When the aneurysm is ruptured, there is also collapse and hypovolemia. The distinction between acutely symptomatic intact aneurysms and ruptured aneurysms is impossible to make on history alone.

Superficial Venous Disease

Patients frequently complain about the unsightly nature of varicose veins, and imbue them with many symptoms. These include aching, itching, and swelling. Symptoms, however, correlate poorly with the apparent severity of the disease. When superficial venous disease is extensive and severe, symptoms are common and include those above with the addition of ulceration.

Deep Venous Disease

Symptoms are usually of swelling, heaviness, and occasionally severe discomfort. The symptoms are usually worse after prolonged standing. There may be a history of deep venous thrombosis or previous abdominal or pelvic surgery with venous damage. Symptoms result from venous hypertension in the limb affected, and this is the final common pathway of both occlusion and incompetence of the deep veins. There may be a history of ulceration even if none is present at the time of examination.

Clinical Examination

Inspection

The general signs of a predisposition to occlusive vascular disease include deposits of fat in the thin skin around the eyes (xanthelasma), and in the corneas themselves (arcus senilis). Patients may have white hair; the fingertips may be tinted yellow with tar from cigarettes, and patients may smell strongly of cigarette smoke. Some of these patients assert that they have stopped smoking. Patients may be short of breath at rest or on minimal exertion because of coexistent cardiac or respiratory disease.

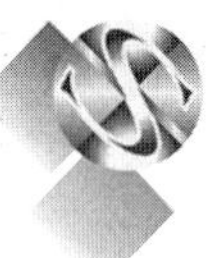

The specific effects of occlusive vascular disease may produce clinical signs apparent on general examination, such as limb swelling ulceration or gangrene. There may be signs of a previous stroke or of severe loss of weight.

Aneurysms may appear as a localized swelling if present in the periphery, for instance, traumatic aneurysms of the femoral, popliteal, or radial artery (Fig. 2.3). There are often very few signs of abdominal aortic aneurysms on general examination, unless the patient is very slim and the abdominal wall may be "draped" across the aneurysm with the patient supine and relaxed. The pressure caused by an aneurysm on adjacent structures may rarely cause related clinical signs (Fig. 2.4).

Palpation: Examination of the Pulses

Lower Limbs

Pulses are normally palpable in the femoral triangle at the midinguinal point, in the popliteal fossa, posterior to the medial malleolus, and on the dorsum of the foot between the first and second metatarsals. In the normal subject, the popliteal pulse is felt by compressing the artery against the tibial plateau anteriorly. This is best done with the patient's leg flexed at the knee. It is particularly important to distinguish aortoiliac disease from infrainguinal disease. In aortoiliac disease the femoral pulses are diminished, whereas in infrainguinal disease the femoral pulses are normal.

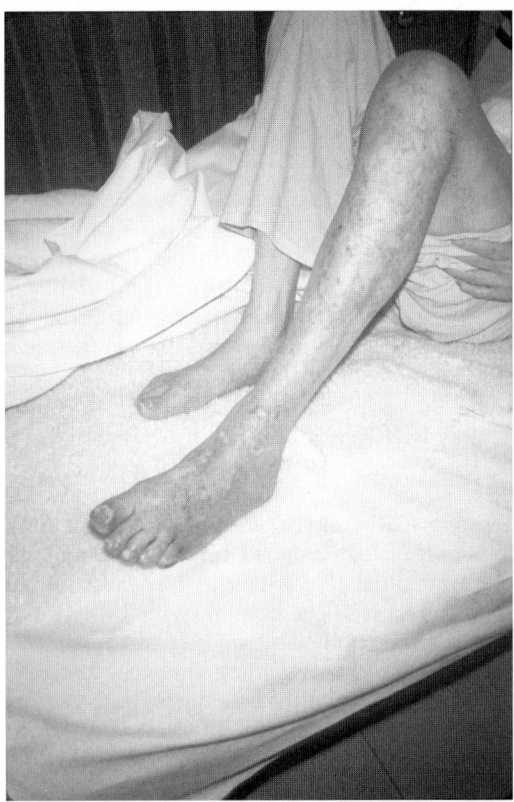

Figure 2.4. Swelling due to venous congestion from a popliteal aneurysm. A popliteal aneurysm caused the swelling of this patient's left leg by pressure on the adjacent popliteal vein. There are also multiple small skin infarcts caused by embolization from the aneurysm.

Upper Limbs

The subclavian pulse is present in the supraclavicular fossa and the axillary artery in the infraclavicular fossa. Thereafter, the brachial artery is usually palpable in the cubital fossa deep to the bicipital aponeurosis. The ulnar pulse is palpable just medial to the tendon of the flexor carpi ulnaris and the radial lateral to the tendon of the flexor carpi radialis on the radial styloid process. A pulse is usually also palpable in the "anatomical snuff box" between the tendons of the extensor pollicis longus and brevis, where it overlies the scaphoid bone.

Neck

The carotid pulse can be felt medial to the muscle belly of sternomastoid. Occasionally

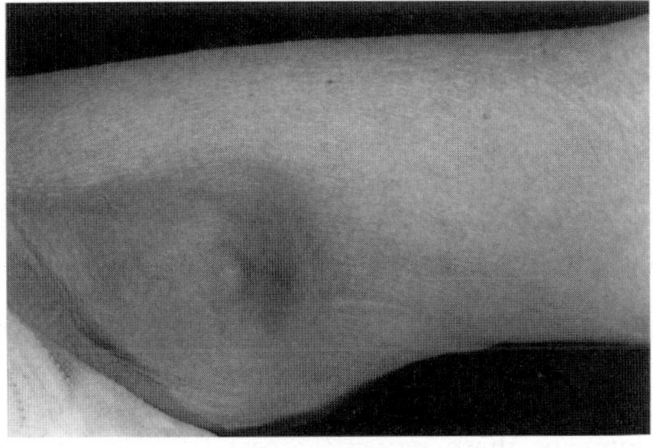

Figure 2.3. This aneurysm of the superficial femoral artery was caused by previous trauma. It presented as a pulsatile swelling of the mid thigh.

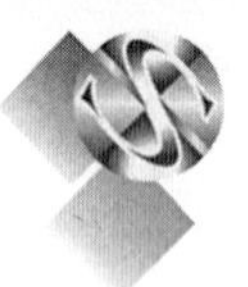

there may be marked tortuosity of the carotid artery in the neck, giving the impression of an aneurysm.

Abdomen

It is usually difficult to feel the normal abdominal aorta without causing the patient discomfort. The aorta is best palpated between the xiphoid and umbilicus. Below the umbilicus, the aorta bifurcates. When aneurysmally dilated the pulse is easier to feel, and may in fact be a presenting symptom.

Auscultation

In each case, palpation of the pulses should be followed by auscultation in the same sites. Where there is a stenosis either at or immediately proximal to the point of examination, a bruit will be heard in time with the cardiac systole. This is particularly relevant in carotid stenosis. Carotid bruits are not very sensitive or specific for carotid stenosis and require confirmation by carotid ultrasound (Magyar et al., 2002). However, a carotid bruit is often indicative of systemic atherosclerosis. Rarely, the bruit of a stenosed renal artery can be heard during auscultation of the abdomen.

Differential Diagnosis of Leg Ulcers

Many vascular patients present with ulcerations. There are three major types of leg ulcers: venous, ischemic, and neuropathic (Table 2.2). Ischemic ulcers tend to be very distal in the vascular tree and painful. Venous stasis ulcers tend to occur in the region of the medial malleolus and have associated brownish discoloration of the skin (lipatodermatosclerosis) and edema. Neuropathic ulcers tend to occur in diabetic patients under pressure points. Patients with diabetes present particular challenges in terms

Table 2.2. Differential diagnosis of leg ulcers

Type of ulcer	Location	Pain	Associated findings
Ischemic	Distal foot	Yes	No pulses
Venous stasis	Medial malleolus	Maybe	Stasis dermatitis
Neurotropic	Pressure points	No	Diabetes

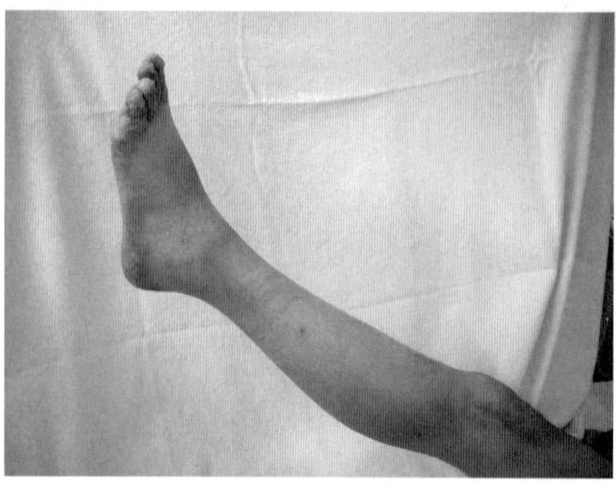

Figure 2.5. Pallor on elevation. The patient's leg is elevated, and the foot displays profound pallor.

of diagnosis and management (Sumpio et al., 2003).

Other Clinical Tests

Capillary Refill

With the patient supine and the great toes together, both toes are gripped by the examiner using one hand and compressed. On release, the toes should change symmetrically from white to pink in less than 5 seconds. Asymmetry suggests arterial disease on the slowest side.

Buerger's Test

This is a test for severe chronic arterial occlusive disease. With the patient supine the straight legs are raised as far as possible. In arterial disease, there is extreme pallor of the feet in this position (Fig. 2.5). The legs are then placed on the examination bench and the patient is told to sit with the legs dependent over the side of the bench. Where there is severe chronic arterial disease, the feet become suffused with a deep ruddy red color, commonly described as "sunset foot." This is caused by ischemic maximal dilation of the arteriolar bed of the skin, allowing the skin to fill with partially oxygenated blood (Fig. 2.6).

Trendelenburg Test

In cases where incompetence of the saphenofemoral junction is suspected as a major

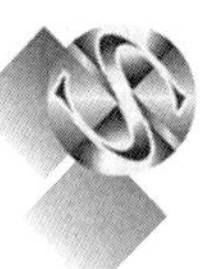

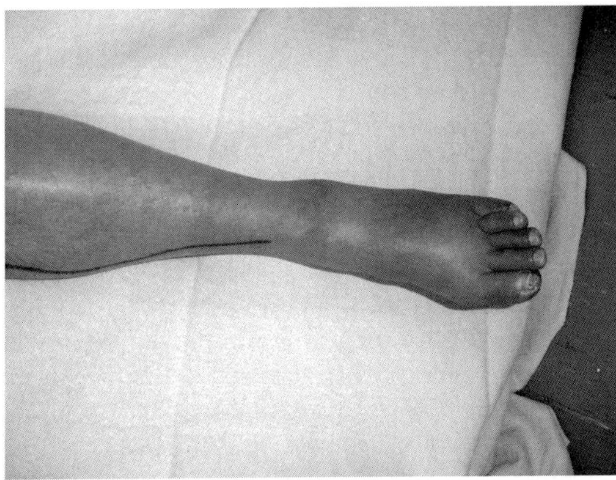

Figure 2.6. Dependent rubor. The leg has been placed dependent over the side of the bed, and is extremely hyperemic.

cause of superficial varicose veins, the patient is asked to lie supine and raise the affected limb to about 45 degrees. Venous blood is "milked" proximally by firm stroking of the leg to empty all of the superficial veins. A tourniquet is applied as proximally as possible to occlude the superficial venous system. The patient is then asked first to sit up and swing the legs over the side of the examination couch, and then to stand. Where saphenofemoral incompetence is the major cause of superficial varicosities, the varicosities will remain collapsed. It is usual for the superficial veins to fill slowly, but rapid filling of the varicosities with the tourniquet in place indicates significant perforator disease distal to the tourniquet. It is possible to localize incompetent perforating veins by repeating the test with the tourniquet just above the knee. In this case calf varicosities will remain collapsed if the guilty perforating vein is between the saphenofemoral junction and the tourniquet. If the incompetent perforating vein is below the knee, the below knee varices will fill rapidly. Although the Trendelenburg method is somewhat insensitive in localizing incompetent perforating veins, it can provide useful clinical information. For more accurate localization of incompetent thigh perforators, and for all those in the calf, it is best to use duplex examination.

Fixed Wave Doppler Examination

A number of small and portable battery-operated machines are available, operating at frequencies between 5 and 10 MHz depending on the depth of penetration required (Fig. 2.7). In each case the signal from the insonation of the examined artery is converted into an audible sound from a built-in speaker. Normally the signal has a "triphasic" sound. Although it is possible to use the Doppler simply to locate an artery, the most common use is to measure the blood pressure at the periphery of a limb. For this, the Doppler machine is used in the same way as a stethoscope when measuring the blood pressure using Korotkoff sounds. A blood pressure cuff is placed around the limb proximal to the artery to be examined. The artery is then insonated and the cuff inflated above the systolic pressure. As the cuff is deflated, the signal returns, and the pressure at which this happens is noted. When the pressure in all the required arteries has been measured, the pressure in the brachial artery is measured using the same technique. The ratio between the ankle pressure and the brachial pressure is known as the ankle–brachial index (ABI). The ABI in normal patients without arterial occlusive disease is greater than 1.

Handheld Doppler examination is also useful in the diagnosis of superficial venous disease

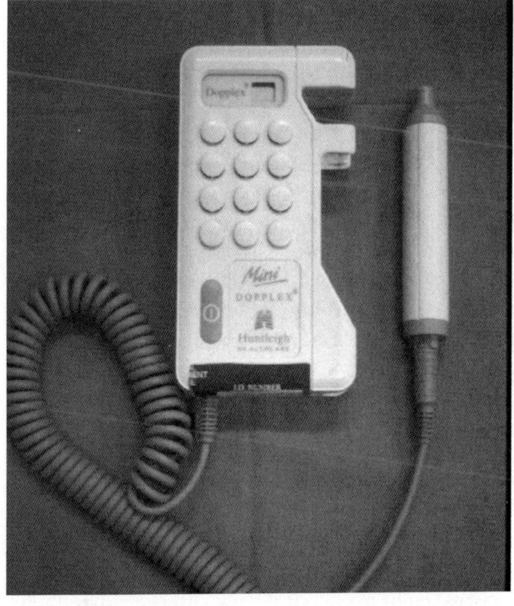

Figure 2.7. An example of the type of handheld Doppler device suitable for use in the clinic.

to confirm the incompetence of the saphenofemoral or saphenopopliteal junctions, and to localize incompetent perforating veins. At each of the saphenous junctions, there is physiological retrograde flow into the superficial system of under 1 second' duration, which is audible using a handheld Doppler machine. If the reflux is of longer duration, it is indicative of pathological incompetence of the junction. With an experienced operator, it is possible to localize incompetent perforating veins.

Clinical Examination of Specific Conditions

Chronic Lower Limb Ischemia

In mild disease the legs may appear normal to inspection, but capillary return is delayed and the feet may be cool to touch. Distal pulses are be either weak and difficult to feel or absent. With increasing severity, the legs may be hairless below the knee, and the toes cyanotic. As ischemia progresses, more proximal pulses may disappear and ulcers may appear on or between the toes. Buerger's test becomes positive. Eventually more proximal painful ulcers over the lower leg, and digital gangrene signals very severe occlusive disease.

Acute Lower Limb Ischemia

Where there is thrombosis of a collateralized chronic stenosis, the signs of acute ischemia may be less severe than in cases of embolus (vide supra). In these less severe cases, the acute onset of the symptoms may be the most obvious clue. The limb may appear normal to inspection but have reduced capillary return, pale rapidly on elevation, and have slightly altered sensation on formal testing. There may be some weakness, principally of the anterior muscle groups of the lower leg. With increasing ischemia, the signs of pallor and weakness increase, and there may be complete paralysis of the foot and toe dorsiflexor muscle groups. In these cases, the foot usually lies at rest in equinovarus due to paralysis of the peroneal muscles. In severe acute ischemia, such as that caused by embolism, the skin becomes mottled with blue blotches on a background of sallow white. If the blotches blanche on finger pressure (unfixed mottling), it may still be possible to save the leg if immediate action is taken to revascularize it. Where the mottling is fixed, that is, it fails to blanche on pressure, it is too late to save the limb. Muscle ischemia and impending necrosis in these severe cases cause the muscles to swell and become tender. This is often best seen in the anterior muscle compartment where the tenderness is often exquisite and the compartment is almost stone hard to palpation. Examination of the pulses allows approximate localization of the level of disease. The presence of normal pulses on the opposite extremity supports the diagnosis of acute embolic disease.

Mesenteric Ischemia

In chronic cases there are often few signs on examination of the abdomen, but signs of weight loss and systemic vascular disease are present. Where the disease is acute, the abdomen can feel curiously doughy in the early stage and is diffusely tender. Bowel sounds may still be present. As time passes and transmural infarction supervenes, peritoneal signs develop.

Upper Limb Ischemia

Chronic arterial occlusive disease seldom affects the upper limb except as part of rare conditions affecting the aortic arch and subclavian arteries. Upper limb ischemia is usually due to embolism. The commonest embolic source in these cases is the myocardium in atrial fibrillation or following myocardial infarction. Other sources include proximal stenoses in the aortic arch and subclavian arteries (Fig. 2.8). The clinical signs of acute upper limb ischemia are the same as in the lower limb: sensory alteration, paresthesia, weakness, and muscle tenderness. It is uncommon for the ischemia to be so severe as to lead to irreversible change because of the rich collateral supply in the arm. In intravenous drug abusers, intraarterial injection of illicit medications "cut" with insoluble excipients may lead to extensive acute occlusion of small distal vessels (Fig. 2.9). Patients often present following deliberate or accidental intraarterial injection, with a short history of almost overwhelming pain together with exquisite muscle tenderness and forearm muscles stone hard to touch. The skin

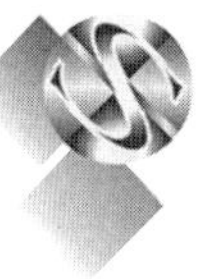

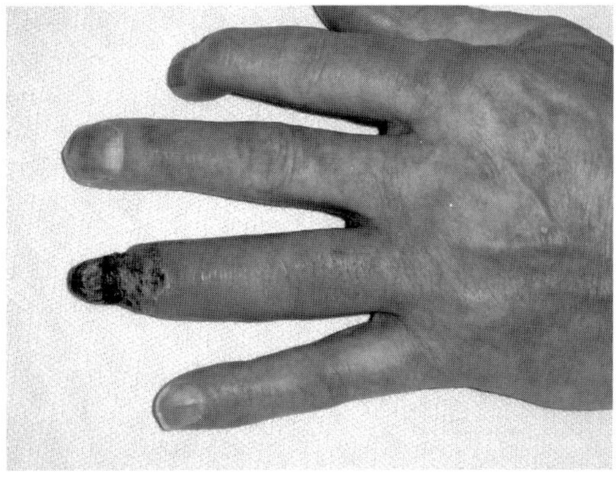

Figure 2.8. Gangrene from an arterial embolus. The distal aspect of the digit is gangrenous secondary to an embolus arising from a subclavian stenosis.

of the forearm and hand is fixed and mottled and the hand clawed.

Chronic Venous Disease

Inspection with the patient standing is one of the most important aspects of the examination of chronic venous disease. The dilated veins of superficial disease are frequently obvious. Other signs of importance include swelling, hemosiderosis of the skin of the malleolar area, lipodermatosclerosis, atrophie blanche, and ulceration (Fig. 2.10). Deep venous disease may be less obvious and present simply with chronic swelling of the limb. In later stages, all of the above signs may be present.

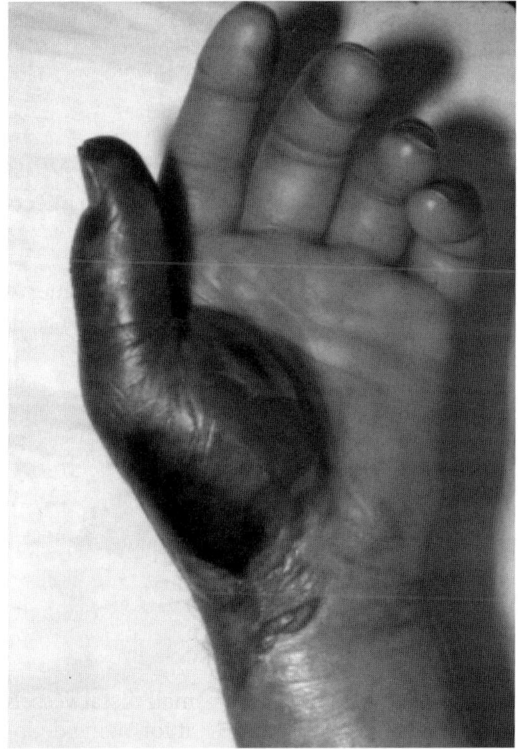

Figure 2.9. Gangrene from drug injection. Injection into the radial artery led to gangrene to the thumb and thenar eminence.

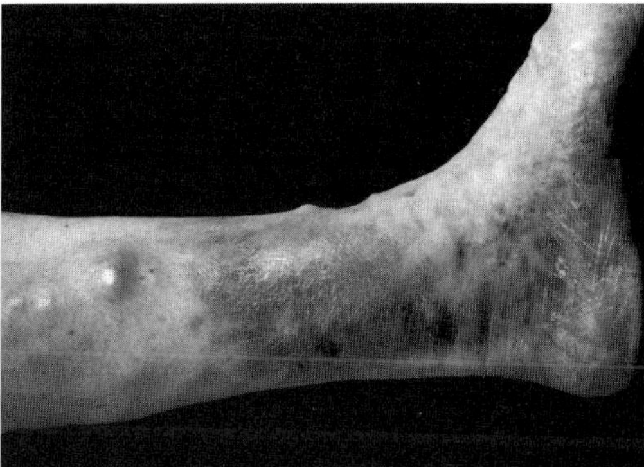

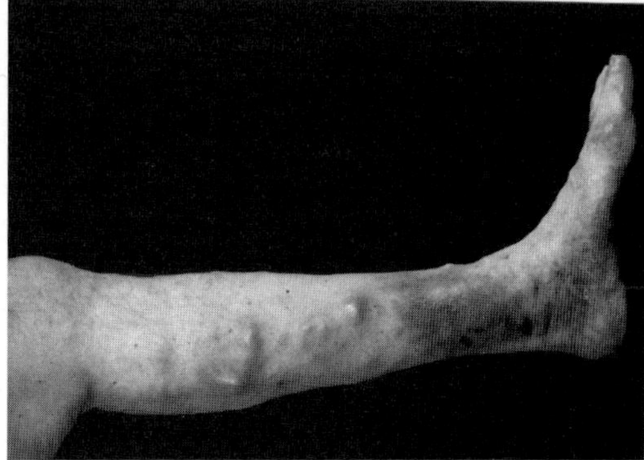

Figure 2.10. Chronic venous insufficiency. The limbs demonstrate the brownish discoloration associated with lipatodermatosclerosis. Varicosities are also present.

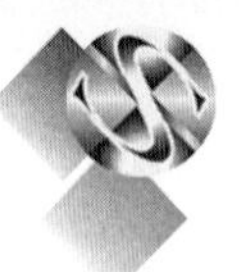
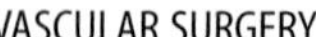

Conclusion

Clinical evaluation of the patient with vascular disease is of the utmost importance. Many clues about a patient's temperament, the disease, and expectations of treatment can be obtained from a thorough interview. Assessing a patient's risk factors for vascular disease not only helps the physician better understand the patient's chief complaint but also directs the preoperative workup of the patient. Despite the recent advances in vascular radiology, nothing replaces an excellent physical examination, which can shed light on the clinical extent of a patient's disease process. Finally, when radiological studies may take valuable time, there are several bedside tests that can be performed rapidly, allowing a vascular surgeon to make immediate treatment decisions.

References

Magyar MT, Nam EM, Csiba L, Ritter MA, Ringelstein EB, Droste DW. (2002) Neurol Res 24:705–8.

Sumpio BE, Lee T, Blume PA. (2003) Clin Podiatr Med Surg 20:689–708.

3

Noninvasive Vascular Examination

Colleen M. Brophy

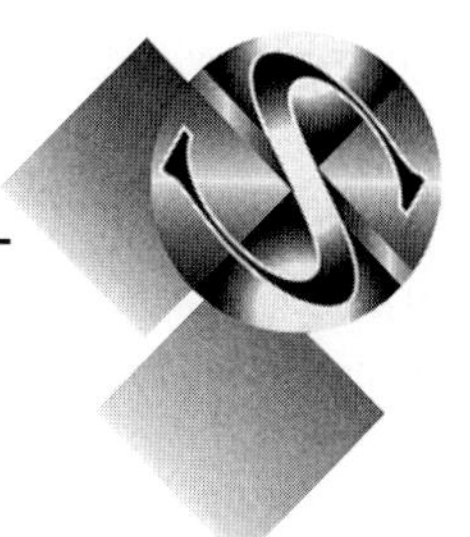

The noninvasive vascular laboratory assists with the diagnosis of peripheral arterial disease. In general, two basic approaches are used: (1) indirect measures that characterize the functional severity of the disease, such as segmental pressures, Doppler waveform analyses, plethysmography, and skin perfusion pressures; and (2) direct measures that characterize the anatomy of the disease using color duplex imaging. These studies are used to accurately diagnose the location and extent of peripheral arterial disease, assist with the planning of therapeutic options for the disease, and follow the outcomes of peripheral vascular interventions.

Indirect Evaluation of Arterial Disease

Ankle-Brachial Index

In patients without palpable pedal pulses, the next step in the clinical evaluation is to perform a Doppler analysis. This is usually performed in the clinic or at the bedside using a handheld Doppler device. The probe is placed at an angle (Fig. 3.1) over the dorsalis pedis and posterior tibial arteries to determine if a signal can be obtained. The complete absence of Doppler signals suggests significant peripheral arterial disease. Approximately 10% of the normal population does not have a dorsalis pedis artery; hence, the absence of a dorsalis pedis signal alone is not a significant finding. It is important to place the probe directly over the artery but at a 45- to 60-degree angle to obtain the best signal. Doppler signals can be used to assess the severity of the disease. A blood pressure cuff is inflated just above the ankle and a Doppler signal is listened for while the cuff is deflated. The highest pressure in which a signal is heard (dorsalis pedis compared to posterior tibial) is the ankle index. A similar approach with a blood pressure cuff on the upper arm and a Doppler probe on the brachial artery is used to determine the brachial index. The ratio of the ankle to the brachial index represents the ankle–brachial index (ABI). The ABI is usually 1 or greater. An ABI of 0.5 to 0.8 is consistent with claudication, and less than 0.4 is consistent with critical limb ischemia. Diabetic patients often develop medial calcinosis. Simply stated, the medial wall of the vessels become calcified ("bone-like") and cannot be compressed by a blood pressure cuff. Thus, the ABI in a diabetic patient may be falsely elevated, and other studies are needed to accurately assess the peripheral vascular status. In general, however, the ABI is a useful screening test for peripheral vascular disease.

Segmental Limb Pressures

Segmental limb pressures assist with determining the location of disease by measuring the pressure in the upper thigh, lower thigh, below the knee, just above the ankle, and at the transmetatarsal level (Figs. 3.2 and 3.3). Again using

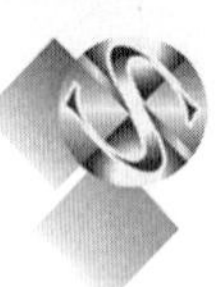

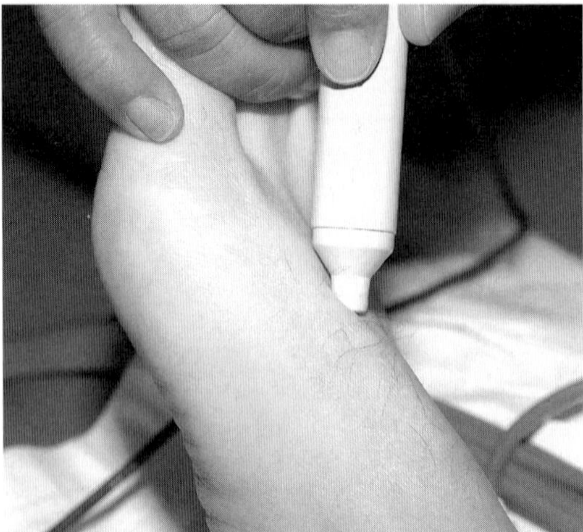

Figure 3.1. Doppler signals are best obtained by holding the Doppler probe at an angle over the artery that is being insonated.

a Doppler, an arterial signal is found at the dorsalis pedis or posterior tibial artery, the cuff is inflated until no signal is heard, and then deflated until the signal resumes. The systolic pressure is recorded for each cuff at each location. A gradient (decrease) in pressure greater than 20 mm Hg between adjacent levels suggests arterial occlusive disease in the vessel between the two cuffs (Fig. 3.3). An arterial pressure in the thigh that is less than that in the arm suggests aortoiliac occlusive disease. A drop in pressure between the upper thigh and lower thigh cuffs suggests superficial femoral artery

disease. It is important to make a distinction between aortoiliac and infrainguinal disease because the overall approach is somewhat different.

An additional useful measurement, particularly in diabetic patients, is to measure the digital pressures. The digital arteries are less likely to be affected by medial calcification and hence provide useful information when the ABI is falsely elevated. Digital pressures are measured by placing a pneumatic cuff around the digit and measuring a plethysmographic arterial waveform using a photoelectrode on the end of the digit. In general, a normal toe pressure is 80% to 90% of the brachial pressure (normal toe–brachial index is 0.8 to 0.9). A toe pressure less than 38 mm Hg has been correlated with impaired forefoot wound healing (Vitti et al., 1994).

In patients with symptoms consistent with claudication but relatively normal indices, exercise testing should be performed. A standard exercise test involves measuring the ABI at rest followed by walking on a treadmill at 2 miles/ hour at a 10% to 15% incline for 5 minutes. The ABI is recorded 1 minute after exercise. Normally, after exercise, there is a slight increase or no difference in the ABI. If the ABI decreases after exercise, this is consistent with claudication.

Pulse Volume Recording

Pulse volume recordings (PVRs) are a plethysmographic measure of limb perfusion.

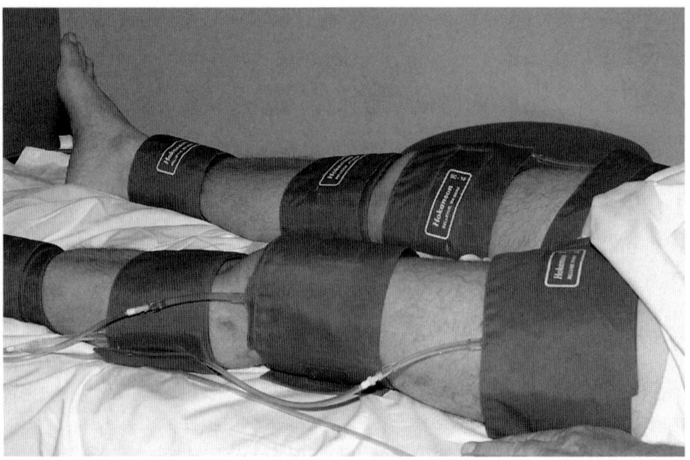

Figure 3.2. Segmental limb pressures are measured by placing the cuffs along the extremity.

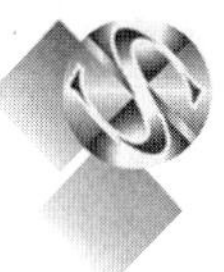

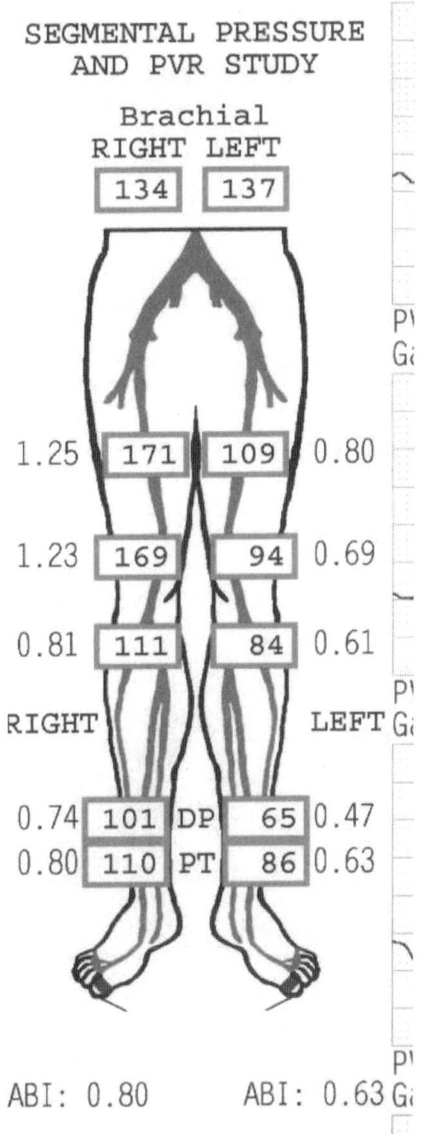

Figure 3.3. Segmental limb pressures show a low high-thigh pressure, indicating iliac disease, and a drop-off between the high-thigh and low-thigh pressures, indicating superficial femoral artery disease on the left side. On the right side there is a drop-off between the pressures in the low thigh and popliteal, indicating distal superficial femoral artery/popliteal artery disease. ABI, ankle–brachial index; Dorsaus Pedis (DP), Posterior Tibial (PT), prothrombin time; PVR, pulse volume recording.

Plethysmography is essentially a measurement of volume. In general, the same cuffs are used to obtain segmental limb pressures and PVRs. The cuff is inflated and the volume shift that occurs with the cardiac cycle in that limb segment is recorded as a waveform. The PVRs do not provide quantitative data but can be analyzed in a qualitative manner. In normal patients there is a brisk upstroke, rapid decline, and dicrotic notch in the waveform. In the presence of peripheral arterial disease, the waveform becomes broader with a decreased amplitude. A PVR tracing that is flat at the forefoot (transmetatarsal) level is consistent with significant peripheral vascular diseases and suggests that revascularization will be required for any forefoot lesion to heal.

Doppler Waveform Analysis

Similar to PVRs, the Doppler waveform can be analyzed to determine if there is disease. Instead of an audio signal, a digital signal is converted to a tracing. Normally the waveform is triphasic (Fig. 3.4). With moderate disease the reverse flow component is lost and the waveform is monophasic. With severe disease, the waveform is blunted and/or absent.

Skin Perfusion Pressure

The skin perfusion pressure (SPP) is an additional noninvasive vascular evaluation that is useful to determine which foot ulcers will heal with local wound care or minor amputation and which will require revascularization or major amputation. An SPP of less than 30 mm Hg can predict failure of forefoot wound healing with

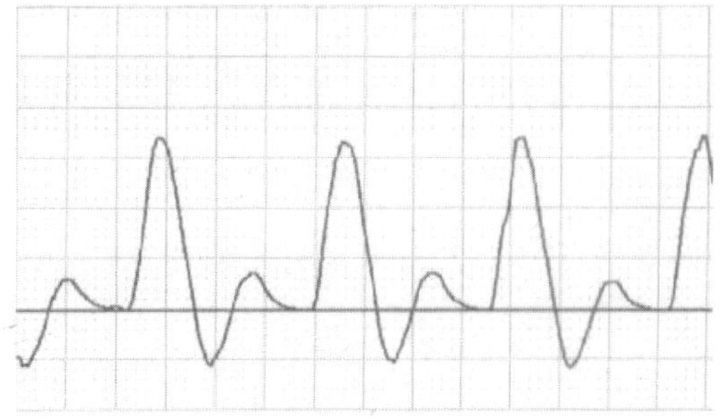

Figure 3.4. Normal triphasic Doppler waveform.

Table 3.1. Noninvasive measurements consistent with impaired wound healing

Ankle–brachial index (ABI)	<0.3–0.4
Toe pressure	<35–40 mm Hg
Skin perfusion pressure	<30 mm Hg
Pulse volume recording (PVR)	Flat forefoot tracing

an accuracy of 80% (Castronuovo et al., 1997). Skin perfusion pressure has largely replaced transcutaneous oximetry.

What Wounds Will Heal?

The aggregate measurements that are consistent with impaired wound healing are listed in Table 3.1. However, it is ultimately the clinical response to wound care that is the most important factor. If debridement and wound care leads to consistently unhealthy appearing wounds, angiography and revascularization should be considered. If good wound care leads to healthy granulation tissue, further evaluation is likely unnecessary.

Direct Evaluation of Arterial Disease

Color duplex imaging or "duplex" imaging incorporates real-time B-mode imaging and pulsed Doppler spectral analysis (Fig. 3.5). B-mode imaging directly views the blood vessel and provides anatomical detail of the vessel. This modality can analyze plaque characteristics, identify thrombus and the intimal flaps, and measure vessel diameter (to detect aneurysms and pseudoaneurysms).

B-mode imaging is also used to localize areas of stenosis so that Doppler velocities can be determined. Velocity analyses are an indirect measure of the degree of stenosis. For carotid artery analyses, the degree of stenosis is estimated based on the peak systolic velocity (PSV), end-diastolic velocity (EDV), and the ratio of the PSV at the stenosis to the velocity in the common carotid artery (V_r). In general a V_r greater than 4 is indicative of clinically significant stenosis (Table 3.2).

Infrainguinal graft surveillance can be performed with duplex imaging. Because most

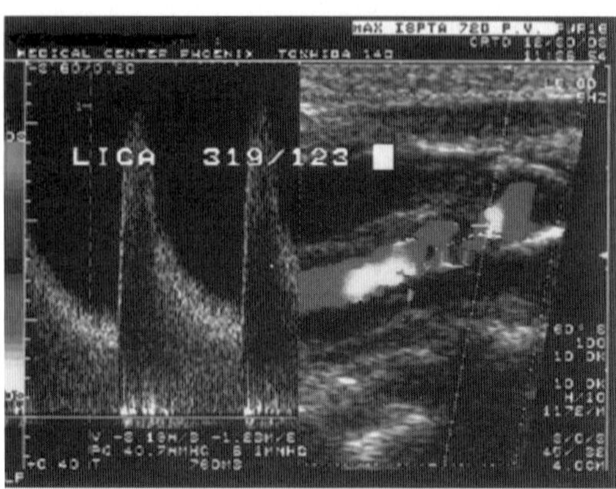

Figure 3.5. Color duplex image of a high-grade carotid stenosis with a peak systolic velocity of 319 and end-diastolic velocity of 123.

abnormalities occur in the first 2 years after implantation, graft surveillance is most important in this time frame. A PSV greater than 150 to 200 cm/second is considered abnormal. In addition, the ratio of the velocity at the stenosis to the normal proximal velocity is used to determine the degree of stenosis (V_r). In addition, high EDVs (>100 cm/second) are also suggestive of high-grade stenoses. Although the high-velocity criteria (PSV, EDV, V_r) are the most accurate to assess the risk of graft thrombosis, low-velocity criteria are also helpful. The graft flow velocity (GFV) should normally exceed 45 cm/second. The velocities are used to stratify the risk of thrombosis (Table 3.3) (Mills, 2001). Prophylactic graft revision should be considered in grafts with a high risk of thrombosis.

Duplex examination is also useful for the diagnosis of popliteal artery aneurysm. This condition should be suspected if a widened popliteal pulse is palpated. An arterial diameter

Table 3.2. Doppler velocity criteria for carotid stenosis

Stenosis (%)	PSV	EDV (cm/sec)	V_r
Normal	<123	<140	<4.0
1–15	<123	<140	<4.0
16–49	<123	<140	<4.0
50–79	>123	<140	<4.0
80–99	>123	>140	>4.0

EDV, end-diastolic velocity; PSV, peak systolic velocity; V_r, velocity ratio.

Table 3.3. Risk stratification for graft thrombosis

Category	PSV (cm/sec)	V_r	EDV (cm/sec)	GFV (cm/sec)
Highest risk	>300	>3.5	>100	<45
High risk	>300	>3.5	<100	>45
Intermediate risk	180–300	>2.0	<100	>45
Low risk	<180	<2.0	<100	>45

EDV, end-diastolic velocity; GFV, graft flow velocity; PSV, peak systolic velocity; V_r, velocity ratio.

greater than 10 mm is considered abnormal. Bilateral aneurysms are seen in about 50% of cases, and proximal aneurysms occur in approximately 30% to 50% of patients. Consequently, it is imperative that aneurysms at other locations be excluded, with abdominal aortic aneurysms and femoral aneurysms the most common.

Conclusion

Noninvasive vascular laboratory tests complement the clinical evaluation in determining the appropriate therapeutic approaches to patients with peripheral vascular disease. The specific laboratory tests should be tailored to the individual patient's diagnoses. The laboratory provides noninvasive information on both functional and anatomical aspects of vascular disease.

References

Castronuovo JJ Jr, Adera HM, Smiell JM, Price RM. (1997) J Vasc Surg 26:629–37.
Mills JL Sr. (2001) Semin Vasc Surg 14:169–76.
Vitti MJ, Robinson DV, Hauer-Jensen M, et al. (1994) Ann Vasc Surg 8:99–106.

4

Radiological Investigations

Steven M. Thomas, Kong T. Tan, and Mark F. Fillinger

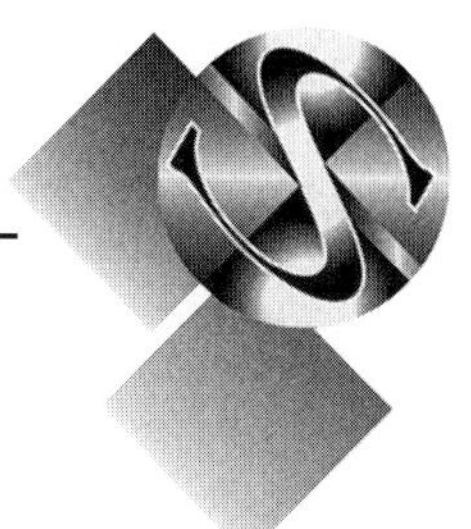

This chapter offers an overview of the available imaging techniques used in vascular radiological practice for the investigation of vascular diseases and how they can be used for a range of common vascular conditions. This discussion emphasizes the move away from invasive techniques and toward noninvasive techniques for the diagnosis of vascular diseases. We then describe the range of endovascular techniques currently required for the investigation and treatment of vascular disease. The most important contemporary approaches and therapies are described, showing the important role these techniques now play in the management of a range of vascular disease processes. This discussion demonstrates how the area of endovascular intervention remains at the forefront of developments in minimally invasive techniques to treat vascular disease. Approaches for specific manifestations of peripheral vascular disease are not discussed, but the Trans Atlantic Inter-Society Consensus (TASC) document is recommended as an overview of endovascular intervention in the management of specific aspects of peripheral arterial disease (Dormandy and Rutherford, 2000).

Controversies

The following controversies currently exist in the field of vascular radiology:

- Conventional diagnostic catheter angiography is likely to be made obsolete by noninvasive vascular imaging.

- When considering endovascular treatment of carotid artery stenosis, the current limitations of noninvasive testing mean that catheter arch angiography is required to assess the arch vessels and the whole of the carotid artery.

- Computed tomography (CT) pulmonary angiography has resulted in little need for conventional pulmonary angiography in the diagnosis of pulmonary embolic disease.

- Arterial closure devices enhance patient throughput, and this may offset the increase in cost from their use. However, they can produce serious complications.

- There is little evidence that primary stenting is superior to primary angioplasty alone in the treatment of arterial occlusive disease in the peripheral circulation.

- Following endovascular aneurysm repair (EVAR) for abdominal aortic aneurysms (AAAs), long-term costs of stent-graft surveillance, and secondary treatment, may outweigh the short-term benefits of EVAR.

Radiological Investigations and Endovascular Approaches

The first vascular imaging technique was described at the end of the 19th century shortly after the discovery of the x-ray. This technique, described by Haschek and Lindenthal, involved

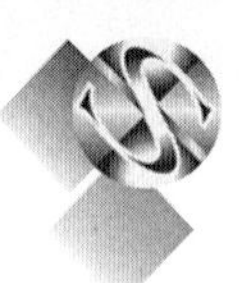

the injection of a chalk-based contrast agent into the vein of an amputated hand. In vivo vascular imaging was first described in the 1920s using agents such as lipiodol, strontium bromide, sodium iodide, and Selectan. The contrast agents were usually introduced by a catheter, following exposure of the vessel used for catheterization, or by percutaneous needle puncture to directly inject contrast into the vessel. Translumbar aortography used this type of technique as early as the 1930s. However, it was developments from the mid–20th century that brought angiography and subsequently vascular intervention to the forefront in vascular diagnosis and treatment. The first of these was the introduction of the Seldinger technique in the 1950s that allowed safe percutaneous access to vascular structures. There then followed significant improvements in the range of available catheters to aid in gaining access to the different vascular beds, and rapid film changers allowed high-quality images to be obtained of all the major vascular beds. As a result, vascular imaging became a major branch of diagnostic medicine. However, arteriography remained an uncomfortable, if not painful, experience because of the use of conventional ionic contrast agents. The introduction of digital subtraction angiography (DSA) and nonionic contrast agents in the last two decades of the 20th century made arteriography much more acceptable to patients and their doctors. Digital subtraction angiography allowed smaller amounts of contrast to be used, and the newer contrast agents rarely produced intense heat or pain. The combination produced fewer systemic side effects as well.

At the same time, attention was directed toward less invasive therapeutic interventions, such as Dotter's technique of sequential dilation for atherosclerotic occlusive lesions. The development of the balloon angioplasty catheter, first described by Gruntzig and Hopff in 1974, heralded an era in which a range of manifestations of arterial occlusive disease became amenable to treatment using percutaneous vascular interventional techniques. There followed developments of a range of techniques for treating arterial occlusive disease such as arterial stents, atherectomy catheters, lasers, and thrombolysis. From these, implantable devices such as inferior vena cava (IVC) filters and stent grafts for aneurysmal disease were developed. All these devices broadened the range of conditions amenable to treatment using interventional vascular radiological techniques.

Improvements in the design of catheters and other devices have resulted in smaller caliber catheters and introduction sheaths. These along with the introduction of closure devices to seal the access site puncture allowed the development of day case ("same day") arterial procedures for both diagnosis and intervention. Despite these improvements, developments in other noninvasive imaging modalities meant that for arterial imaging and diagnosis, the use of what remains an invasive technique is required less frequently. Whereas arteriography was once a first-line investigation, noninvasive techniques such as ultrasound, radionuclide imaging, CT, and magnetic resonance imaging (MRI) now have a much wider role to play in both general diagnostic radiology and in the radiological investigation of vascular disease. Not only are these techniques safer, they also have the potential for a greater diagnostic yield because of the additional information that can often be obtained using these techniques. As a result of improvements in these noninvasive vascular imaging techniques, it is possible that the need for conventional diagnostic catheter angiography will become obsolete. However, at present, despite the reduced requirement for angiography for general diagnostic work, there remains a role for angiography in the investigation of vascular disease, either as a first-line investigation or following other imaging investigations. Also angiography remains paramount as part of all percutaneous endovascular interventional techniques.

Imaging Modalities

The imaging techniques available for the investigation of vascular diseases are best divided into invasive (i.e., catheter angiography) and noninvasive techniques. The following is a brief description of the commonly used modalities.

Catheter Angiography

Catheter angiography is an x-ray investigation in which a contrast agent is injected into the vascular system via a catheter, and sequential x-ray exposures are performed. The x-ray receiver can

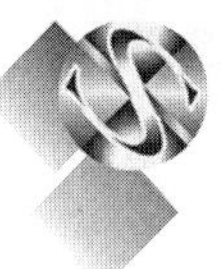

be plain x-ray film (older machines), but are now almost universally digital systems, using an image intensifier or a flat panel detector. Older machines using cut plain x-ray films were cumbersome and difficult to operate. In addition, the postprocessing facilities were very limited. In contrast, digital systems are easy to operate, require lower contrast dosage, produce better contrast resolution, have real-time display, and have facilities for image manipulations, such as pixel shifting and digital subtraction angiography.

Contrast Agents

The primary aim of the contrast agent is to allow imaging of vessel anatomy and morphology. During fluoroscopy, x-ray contrast agents act by changing the attenuation between tissues. Iodinated agents and gadolinium have a higher density than surrounding tissue, whereas carbon dioxide has a lower density.

Iodinated Contrast Agents

The most widely used contrast agents for catheter angiography are the water-soluble iodine-based agents. They can be divided into ionic and the newer nonionic agents. Nonionic agents have the advantage of considerably reducing the risk of adverse reactions to contrast, but are more expensive. In the United Kingdom the low-osmolar nonionic agents are used almost exclusively for intravascular procedures. These agents are denser than blood, and the commonly used strength for diagnostic and interventional work is 300 mg of iodine per milliliter of contrast. For hand injections, this strength of contrast is usually diluted 50:50 with saline. Patients with a previous history of adverse reactions to these contrast media, a strong history of allergic disease, or a hypersensitivity to iodine are at risk of developing a severe allergic reaction to these contrast agents. Other investigative modalities that do not require iodinated contrast media such as MRI or ultrasound should be considered, or alternative non–iodine-based contrast such as carbon dioxide (CO_2) or gadolinium, as described below. The other major problem with iodinated contrast is nephrotoxicity. Overall, contrast-induced nephropathy occurs in approximately 5% of all procedures requiring iodinated contrast media. For the majority, the effect is temporary. However, in high-risk patients the incidence of contrast-induced nephropathy is around 20% to 30%, and in a significant number of cases the effect is permanent and nonreversible. High-risk groups are those patients with preexisting renal impairment, diabetes mellitus, dehydration, on nephrotoxic drugs, and a history of multiple myeloma. These patients should be well hydrated prior to the procedure, if necessary by the administration of intravenous saline, and their renal function should be checked 48 hours postprocedure. Recently, some studies involving a small number of patients suggest that acetylcysteine and calcium channel blockers may reduce the incidence of contrast-induced nephropathy (Kay et al., 2003). There is also evidence that at-risk patients, particularly those with diabetes mellitus, have a lower incidence of contrast-induced nephropathy following the use of recently introduced iso-osmolar contrast agents (Aspelin et al., 2003). There is also a risk of potentially fatal lactic acidosis if a patient taking metformin develops acute renal impairment following the administration of iodinated contrast. Ideally metformin should be discontinued at the time of, or prior to, the procedure and withheld for 48 hours subsequent to the procedure and reinstituted only after renal function has been reevaluated and found to be normal.

Other Agents

Mainly because of the risk of nephrotoxicity with iodine-based agents, CO_2 has recently been advocated as a vascular contrast media for patients with renal impairment. It can also be used when there are contraindications to iodinated contrast such as a history of iodine or contrast allergy. Minor alterations in techniques and software are required for CO_2 angiography. Although dedicated CO_2 pump injectors are available, these are expensive to purchase. Cheaper alternative techniques, not requiring a dedicated pump injector, have been described and used with complete safety if appropriate measures are utilized (Snow and Rice, 1999). Stacking software is required to overcome fragmentation of the CO_2 gas column by the flowing blood (Fig. 4.1). For adequate imaging of the tibial and distal arteries, elevation of the feet by

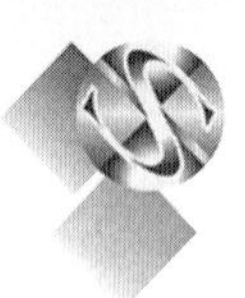

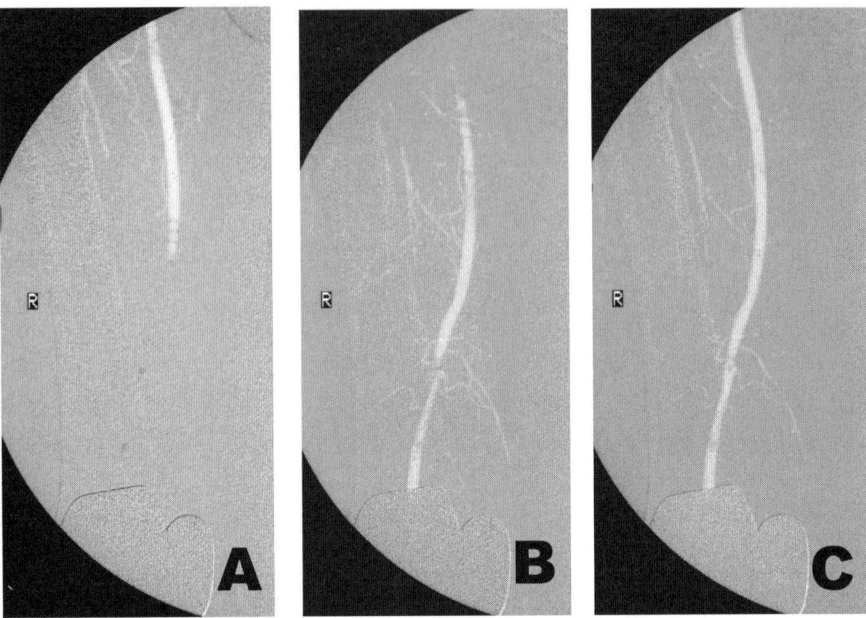

Figure 4.1. Carbon dioxide angiography showing the application of stacking software to remove the beading effect seen in panels A and B.

10 to 20 degrees may be necessary. Unlike iodine-based agents, CO_2 can be administered in large quantity, even in patients with pulmonary disease, without any adverse effect. The CO_2 gas displaces the blood and appears radiolucent in relation to surround tissue (negative contrast agent). Unfortunately, due to its low density, CO_2 angiography has a lower contrast resolution compared to iodine-based agents and hence produces a poorer image quality, particularly in the small peripheral vessels. Furthermore, CO_2 gas can cause the vapor lock phenomenon, a condition in which the gas is collected over the most anterior aspect of an artery, in particular the aorta, causing poor visualization of the mesenteric arteries and producing temporary abdominal pain, thought to be secondary to bowel ischemia. Finally, CO_2 angiography is contraindicated for "above-diaphragm" angiography, because of the risk of cerebral embolization.

Gadolinium chelate, an MRI contrast agent, can also be used as an intravascular contrast media. However, it is a poor radiographic contrast agent, and it should not be used in patients with renal impairment, as there is evidence that at the doses required for conventional angiography (as opposed to MRI) it is potentially more nephrotoxic than iodinated contrast (Thomsen et al., 2002). It can be useful in patients with other contraindications to iodinated agents, utilized as a problem solver to answer specific questions that cannot adequately be defined by CO_2 angiography. Because of dose limitations (maximum 0.3 mmol/kg), careful planning is required prior to its use.

Even with the introduction of smaller catheters and safer contrast agent, the role of contrast catheter angiography as the primary investigation tool of vascular diseases is diminishing due to its many drawbacks (Table 4.1). In the future, it will be employed mainly as part of an interventional procedure or in special diagnostic situations.

Computed Tomography

Until relatively recently, the images obtained from CT examinations were of suboptimal quality for the assessment of most vascular diseases except aneurysmal conditions. This was due to the long examination time (minutes) and thick slice width (5 to 10 mm); hence, images were subjected to movement artifacts and were

Table 4.1. Complications of angiography

Contrast medium–related complications
  Minor adverse reactions: common, but rarely life
    threatening (e.g., urticaria, nausea)
  Major adverse reactions: rare, but serious
    (idiosyncratic anaphylactoid reactions)
  Local vascular changes (e.g., effects on red
    cells/coagulation)
  Systemic vascular changes (e.g., increases in blood
    volume)
  Individual organ toxicity (e.g., renal)
Access site complications
  Hemorrhage
  Intramural or perivascular injection of contrast
  Vascular thrombosis (following dissection or local
    trauma)
  Peripheral embolization
  Vascular stenosis or occlusion
  Pseudoaneurysm formation
  Arteriovenous fistula
  Local infection
  Nerve damage
  Damage to other local structures
Catheter and general complications
  Air embolism
  Catheter thrombus embolization
  Dissection or perforation of vessels
  Organ ischemia or infarction secondary to spasm,
    dissection, or embolization
  Fracture and loss of guidewire or catheter fragments
  Catheter knot formation
  Mistaken injection of toxic material (e.g., skin
    cleansing agent)
  Vasovagal reactions
  Adverse reaction to local anesthetic or other drugs

have multiple banks of detectors (up to 64), allowing several slices to be acquired with each revolution of the scanner. The volumetric data obtained from recent scanners can be processed and displayed as multiplanar reformats (MPRs), maximum intensity projections (MIPs), or surface shaded displayed (SSD) (Fig. 4.2). Details about these reconstructions are beyond the scope of this chapter, but it is probably fair to say that MPR is most frequently used clinically.

With the new generation of multidetector scanners, the best spatial resolution of the images obtained is around 0.5 mm, which is adequate for assessing most vascular systems. However, as with contrast angiography, the main limitation of CT examinations is the requirement of large volumes (100 to 150 mL) of potentially nephrotoxic iodine-based contrast agent even with the new generation machines. Alternative contrast agents such as gadolinium can be used for CT, but produce less contrast and are more expensive.

Currently, the main roles of CT in relation to vascular diseases are (1) diagnosis of aortic

of low spatial resolution. These shortcomings prohibited the high-quality reconstruction often necessary for vascular studies. However, the introduction of spiral/helical CT shortened the examination time dramatically to less than 30 seconds and allowed the use of thin collimation (i.e., slice thickness). This short acquisition time meant the examination could be performed in a single breath-hold, reducing the motion artifact that was frequently encountered with older scanners. Thin collimation in turn improved spatial resolution, further enhancing image quality. These factors were further improved with the introduction of multislice/detector spiral CT. In comparison to the first-generation spiral CT scanners that have a single bank of x-ray detector, multidetector scanners

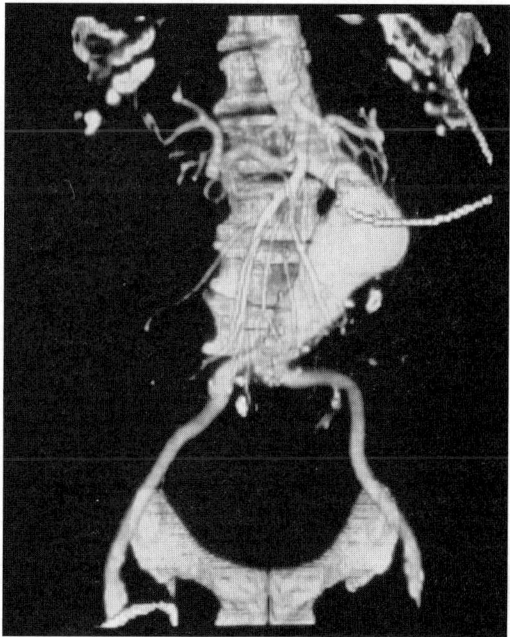

Figure 4.2. Surface shaded reconstruction showing the relationship of an infrarenal abdominal aortic aneurysm to the bony landmarks.

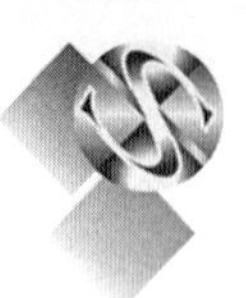

aneurysms, (2) assessment for open or endovascular treatment of aortic aneurysm, (3) endovascular stent graft surveillance, and (4) vascular trauma. Although CT provides accurate imaging of visceral and peripheral arteries, magnetic resonance angiography (MRA), which has none of the disadvantages of CT (i.e., nephrotoxic contrast agent and ionizing radiation), is more widely accepted by clinicians. Because magnetic resonance provides poor visualization of calcified arteries, a combination of MRA and noncontrast CT is often required in these cases.

Magnetic Resonance Angiography

Prior to the advent of gadolinium-enhanced three-dimensional (3D) MRA by Prince and coworkers, MRA played a small role in the investigations of vascular diseases, mainly because the images obtained were of poor quality due to movement and turbulence-induced artifacts (Prince et al., 1993). The use of gadolinium chelate as a contrast agent shortens the examination time significantly, allowing the examination to be performed in a single breath-hold, reducing movement artifacts. In addition, gadolinium-enhanced MRA is not susceptible to the flow artifacts that plague noncontrast MRA. The data range in 3D MRA is acquired as a continuous volume, and this allows 3D reconstruction of the images, producing images comparable to catheter angiography. The resolution limit of current MR scanners is approximately 1 mm, which is adequate for the imaging of most arteries, including the pedal vessels. Visualization of smaller vessels is software dependent, however, and MR images of distal vessels are limited by contrast issues, as the gadolinium dilutes as it travels distally and enhances the veins soon after the distal arteries. Despite these issues, MRA of the infrainguinal vessels can be performed with adequate quality for planning distal bypasses in centers with very high quality MRI.

The main advantage of MRA, in relation to CT, is the use of gadolinium as a contrast agent, which is safe and does not cause renal impairment, except in rare cases. The current limitations of MRA are high cost, lack of availability, patient claustrophobia, narrow range of field of view (for example, it is unable to image the entire aorta in one continuous acquisition), and

poor display of intraluminal thrombus and calcification of the arterial wall. The latter two limitations are important to consider in endovascular procedures, such as aneurysm stent grafting. In addition, MRA has the tendency to over-grade the degree of stenosis. Hence, in most units, confirmatory catheter angiography is routinely performed prior to intervention in cases where the MRA has shown significant stenotic disease.

Currently, the main roles of MR are for the investigations of aortoiliac disease, visceral arteries, and extent of arteriovenous malformations. In addition, as it involves no ionizing radiation, MR is the most appropriate imaging modality for young patients requiring long-term follow-up, such as those with aortic dissection, aortic root replacement surgery, or aortic coarctation. Although MR is not widely used at the moment as the primary imaging modality for vascular disease, with further advances in software and hardware designs expected in the future, it will become an ideal imaging tool.

Radiation Safety

X-rays are an ionizing radiation, interacting with water molecules, producing radicals that cause cellular damage and death. The effect can be immediate, for example, skin necrosis, or late, such as genetic mutation or cancer formation. It is important to bear in mind that radiation exposure is cumulative and permanent; hence, it is prudent that the exposure to x-rays be minimized. There are several simple methods to reduce the exposure to both patients and operators:

1. Radiation exposure is proportional to fluoroscopy time, and hence the most effective way to reduce exposure is to reduce the fluoroscopy time. Use pulse mode rather than continuous mode when possible and plan cases in advance to obtain only the necessary views.

2. Increase the distance from the source. Exposure decreases with the square of the distance from the source (inverse square law).

3. Use lower magnification and careful collimation.

4. Use posterior-anterior imaging, that is, the x-ray source is from the posterior of a supine patient.
5. Position the image intensifier as close as possible to the patient to reduce scatter.
6. Use protective barriers such as table aprons, lead glass shields, as well as the usual lead apron, thyroid shield, and glasses.

The use of dosimeter badges by all persons working with ionizing radiation is mandatory. In the United Kingdom, the badge must be positioned at waist level under the lead apron. Additional badges can be worn (such as on the fingers or forehead) for specific exposed areas. In the United States, badges are required either outside the apron at the neck level, beneath the lead apron, as in the U.K., or in both locations (with finger badge an option). In the U.K. and U.S., no individual working in the controlled area should receive doses in excess of (1) 20 mSv/year to the body, (2) 150 mSv/year to the lens, and (3) 500 mSv/year to hands or forearm. Finally, although the use of dosimeters is mandated, it is the responsibility of the operator to wear and use them correctly.

Investigations of Vascular Diseases

This section is divided into system-based categories. Common conditions and appropriate investigations for each system are discussed.

Peripheral Vascular Disease (Lower Limb)

This is the most common of all vascular conditions, accounting for the majority of the work load in any vascular unit. Clinically, this condition is best divided into two subcategories: (1) patients with symptoms of claudication without any tissue loss or rest pain; and (2) patients with rest pain or tissue loss, suggesting limb-threatening ischemia. In those patients with symptoms that are severe enough to warrant intervention, further investigation is justified. However, most claudicants do not require intervention and are treated conservatively, and thus further imaging is not necessary. In most cases,

duplex examination is adequate as a first-line investigation for the demonstration of the external iliac arteries, femoral arteries, and even as distally as the tibial trifurcation. Conventional catheter angiography, MRA, or CT angiography can be performed if the examination is of suboptimal quality or if the assessment of distal arteries is required, for example in cases where distal bypass surgery is considered. This depends on staff expertise and equipment availability in individual centers. In some centers distal bypass decisions can be based on duplex arterial mapping, MRA or even CT angiography (CTA), but currently most units still depend on catheter angiography. In patients with suspected aortoiliac disease, duplex examination is more difficult due to anatomical constraints. In this situation, MRA or CTA is generally preferred. If these two options are not available, an angiogram can be performed via a catheter that is positioned in the distal abdominal aorta. If brachial or radial artery access is used, access should be obtained from the left arm to minimize the risk of embolic complications to the cerebral circulation.

Catheter angiography is useful to diagnose vasculitic conditions such as thromboangiitis obliterans (Buerger disease). This condition classically affects small and medium-size arteries and veins of the lower limbs in young smokers with a typical angiographic appearance. In patients with blue digit syndrome, catheter angiography may show the source of emboli, typically atherosclerotic plaques in the aorta or iliac arteries. However, CT or other noninvasive modalities are preferred for the initial evaluation in blue digit syndrome, because the catheter-based modalities carry the risk of further atheroemboli.

Finally, although conventional catheter angiography plays an ever-diminishing role as the primary diagnostic tool in the investigation of peripheral vascular disease (PVD), it still has a few advantages in comparison to noninvasive techniques. Direct pressure measurement can be performed in equivocal stenosis (>10 mm Hg systolic gradient is considered significant), with the use of enhanced gradients in cases of possible "subcritical" stenosis [by the use of distal vasodilators such as glyceryl trinitrate (nitroglycerin in the U.S.) or papaverine], as well as allowing intervention to be performed in the same sitting.

Upper Limb Vascular Diseases

Upper limb vascular diseases are far less frequently encountered than those of the lower limb. These can usually be attributed to subclavian steal syndrome, embolic disease, or blue digit syndrome (distal embolization), and rarely due to diffuse atherosclerotic disease commonly seen in the lower limbs. Duplex ultrasonography is useful as a preliminary test. Although it is anatomically not possible to visualize the first part of the subclavian artery directly, waveform analysis of flow in the distal segments may reveal changes (such as damped signal or spectral broadening) that are suggestive of proximal occlusion or stenosis. In addition, duplex examination may detect flow reversal in the vertebral artery, which suggests a steal phenomenon and is a good indication of significant ipsilateral proximal subclavian artery stenosis or occlusion. Magnetic resonance angiography is widely accepted for the visualization of arch vessels, but aortic pulsation artifact may obscure anatomical detail at the origins of the great vessels. Computed tomography angiography is useful but subjected to beam-hardening artifacts from the thoracic cage and contrast in the venous system, both of which are in close proximity to the arteries of interest. Ultimately, catheter angiography is still the definitive test for the investigations of patients with upper limb ischemia. It is pertinent that a flush aortic arch angiogram is performed in two planes (left and right anterior oblique), as origin disease is frequently missed if only one projection is obtained.

A rare cause of upper limb ischemia is Takayasu arteritis (pulseless disease), a condition most commonly seen in young female Asians. It is a granulomatous disease involving major arteries, in particular the aortic branches and pulmonary arteries. Clinically, the patient is systemically unwell with symptoms and signs of limb ischemia or renovascular hypertension. Radiological features suggestive of the condition are enhancing thickened arterial wall on CT, segmental stenotic or occlusive disease of major arteries, and aneurysm formations.

Carotid Arteries

Duplex ultrasonography examination is the preliminary test for patients with suspected carotid artery stenosis in whom intervention is considered appropriate (see Chapter 3). The procedure is relatively easy to perform with good accuracy in experienced hands. In addition, it provides morphological assessment of the plaque. Hence, in many vascular centers, duplex examination is the sole radiological investigation prior to carotid endarterectomy. However, when endovascular treatment is an option, it is important that the entire carotid artery is assessed for synchronous stenotic disease, tortuosity, and a favorable angle of origin of the vessel to be treated (Fig. 4.3). These factors determine if endovascular treatment is feasible. Unfortunately, duplex examination cannot answer all these questions, and in our unit we presently rely on conventional arch aortography for full assessment (selective catheterization should not be required). However, it is likely that as improvements in MRA and CTA continue to be made, the full characterization of carotid stenosis, the arch vessels, and cerebral circulations will be of sufficient quality to eliminate the requirements for catheter angiography to determine whether a patient is a good candidate for endovascular intervention.

Carotid body tumor is a rare condition that classically presents as a painless pulsatile mass below the angle of the jaw, and is laterally mobile but fixed vertically. Approximately 10% of cases are bilateral. The typical ultrasonic feature is an oval mass splaying the carotid internal and external carotid arteries. This mass enhances avidly on CT or MR examinations.

Pulmonary Arteries

There are few medical conditions that require the imaging of the pulmonary vasculature. Most frequently this is required for suspected acute pulmonary embolic (PE) disease or as part of the investigation of pulmonary hypertension, to exclude chronic thromboembolism. In the majority of cases with suspected acute PE, the initial investigations should consist of a chest radiograph and a radionuclide ventilation-perfusion (V/Q) scan or a CTA. Unfortunately, up to 50% of V/Q scans are of no diagnostic value, and in these circumstances supplementary investigations are required. Previously, catheter angiography was the imaging modality of choice, but with the advent of spiral CT the role of catheter angiography is limited to situations such as massive PE, where immediate

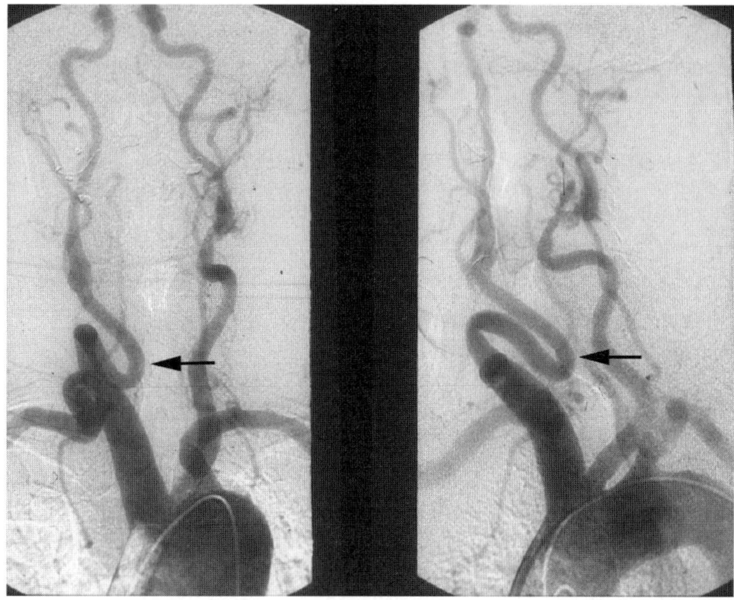

Figure 4.3. Tortuous common and internal carotid arteries (arrow), a contraindication to carotid artery stenting.

intervention may be required. Although CTA is undoubtedly accurate for the diagnosis of moderate to large emboli, it is limited by its inability to reliably diagnose subsegmental embolism, particularly with the older single-slice spiral scanners. However, the clinical significance of subsegmental PE is uncertain and may have only minimal impact in the long-term outcome. The results of ongoing outcome studies where patients are managed on the basis of multidetector/slice helical CT findings are eagerly awaited.

Magnetic resonance angiography has not been thoroughly evaluated as a tool for the diagnosis of PE, but a recent study showed that it has reasonable accuracy in comparison to catheter angiography (Haage et al., 2003). However MRA, as with CTA, is limited by the poor visualization of subsegmental arteries, and resolution tends to be approximately half that of CT in most institutions. Magnetic resonance angiography is unlikely to be widely used for the diagnosis of PE until further data are available (Haage et al., 2003).

In certain situations, the catheter pulmonary angiogram remains the investigation of choice. Patients with acute massive PE and cardiorespiratory instability should proceed directly to catheter angiogram, where treatment such as thrombectomy or thrombolysis can be adminis-

tered immediately following the confirmation of the diagnosis. Furthermore, it is possible to insert an IVC filter at the same time to prevent further embolism, if this remains a risk. Pulmonary angiography is also indicated in patients in whom noninvasive diagnostic tests remain inconclusive and a reasonable suspicion for PE exists. In this situation, pulmonary angiography is aimed at excluding PE, thus allowing withdrawal of anticoagulant therapy with its inherent bleeding risk. In patients in whom the consequence of bleeding is unforgiving, for instance following recent neurosurgery, pulmonary angiography can provide a definitive diagnosis. The disadvantages of pulmonary angiography are that it is invasive and uses nephrotoxic contrast agents. Nevertheless, the safety of this technique has improved dramatically over the past 10 years. Current estimates of mortality and morbidity are around 0.03% and 0.47%, respectively, in experienced hands.

Pulmonary arteriovenous malformation (AVM) is a rare condition in which there is an abnormal large vascular communication between the pulmonary artery and vein. This allows shunting of blood from the pulmonary circulation to the systemic circulation and hence the risk of complications such as cerebrovascular accident and cerebral abscess. The

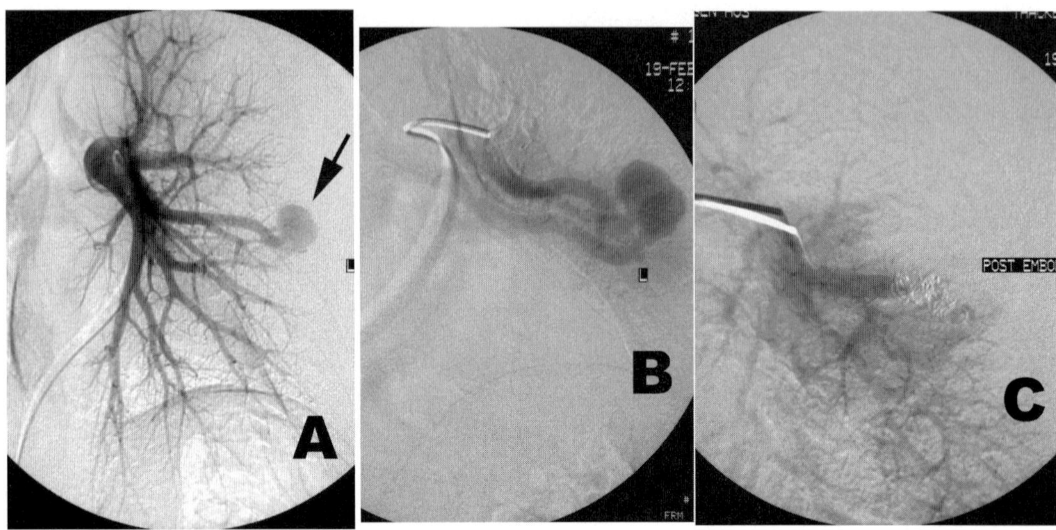

Figure 4.4. Coil embolization of pulmonary arteriovenous malformation (AVM). A: Pulmonary angiogram shows an AVM in the periphery of left lobe (arrow). B: Selective angiogram demonstrates the characteristic early draining vein. C: Angiographic appearance after successful embolization.

AVM can be solitary (40% of cases) or multiple, often associated with hereditary hemorrhagic telangiectasia (Rendu-Osler-Weber syndrome). Diagnosis can be reliably confirmed by CT or MR examinations, showing a vascular mass with a large feeding artery and draining vein (Fig. 4.4). Catheter angiogram is indicated only as a part of the current treatment of choice, i.e., embolotherapy.

Mesenteric Arteries

The main indications for the investigation of mesenteric arteries are gastrointestinal (GI) bleeding, intestinal angina, and mesenteric artery aneurysms or pseudoaneurysms. For GI bleeding, endoscopy is the first-line investigation. If the bleeding site or cause is not identified (up to 40% of endoscopic examinations), the patient should have a radionuclide test if the hemorrhage is not life threatening, or urgent selective catheter angiography if the patient is hemodynamically unstable and actively bleeding. Radionuclide investigations are more sensitive than catheter angiography for the investigation of GI bleeding (isotope remains in the vascular system far longer than contrast agent), but less accurate in identifying the exact anatomical site or the nature of the disease.

Technetium 99m (^{99m}Tc) sulfur colloid or ^{99m}Tc-labeled erythrocytes are used to localize mild-to-moderate intermittent bleeding, particularly in the lower GI tract, and ^{99m}Tc pertechnetate is used to detect Meckel's diverticulum. Selective catheter angiography may reveal the exact site of hemorrhage but this is highly dependent on the timing of the procedure. Many investigations turn out to be false negatives (reported accuracy of 40% to 90%), as the patients are not actively bleeding at the time of investigation. Nonetheless, the tests may still show areas of abnormal vascularity such as angiodysplasia. In addition, endovascular treatment such as embolization or vasopressin infusion may be initiated, and, it is hoped, avoid the high morbidity and mortality (up to 30%) of emergency surgery. The treatment may permanently stop the bleeding or allow a window of opportunity to stabilize the patient prior to definitive surgical resection if deemed necessary.

Although atheromatous disease of the mesenteric arteries is common, mesenteric angina is a rare entity. This is because there are numerous large collaterals between the mesenteric arteries, and hence the symptoms of mesenteric angina only manifest if there is severe stenosis or occlusion in two of the three mesenteric arteries (celiac, superior mesenteric, and infe-

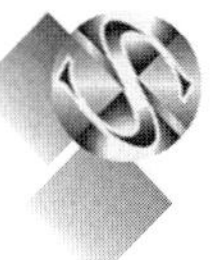

rior mesenteric arteries). The first-line investigation should be duplex ultrasonography, as it has excellent diagnostic value in many institutions. The origins of celiac and superior mesenteric artery are relatively straightforward to assess. However, the inferior mesenteric artery is frequently not seen due to overlying bowel gas. Because of this, many radiologists prefer MRA as the primary investigational modality for this condition. The 3D acquisition allows accurate assessment of the ostial disease with sensitivity and specificity comparable to that of catheter angiography. Computed tomography angiography is also being used as an adjunctive diagnostic modality in some institutions, primarily to aid in evaluation of calcific aortic plaque that is not seen well on MRA, but may have a substantial impact on the approach to surgical intervention. Currently, catheter angiography is usually reserved for cases in which other imaging modalities are equivocal, or when endovascular intervention is considered.

Mesenteric artery aneurysm is an uncommon condition, and is best assessed with cross-sectional studies such as CT. This allows the identification of the vessel of origin, the size of the aneurysm, and the mass effect on the surrounding structure. Catheter angiography can then be performed as part of the embolization treatment or for evaluation of potential aneurysms in the mesenteric arcades.

Renal Arteries

The main indications for imaging of the renal arteries are (1) diagnosis of renal artery stenosis, most commonly atherosclerotic or fibromuscular dysplasia (FMD); and (2) evaluation of potential live renal donors. Although conventional catheter angiography is still considered the gold standard, it involves the use of nephrotoxic contrast agent in a group of patients with a high incidence of preexisting renal impairment, and hence is employed only in cases where other tests are unavailable or inconclusive. In many institutions MRA is currently the investigation of choice in patients with suspected renovascular disease, primarily due to the lack of nephrotoxicity with gadolinium-chelate. It has high sensitivity and specificity for the assessment of ostial disease, but is unproven for distal stenosis such as in FMD. In our unit,

patients with suspected FMD have MRA as the first-line investigation, followed by catheter angiography if the MRA is of suboptimal quality or there is strong clinical suspicion of FMD. Although CTA is accurate for assessing renal artery stenosis, it is subjected to a similar drawback as catheter angiography, that is, requiring iodinated contrast media and ionizing radiation. Duplex examination is the initial imaging modality of choice in many institutions due to its low cost and relatively high accuracy for renal artery stenosis, but it is more prone to missing duplicate renal arteries, and it is highly operator- and patient-dependent, with up to a 15% technical failure rate.

With the current shortage of cadaver renal donors, living-related renal transplant surgery has become a common procedure. Previously, the donors had to undergo catheter angiography, ultrasonography, and intravenous urography as part of the assessment. Currently, MR is the imaging method of choice as it provides the most comprehensive and accurate assessment of the donor in one sitting. It allows anatomical and morphological evaluation of the renal parenchyma, veins, arteries, and ureters with confidence. In addition, it may show other intraabdominal pathologies such as adrenal or pelvic masses. Computed tomography angiography with 3D reconstruction can also be used in patients who are known to have normal renal function, as is true for most potential renal donors.

Aortic Aneurysms and Dissections

The conventional treatment for patients with aneurysmal disease of the aorta is surgical. Patients with abdominal aortic aneurysms (AAAs) or thoracic aortic aneurysms of greater than 5.5 or 6.5 cm in diameter, respectively, are generally best treated, depending on the patient's fitness for surgery, because of the increasing risk of rupture above these sizes. In most cases, CT examination alone is adequate to provide all the information needed prior to open surgical repair. Computed tomography shows the relation of visceral arteries to the aneurysm sac, the size and extent of the aneurysm, and other conditions that may preclude surgical repair, such as horseshoe kidney. In the early 1990s endovascular aneurysm repair (EVAR) revived the role of catheter

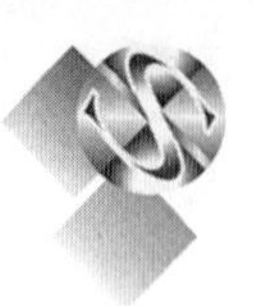

angiography for the assessment of aortic aneurysms. Catheter angiography began to diminish again, however, as spiral CT with 3D reconstruction and specialized software in the mid-1990s allowed high-quality reconstructions not previously possible. Accurate preoperative imaging is crucial to ensure proper selection of patients, stent-graft types, and potential intraoperative adjuncts such as coil embolization, iliac angioplasty, renal stenting, femoral endarterectomy, and iliac conduits. To eliminate the need for catheter angiography preoperatively, work focused on 3D reconstruction of CT and MR data, with specialized software for detailed measurements and even endograft simulations preoperatively. Currently, CT or MR with 3D reconstruction and computer-aided measurement, planning, and simulation is the standard for imaging prior to EVAR, with measurement accuracy and outcomes equal or superior to catheter angiography and without the morbidity or expense (Broeders et al., 1997; Fillinger, 1999, 2000). The main disadvantages of MR are the difficulty in visualizing thrombus and calcification, important points to be considered, as thrombus in the neck of the aneurysm may preclude endovascular repair. Nevertheless, future advances in MR technologies are expected to resolve these problems.

Although the technical success of stent-graft implantation is well established, only modest data are available for midterm results, and data on long-term efficacy and safety are not yet established. The goals of postprocedure imaging are to (1) confirm appropriate stent-graft placement, (2) assess the effectiveness of aneurysm exclusion, (3) follow the aneurysm sac size, and (4) detect device failure and/or migration. Because late complications have been observed, lifelong follow-up is felt to be essential at the present time. The current imaging strategy should include plain radiographs of the stent graft in four projections (anterior-posterior, lateral, and two obliques) and CT angiography at 1, 6, and 12 months postoperative, and then annually. More or less frequent imaging may be recommended depending on the imaging results (e.g., endoleak or migration), type of stent graft, and manufacturer recommendations. Plain radiographs are an excellent and inexpensive means to assess the metallic stent-graft frame for structural failure, angulation, and kinking. Plain radiographs have typically

been recommended for establishing migration, but this is best performed on CT. Triple-phase CT examinations (nonenhanced, arterial phase, and delayed "venous" phase) allow serial measurements of aneurysm sac diameters, monitoring of the integrity and position of the device, and detection of an endoleak (reperfusion of the aneurysm sac) (Fillinger, 1999). Three-dimensional reconstruction with volume measurements is the most sensitive method for detecting aneurysm sac size changes, but requires expertise in image segmentation or outsourcing to a commercial entity. It may allow earlier detection of problems that require intervention after EVAR or earlier reassurance to the patient and less frequent surveillance in successful repairs (Fillinger, 1999; Kay et al., 2003). Duplex ultrasound is a useful adjunct for the detection of endoleak, without the risk of contrast nephrotoxicity and ionizing radiation. However, it may not show the source of endoleak and is unable to assess stent-graft integrity accurately. Three-phase contrast-enhanced MRA serves as an attractive alternative to CTA in patients with renal impairment and relative contraindications to iodinated contrast media. There is evidence that it is superior to CT in depicting small type 2 (collateral) endoleaks. Unfortunately, it is not suitable for stainless steel devices, which cause severe image degradation secondary to metal artifacts. Currently, the role of catheter angiography is to characterize endoleaks (inflow and outflow channels) detected by the noninvasive tests or to further evaluate sacs that appear to have enlarged without an endoleak.

Aortic dissection is a condition in which a spontaneous tear of the tunica intima allows circulating blood to gain access to the tunica media, splitting it longitudinally. The objective of imaging is not only to diagnose the condition but also to localize the site of entry, assess the extent of dissection, and identify associated complications. The potential complications that may occur are occlusion of major aortic branches such as coronary and visceral arteries; aortic valve insufficiency; rupture into the pericardial sac, mediastinum, or pleural cavity; and aneurysm formation in the long-term. At present, the imaging modality of choice for acute dissection is CT angiography. It has excellent sensitivity and specificity in comparison to catheter angiography, which is considered the

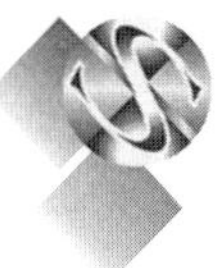

standard of reference. However, it is vital that the examination be performed in the arterial phase of contrast enhancement, as failure to do so may lead to misinterpretation of a dissection as an aneurysm. Transesophageal ultrasonic examination is a useful adjunct, showing the presence or absence of aortic valve incompetence and pericardial effusion, and confirming the presence of the intimal flap. Magnetic resonance is as accurate as CT, if not more so, in diagnosing acute dissection. However, it is rarely employed because of the lack of immediate availability, the delay from bedside to scanner, the long examination time, the limited access to the patient, and the restricted monitoring of vital signs, which is especially problematic in these often hemodynamically unstable patients.

Vascular Trauma

Vascular injuries can occur in a number of ways, such as motor vehicle accidents, knife or gunshot wounds, or iatrogenically. In most cases, the history and clinical features provide the diagnosis. Hemodynamically unstable patients usually proceed immediately to the operating room for control of the hemorrhage. If the patient is stable enough, imaging can be used to confirm hemorrhage or injury, localize the site, and assess the severity. In addition, treatment options can be planned from the information acquired, and in some cases catheter-based therapeutic intervention can be performed. Direct vascular injuries in a stable patient are often best investigated initially by CT examination. One major advantage of contrast-enhanced CT over ultrasound is the ability to identify the exact site of bleeding and potentially help plan the approach for surgical or endovascular intervention.

Aortic injury occurs most often following a rapid deceleration injury, and the vast majority of cases are due to motor vehicle accidents. Complete rupture accounts for 85% of cases, and most patients do not survive. The remaining 15% have incomplete rupture (contained rupture) and they require immediate treatment, as half of them will progress to complete rupture within 24 hours. The most common site of injury (90%) is at the aortic isthmus, just distal to the left subclavian artery. The prelimi-

nary investigation is a chest radiograph. It may show features suggestive of transection, such as a widened mediastinum, apical cap, and displacement of the trachea, left main bronchus, or nasogastric tube. A normal chest x-ray does not exclude transection, but will diagnose conditions such as pneumothorax or hydrothorax. Arterial phase contrast-enhanced spiral CT with fine collimation is the most widely used modality for the imaging of aortic transection. Features of aortic injury are the presence of an abrupt change in aortic contour, false aneurysm, intimal flap, or extravasation of contrast. Mediastinal hematoma is a frequent finding in traumatic chest injury, but in the majority of cases, the source of hematoma is the azygos or hemiazygos veins and paraspinal and intercostals vessels rather than aortic injuries. Although catheter angiography is still considered the standard of reference for investigation of aortic transection, it is employed only when the CT examination is equivocal or as part of the endovascular treatment. When performing catheter angiography, it is vital that at least two projections of the arch and descending aorta be obtained prior to pronouncing the investigation normal. In addition, an awareness of ductus diverticulum is required. This is the vestigial remnant of the ductus arteriosus and is present in approximately 10% of the population. This anatomical variant appears as a small bulge on the medial wall of the aorta, just inferior to the origin of the left subclavian artery, and is frequently misinterpreted as a false aneurysm.

Conclusion

We have presented an overview of available imaging techniques in use in vascular radiological practice, emphasizing the move away from invasive techniques and toward noninvasive techniques for diagnosis of vascular diseases. The most important contemporary approaches and therapies have also been described, showing the important role these techniques now play in the management of a range of vascular disease processes.

References

Aspelin P, Aubry P, Fransson SG, Strasser R, Willenbrock R, Berg KJ. (2003) N Engl J Med 348:491–9.

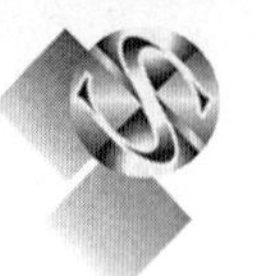

Broeders IA, Blankensteijn JD, Olree M, Mali W, Eikelboom BC. (1997) J Endovasc Surg 4:252–61.

Dormandy JA, Rutherford RB. (2000) J Vasc Surg 31:S1–S296.

Fillinger MF. (1999) Surg Clin North Am 79:451–75.

Fillinger MF. (2000) Semin Vasc Surg 13:247–63.

Haage P, Piroth W, Krombach G, et al. (2003) Am J Respir Crit Care Med 167:729–34.

Kay J, Chow WH, Chan TM, et al. (2003) JAMA 289:553–8.

Prince MR, Yucel EK, Kaufman JA, Harrison DC, Geller SC. (1993) J Magn Reson Imaging 3:877–81.

Snow TM, Rice HA. (1999) Clin Radiol 54:842–4.

Thomsen HS, Almen T, Morcos SK. (2002) Eur Radiol 12:2600–5.

5

Bleeding and Clotting Disorders

Vivienne J. Halpern and Frank C.T. Smith

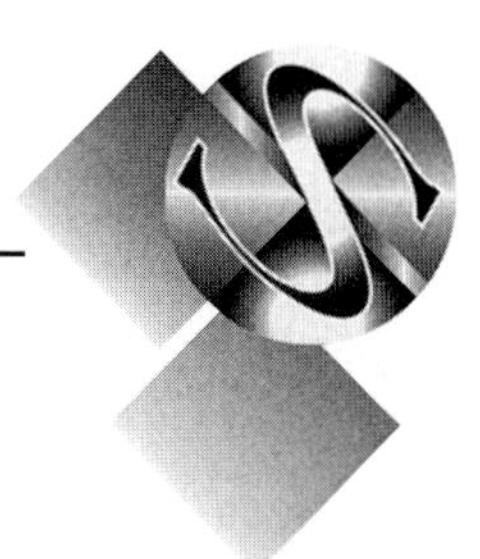

Bleeding and clotting disorders have major implications for the effective management of vascular patients. Such disorders can influence disease progression, perioperative complications, graft patency, limb salvage, and wound healing. Most of these disorders are relatively rare, and diagnosis requires an index of clinical suspicion combined with a need to obtain a relevant medical history and appropriate specialized investigations. Correct and timely treatment may help prevent some of the complications associated with these disorders. This chapter reviews the presentation, diagnosis, and management of some of the more common disorders. Medications frequently associated with abnormal bleeding or clotting are also discussed.

History, Physical and Laboratory Evaluation

Recognition of a patient with a bleeding or clotting disorder involves taking an adequate history. A screening questionnaire, such as that provided in Table 5.1 is useful and may help to direct further investigation. Obtaining a history of mucosal bleeding involving epistaxis, gum bleeding, or menorrhagia may be more consistent with platelet disorders (thrombocytopenia, von Willebrand disease, etc.) than, for instance, bleeding into a joint or muscle, which occurs more commonly with hemophilia. Patients with a history of myeloproliferative, myelodysplastic, and lymphoproliferative disorders may also have increased bleeding through several mechanisms, which may not appear in routine preoperative testing. Renal failure predisposes to bleeding tendencies based on platelet dysfunction, whereas, for instance, recent splenectomy may induce thrombocythemia predisposing to abnormal clotting. An abnormal history of clotting, such as multiple episodes of deep venous thrombosis (DVT), may warrant screening for thrombophilia.

Medications can influence both bleeding and clotting. Commonly used drugs such as aspirin and other nonsteroidal antiinflammatory drugs (NSAIDs) affect platelet function, as do Aggrenox and Plavix. Herbal remedies and various vitamin combinations may also increase bleeding risks (Table 5.2). Furthermore, malnutrition and vitamin deficiencies, such as vitamin C deficiency, may contribute to abnormal bleeding tendencies. Estrogen or estrogen-like medications including phytoestrogens predispose to thrombotic episodes. PC-SPES is an herbal preparation with several components used for treatment of prostate carcinoma. It contains phytoestrogens, which may induce thrombosis. However, it also contains Baikal skull cap (*Scutellaria baicalensis georgi*), which is a coumarin (a naturally occurring group of substances, structurally similar to warfarin). These examples illustrate the importance of querying the use of herbal medications as well as more conventional pharmacotherapies when

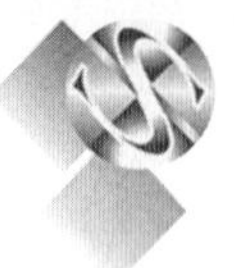
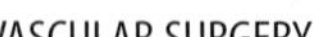

Table 5.1. Screening survey for abnormal bleeding or clotting

Do you suffer from a bleeding disorder?
Do you have bleeding from the gums or from the nose?
Have you ever coughed up or vomited blood?
Do you notice easy or spontaneous bruising or does it take you a long time to stop bleeding when cut?
Do you have excessive bleeding with menstrual cycles?
Have you had any blood in the urine or with stools?
Have you had any bleeding into muscles or joints?
Have you had a tooth extraction or any other procedure after which bleeding has taken a long time to stop?
Have you needed to receive any blood products, plasma, or vitamin K to help stop bleeding?
Do you have any problems with your liver or kidneys?
Has anyone in your family had any of the above problems?
Have you or anyone in your family had a history of clots in the blood vessels, either artery or veins?
Do you take oral contraceptives?
Do you take aspirin or any medications for pain or arthritis?
Do you take any steroid medications?
Do you take any herbal medications or vitamins?
Do you take Coumadin or other blood thinners?
Do you take any medications to prevent stroke or heart attacks?
Do you have any blood diseases?

Table 5.2. Common medications, herbs, and vitamins associated with increased bleeding

Medication	Mechanism of action	When to stop preoperatively
Medications that may increase bleeding		
Aspirin	Inhibits platelet aggregation via thromboxane B_2	5–7 days before major surgery 3–4 days before minor surgery
Persantine	Inhibits phosphodiesterase to increase cyclic AMP	Omit dose before surgery
Aggrenox	Combined Persantine and aspirin: increased effects of aspirin	As aspirin
Plavix	Irreversible binding to platelet inhibits ADP binding to platelet	Stop 7–10 days before surgery
NSAIDs	Various mechanisms	24 hours prior to surgery
Herbs/vitamins that may increase bleeding		
Feverfew	Used for migraines, ? inhibits platelet aggregation via thromboxane B_2, may be irreversible	Stop at least 1 week before surgery
Garlic	Inhibits platelet function by inhibiting thromboxane synthesis; may be irreversible	Stop at least 7–10 days before surgery
Gingko	Inhibition of platelet activating factor	Stop at least 36 hours prior to surgery
Ginseng	Inhibits platelet aggregation; prolongs PT and PTT; may be irreversible	Minimum of 24 hours prior to surgery
Vitamin E	May decrease platelet adhesiveness; may effect vascular endothelium	Unclear; should stop around 5 days before surgery
Willow bark	Salicylate precursors	Stop 7–10 days before surgery, similar to aspirin
Oil of wintergreen	Affects platelet function	
Meadowsweet flower		

ADP, adenosine diphosphate; AMP, adenosine monophosphate; NSAID, nonsteroidal antiinflammatory drug; PT, prothrombin time; PTT, partial thromboplastin time.

assessing the patient with a bleeding or clotting disorder.

Investigations

Standard preoperative investigations for most vascular surgery patients include prothrombin time (PT), international normalized ratio (INR), activated partial thromboplastin time (aPTT), platelet count, and activated clotting time (ACT). A platelet count of 50,000/µL should ensure adequate hemostasis, whereas a count of 10,000/µL or less may result in spontaneous bleeding. The aPTT evaluates the intrinsic and contact activation pathways of coagulation with the exception of factors VII and XIII. This investigation is used to monitor the effects of treatment with heparin. The extrinsic pathway (factors II, V, VII, and X, and fibrinogen) is evaluated with the PT and INR. These tests are employed to check the effectiveness of oral anticoagulation with warfarin. Additional tests should be directed by the history and clinical picture.

The prevalence of inherited bleeding and clotting disorders is relatively rare. Patients with a recurrent, familial, or juvenile history of DVT; arterial thrombosis at a young age or without evidence of atherosclerosis; or thrombosis in an unusual location, such as mesenteric or cerebral veins, should be assessed for a hypercoagulable state. Recurrent graft failure whether in a bypass or an arteriovenous fistula, when not explained by the presence of an anatomical lesion, may also imply a prothrombotic state. Components of a thrombophilia screen include those listed in Table 5.3 (Donaldson et al., 1990).

Patients with a history of abnormal bleeding, but not requiring medication, should undergo routine preoperative investigations as above. Excessive or prolonged bleeding during surgical procedures where routine preoperative testing of PT, aPTT, and platelet counts was normal may represent a platelet functional abnormality, a dysfibrinogenemia, factor XIII deficiency, vascular endothelial disorders, other mild factor deficiencies (if >25% of factor present), or α-antiplasmin deficiency. Surreptitious use of medication might also be considered. Where abnormal preoperative investigations are encountered, there is a rationale for further tests. A protocol is suggested in Table 5.4.

Table 5.3. Thrombophilia screen

Protein C levels
Protein S levels
Antithrombin III
Factor V Leiden
Activated protein C
Lupus anticoagulant
Anticardiolipin antibody
Antiphospholipid antibody
Homocysteine levels
Prothrombin 20210A mutation
Factor VIII and XI levels

Bleeding Disorders

Bleeding disorders may be secondary to abnormalities of plasma clotting factors, blood vessels, or platelets. Some hemostatic defects involve more than one of these systems.

Table 5.4. Protocol for further investigation of abnormal preoperative blood tests

Repeat abnormal PT/INR, aPTT with 50:50 mix with normal plasma (mixing study)
If then normal, undertake the following investigations:
Normal PT/INR, increased aPTT:
Test for factor deficiency: usually isolated XI, IX, VIII
Increased PT/INR, normal aPTT:
Test for factor deficiency: isolated VII or can be multiple
Test for liver abnormalities
Look for vitamin K deficiency (malnourished patient, patient on prolonged antibiotics)
Increased PT/INR and aPTT:
Test for factor deficiency: isolated X, V, prothrombin, fibrinogen, or can be multiple
If abnormal mixing study, undertake the following investigations:
Normal PT/INR, increased aPTT:
Test for inhibitor activity, especially for XI, IX, VIII
Test for nonspecific inhibitors, e.g., antiphospholipid antibodies
Increased PT/INR, normal aPTT:
Test for factor VII inhibitor
Test for nonspecific inhibitors (rarely cause isolated increase in PT/INR)
Increased PT/INR and aPTT
Test for inhibitors of X, V, prothrombin, fibrinogen
Test for nonspecific inhibitors

aPTT, activated partial thromboplastin time; INR, international normalized ratio; PT, prothrombin time.

In normal hemostasis, the blood vessel constricts in response to injury to reduce bleeding. Circulating platelets adhere to subendothelial collagen that is exposed by injury, promoted by release of tissue factor (TF) from the damaged vessel wall. Platelets bind von Willebrand factor (vWF) at the glycoprotein Ib receptor, stabilizing adhesion. Fibrinogen binds to platelet glycoprotein IIb/IIIa receptors forming bridges between adjacent platelets and causing aggregation. Activated platelets also release potent aggregating agents to recruit more platelets.

Coagulation is initiated through the extrinsic pathway. Exposed endothelium releases TF, which complexes with and activates factor VII. Factor VIIa then activates both the common pathway and the intrinsic pathway. The intrinsic pathway requires factor VIII and factor IX to proceed to the common pathway. Von Willebrand factor also forms a noncovalent bond with factor VIII and is essential for its survival in the circulation. Von Willebrand factor also potentiates factor VIII activity in clot formation and protects it from proteolysis. In the final step of the coagulation pathway, thrombin cleaves fibrinogen to generate fibrin monomers, which then polymerize and link to one another to form a chemically stable clot. Thrombin also feeds back to activate cofactors VIII and V, thereby amplifying the coagulation mechanism. Together platelet aggregates and fibrin form the clot that achieves hemostasis. The coagulation cascade is illustrated in Figure 5.1. Any disruption of these pathways may lead to increased bleeding.

Features in the history and physical examination that may help to differentiate among factor deficiencies, platelet disorders, and endothelial (blood vessel) dysfunction are listed in Table 5.5.

Inherited Disorders of Coagulation

Factor Deficiencies

Hemophilia A and B represent 80% of inherited bleeding diatheses. These are both sex-linked recessive deficiencies affecting mostly males.

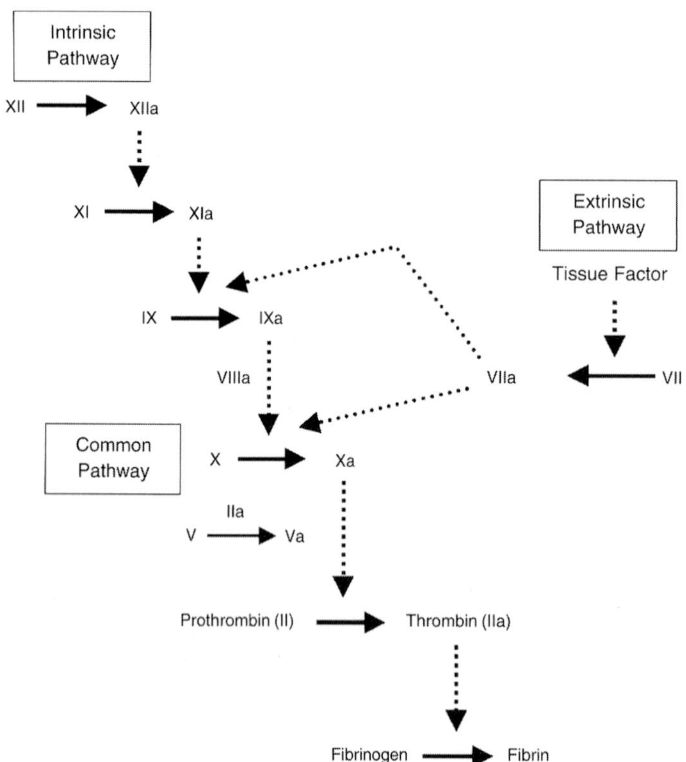

Figure 5.1. The coagulation cascade. Under physiological conditions, tissue factor is not exposed to blood. However, after injury, tissue factor is exposed to blood and activates the extrinsic pathway by acting in concert with activated VII and phospholipids to convert factor IX to IXa and factor X to Xa. The "intrinsic pathway" includes activation of factor XII to XIIa, which activates factor XI to XIa, IX to IXa, and X to Xa. Factor Xa is the active catalytic ingredient of the prothrombinase complex, which includes factor Va and phospholipase and converts prothrombin to thrombin. Thrombin is a protease that cleaves fibrinogen to fibrin. The resulting fibrin monomers polymerize, forming a clot.

Table 5.5. The relationship of factor disorders, platelet and blood vessel (endothelial) dysfunction to aspects of clinical presentation

Clinical picture	Factor disorder	Platelet dysfunction	Endothelial dysfunction
Onset of bleeding	Delayed	Immediate	Immediate
Duration of bleeding	Prolonged	Short	Variable
Precipitant of bleeding	Often spontaneous	Trauma	Variable
Site	Joints, muscle, viscera	Skin, mucous membranes, GI tract	Skin, GI tract
Family history	Usually present (unless factor inhibitor)	Absent	Usually absent
Drug-related	Rarely	Often	Sometimes
Sex predominance	Usually male	Often female	Usually female
Response to focal pressure	No response	Sometimes responds	Responds
Platelet count	Normal	Normal, low, or high	Normal
Prothrombin time	Abnormal in cases of factor II, VII, IX, and X deficiency (and inhibitors)	Normal	Normal
Partial Thromboplastin time	Abnormal with factor VIII or IX deficiency (and inhibitors)	Normal	Normal

GI, gastrointestinal.

They are caused by factor VIII (classic hemophilia) and factor IX (Christmas disease) deficiencies, respectively. Hemophilia A is four to six times more common than hemophilia B. Together they have a prevalence of about 20/100,000 in the United States and 9/100,000 to 15/100,000 in Great Britain.

The risk for bleeding depends on the degree of factor deficiency. At levels less than 1% to 2% of normal (severe disease), spontaneous bleeding is likely to occur and the aPTT is prolonged. Patients may present with spontaneous soft tissue or intramuscular hemorrhage, hemarthroses, hematuria, and spontaneous retroperitoneal bleeding. Patients with mild (>5%) and moderate (1% to 5%) disease usually have bleeding only with injury or surgery. Patients may have increased bleeding with levels above 25%, but these deficiencies are hard to detect as the aPTT will be normal.

Treatment for hemophilia A involves infusion of recombinant factor VIII concentrates of which several are commercially available, the amount depending on the deficiency present. This includes a loading dose and then a maintenance dose for the appropriate period depending on the location of the bleed if spontaneous or perioperative. For milder hemophilia or cases of mild hemorrhage, or if factor VIII concentrates are not available, cryoprecipitate or fresh frozen plasma (FFP) may be used.

The treatment for hemophilia B is similar, using specific factor IX concentrates or factor IX complex transfusion. The factor IX complex contains one unit of factor IX per milligram of protein with varying amounts of other vitamin K–dependent proteins. The concentrates are preferred treatment. Again, loading dose and maintenance doses are administered according to the given situation.

Another factor deficiency (vWF), which can present like hemophilia, occurs in von Willebrand disease (vWD). Overall, this is the most common bleeding disorder with an incidence of up to 1% in some populations. There are three subtypes of VWD, the most severe and uncommon being type 3. In this form, vWF in plasma and platelets is markedly reduced or absent, thereby reducing factor VIII activity to 1% to 10% of normal. Patients can present with spontaneous or severe bleeding. Inheritance is autosomal recessive. Type 1 is the most common type, representing around 70% of cases. vWF is reduced to the range of 20% to 50% with a concomitant reduction of factor VIII activity. The structure of vWF is generally normal in this type, and inheritance is autosomal dominant. Patients usually present with mild to moderate bleeding diatheses, and the levels of vWF do not necessarily correlate with clinical symptoms. This may be because some patients with type 1 VWD have reduced levels of both plasma and platelet vWF, whereas some just have reduced plasma levels.

Type 2 VWD is divided into further subtypes 2A, 2B, 2M, and 2N based on the site of the genetic mutation. Type 2A is the most common and accounts for around 10% of all vWF deficiency cases. Inheritance is autosomal dominant. The largest multimers of vWF are absent, and this leads to a lack of platelet binding. Activity of factor VIII, however, can be near normal in this subgroup. Clinical presentations in this group are therefore variable. In type 2B, patients lack multimers in the plasma but have near-normal levels in platelets. However, these patients are usually thrombocytopenic, which can be made worse with exercise, stress, pregnancy, or advanced age. Levels of factor VIII are low to normal. Presentation is again variable and inheritance is autosomal dominant. Type 2M is very rare and has abnormal multimers as its cause of abnormal coagulation. This has not been well defined in terms of inheritance. Type 2N is inherited as an autosomal-recessive condition and sometimes mimics mild hemophilia. These patients have normal vWF multimers and normal vWF activity but reduced factor VIII activity due to poor binding between vWF and factor VIII. This variant should be considered in the differential diagnosis of factor VIII deficiency, especially if the patient is female and other aspects of the pedigree support autosomal-recessive inheritance rather than sex-linked. Von Willebrand disease may be treated with desmopressin acetate [deamino-8-D-arginine vasopressin (DDAVP)], which probably increases vWF, tissue plasminogen activator (tPA), and factor VIII secretion from stored sources. Some of the subtypes may also require factor replacement. More recent treatments include recombinant factor VIII/vWF concentrates, which reduce risks of transmission of infection.

Other factor deficiencies are quite rare. Factor V deficiency is inherited as an autosomal-recessive trait. It has a wide range of clinical manifestations but seems to have less bleeding associated with it than hemophilia A. Severe factor V deficiency (levels <1% of normal) presents with abnormal bruising, soft tissue hemorrhage, and epistaxis. Bleeding from the umbilical stump at the time of birth is common. Women commonly have abnormally heavy menstrual bleeding and postpartum bleeding. Most cases present in adulthood. Fresh frozen plasma is the mainstay of treatment.

Factor VII deficiency is inherited as an autosomal-recessive disorder and affects males and females equally with an incidence of about 1 in 500,000. Clinical manifestations can be similar to those of hemophilia with severe deficiencies (<1% level) as the factor Va/tissue factor complex is the key initiator of coagulation in vivo. However, about half of patients are asymptomatic, and levels of factor V do not correlate well with clinical manifestations. Interestingly, diminished or defective function of tissue factor has not been documented as a cause of decreased factor VII activity. The most common presentations include easy bruising, soft tissue hemorrhage, and menorrhagia in women. Patients with levels less than 1% of normal may present like hemophiliacs with pathology including intracranial bleeds and hemarthroses. Current treatment in the United States is with FFP, although factor VII concentrates and recombinant factor VII are available in Europe.

Factor X deficiency is transmitted as an autosomal-recessive trait and has an estimated incidence of 1 in 500,000. Usually those with greater than 15% of normal levels do not have severe bleeding, although bleeding with major surgery or trauma may occur. However, with more severe deficiencies, severe bleeding episodes similar to those seen in hemophilia may occur, including hemarthroses, retroperitoneal hematomas, hematuria, pseudotumors, and menorrhagia. Another cause of factor X deficiency is amyloidosis. In this situation, transfusion of factor X is not helpful because of its absorption by the extracellular amyloid. Improvement does not occur unless the amyloidosis resolves, although splenectomy may help by debulking splenic amyloid. Treatment for standard factor X deficiency is with FFP or prothrombin complex concentrates. Pure factor X concentrates are not available for commercial use yet. Concentrations of 10% to 15% give adequate hemostasis. Overtransfusion can lead to thromboembolic events and disseminated intravascular coagulation (DIC).

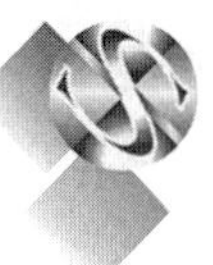

Factor XI deficiency occurs mostly in Ashkenazi Jews with a gene frequency in this population of 4.3%. Bleeding usually occurs with levels ≤20% of normal and usually only after major trauma or surgery. Rarely, there is spontaneous bleeding as seen with hemophilia, although soft tissue hemorrhage, epistaxis, and bleeding after dental extraction and with major surgical procedures may occur. Menorrhagia may occur in females. Bleeding risk is significantly increased in patients taking aspirin. Treatment when necessary is with FFP and with cryoprecipitate-poor plasma. Factor XI concentrates are available.

Fibrinogen Abnormalities

The dysfibrinogenemia are mostly inheritable abnormalities of fibrinogen structure and function. Clinically, many patients are asymptomatic but some present with either bleeding or a thromboembolic event or both. There are multiple different abnormalities too diverse to discuss in detail in this chapter because they have variable inheritance, affect different portions of the molecule, and have different manifestations. Suffice it to say they should be considered in patients with a history of bleeding and abnormal coagulation testing. Inheritable afibrinogenemias and hypofibrinogenemias also exist. Patients present with bleeding episodes in the afibrinogenemias and with hypofibrinogenemias with levels above 50 mg/dL. Afibrinogenemias are inherited as an autosomal-recessive trait but hypofibrinogenemias are less predictable. Bleeding complications when they occur can be severe, with a high incidence of bleeding in the neonatal period. This may result in death in about one third of patients with severe hypo- and afibrinogenemias.

Platelet Disorders

Bernard-Soulier syndrome (glycoprotein Ib-IX deficiency) is a disorder of platelet adhesion and is a relatively rare cause of bleeding. It is characterized by a prolonged bleeding time, large platelets, and thrombocytopenia due to an inability to adhere to vWF in the subendothelial matrix. It presents in infancy or childhood with epistaxis, ecchymosis, and bleeding gums. Treatment is with platelet transfusion. Hormonal control may be helpful with menorrhagia, and DDAVP may be useful for prophylaxis prior to procedures.

Deficiencies of platelet collagen receptors also exist but do not cause significant bleeding, although they may prolong bleeding time.

Disorders of platelet aggregation include a deficiency of IIb/IIIa, known as Glanzmann's thrombasthenia, characterized by a prolonged bleeding time and abnormal clot retraction. It is inherited as an autosomal-recessive trait in clusters of disease. It presents with mucocutaneous bleeding in the neonatal period or in infancy and occasionally as bleeding following circumcision. Epistaxis and purpura are the most common presentation. Severe bleeding with menses may be encountered. If it is unrecognized, significant bleeding with surgery or trauma will occur if the patient is not transfused with normal platelets. Platelet counts and smears are normal, but bleeding times are very prolonged. Platelet aggregation is absent in normal testing except with epinephrine, where it is weak. Platelet secretion is normal with strong agonists like thrombin but is absent with weak stimulators like epinephrine and adenosine diphosphate (ADP). Clot retraction is either absent or reduced. Treatment is undertaken with platelet transfusion if bleeding is present. Leukocyte-depleted platelets may reduce risks with future transfusions. Hormonal therapy is useful with menorrhagia. Regular dental care is important to reduce the risk of gingival bleeding but Amicar (ε-aminocaproic acid) may be valuable in helping to control bleeding after dental extractions.

Disorders of platelet secretion are related to deficiencies in one or more of the four types of platelet granules or to abnormalities in the secretory mechanism. Platelets have four types of granules:

1. Dense or δ granules containing ADP, adenosine triphosphate (ATP), calcium, serotonin, and pyrophosphates
2. α-granules containing a variety of proteins, some of which are obtained from the plasma and others synthesized by megakaryocytes; these include fibrinogen, vWF, albumin, factor V, immunoglobulin G (IgG), fibronectin, and proteinase inhibitors from the plasma and platelet

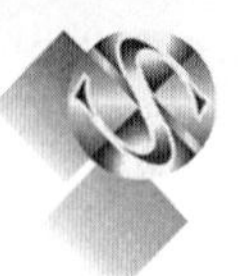

factor-4, β-thromboglobulin, platelet-derived growth factor, and thrombospondin from megakaryocytes

3. Lysosomes containing acid hydrolase
4. Microperoxisomes containing peroxidase activity

Secretory dysfunction usually results in mild to moderate bleeding manifested by easy bruising, menorrhagia, and excessive postoperative or peripartum bleeding. Testing reveals a prolonged bleeding time, a decreased second wave of aggregation with ADP and epinephrine stimulation, and decreased aggregation with collagen. Secretory dysfunction should be differentiated from acquired disorders with acetylsalicylic acid (ASA) use, uremia, and multiple myeloma, and from VWD.

Gray platelet syndrome is an α-granule deficiency. Platelets occur without these granules but with vacuoles and small α-granule precursors containing material that stain positive for vWF and fibrinogen. Additionally, the vacuoles and these precursors contain P-selectin and GIIb-IIIa. These factors indicate the presence of α-granules, but the normal proteins they contain cannot be packaged. Other granules are present in normal quantity. Patients have a history of mild to moderate mucocutaneous bleeding. They have prolonged bleeding times with moderate thrombocytopenia (60,000 to 100,000), reticular fibrosis of the bone marrow, and large platelets that appear gray on Wright-stained blood smears–hence the name. Platelet aggregation studies are variable. Treatment requires transfusion of normal platelets and at least one patient responded to DDAVP. The Quebec platelet disorder is extremely rare and again involves α-granules that appear grossly normal but are deficient in many of the proteins normally seen including factor V, fibrinogen, vWF, and fibronectin. Patients present similarly to the gray platelet syndrome and are treated the same way.

Dense granule deficiency or δ-storage pool disease is a heterogeneous group of disorders, which can be divided into deficiency states associated with albinism and those in otherwise normal patients. With albinism, the disease is related to a qualitative deficiency in these granules. In nonalbinos, the number of granules is near normal. In some of these nonalbino patients it is associated with a variable deficiency of α-granules. The content of lysosomal hydrolase is normal, but thrombin-induced acid hydrolase secretion is impaired, which can only be corrected with ADP. Patients present with mild to moderate bleeding. Platelet counts are usually normal, but bleeding times are prolonged. The quantity of thromboxane B_2, a metabolite of thromboxane A_1, is reduced. Secondary aggregation induced by ADP and epinephrine is reduced. Collagen-induced aggregation is abnormal at low concentrations of collagen but is normal with high concentrations. Therapy requires transfusions of normal platelets if there is massive bleeding. Otherwise, DDAVP is the initial treatment and cryoprecipitate can also be used. In one study, prednisolone seemed to reduce bleeding in patients with inherited platelet disorders but not in patients with thrombasthenia or ASA use.

Platelet function in patients with inherited disorders of platelet secretion resembles that of patients receiving platelet function inhibitors like ASA. These disorders are a heterogeneous collection of abnormalities of secretion-response adhesion. In families where these disorders have been noted, the pattern appears to be autosomal dominant. A prolonged bleeding time and marked impairment of aggregation and secretion in response to ADP, epinephrine, and low concentrations of collagen occur. Stronger agonists like high levels of collagen, however, may induce a near-normal or normal response. Treatment is the same as that for patients with platelet storage disorders.

Vascular Defects

Inheritable conditions that lead to defects in the vascular bed include Marfan's syndrome and Osler-Weber-Rendu disease. These may increase bleeding through mechanisms that are not entirely clear.

Acquired Disorders of Coagulation

This group of disorders includes factor inhibitors as well as acquired diseases that affect platelet and endothelial function. Factor inhibitory proteins can be classified as neutralizing, nonneutralizing, or altering. They are

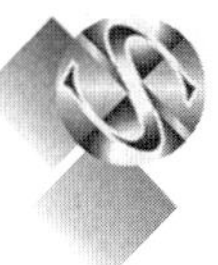

usually autoantibodies. The most common factor inhibitor is factor VIII, often referred to as acquired hemophilia, but inhibitors have been found to thrombin and prothrombin, fibrinogen, thrombin and prothrombin, fibrinogen, vWF, and factors V, VII, IX, X, and XI as well (Fig. 5.1). These are seen in response to inflammatory diseases such as rheumatoid arthritis and other autoimmune diseases like systemic lupus erythematosus (SLE) and Sjögren's syndrome and even inflammatory bowel syndrome. They also appear during pregnancy and the puerperium, as well as with various tumors. They may be associated with a variety of medications including aminoglycosides, penicillins, valorous acid, etc. They are also seen with cirrhosis and major surgery.

Interestingly, factors V and X and thrombin inhibitors have been seen following the use of topical thrombin and fibrin glue, usually after multiple exposures. Not only can this lead to perioperative bleeding, but also inhibitors of factor X can interfere with monitoring of low-molecular-weight heparin (LMWH) anticoagulation with the antifactor Xa assay.

Factor inhibitors may lead to increased bleeding and, rarely, spontaneous bleeding. Most conditions are initially detected as a prolongation of one or more of the coagulation screening tests—PT/INR/aPTT—or thrombin time. To differentiate between the different types of inhibitors, a clotting study should be done on a 1:1 mixture of the patient's plasma with normal plasma. A lack of correction of clotting time indicates a neutralizing antibody. Vigilance in testing is essential because at body temperature some studies initially correct and then return to a prolonged state after an hour. This is particularly true of factor V and VIII inhibitors.

If the mixing study corrects, this suggests the presence of a nonneutralizing antibody that may facilitate clearance of the clotting factor from circulation. The antibody should be isolated to differentiate its presence from a deficiency of the factor.

Treatment of bleeding includes infusion of factors to levels that overwhelm the antibodies and return the coagulation profile to normal. Long-term treatment includes immunosuppression with steroids or other agents and plasmapheresis with immunoabsorption with Ig-Therasorb. The latter can be used in conjunction with transfusion.

Hypercoagulable States

Like bleeding disorders, these states can be categorized as inherited or acquired (Table 5.6). Hyperhomocystinemia, however, can be either inherited or acquired. Indications for thrombophilia screening have already been outlined and the components of such a screen are referred to in Table 5.3. For most of the hypercoagulable states, treatment involves the use of LMWH or unfractionated heparin with conversion to oral warfarin. Often, if the patient has already had a thrombotic episode, anticoagulation is undertaken for life.

Table 5.6. Differential diagnosis for hypercoagulable states

Inherited (primary)
- Protein C and S deficiencies
- Antithrombin III deficiency
- Factor V Leiden mutation leading to activated protein C resistance
- Prothrombin 20210A gene mutation
- Heparin cofactor II deficiency and other heparin binding proteins
- Cystathionine synthase deficiency (hyperhomocystinemia)
- Dysfibrinogenemia
- Dys- and hypoplasminogenemia

Acquired (secondary)
- Cancer
- Pregnancy
- Oral contraceptives and other hormone replacement therapy (HRT)
- Myeloproliferative disorders
- Hyperlipidemia
- Diabetes mellitus
- Vasculitis
- Antiphospholipid syndrome (lupus anticoagulant, anticardiolipin antibodies)
- Postoperative states/trauma
- Immobilization
- Nephrotic syndrome
- Congestive heart failure
- Increased levels of factor VII and fibrinogen
- Obesity
- Heparin thrombocytopenia
- Anticancer drugs (bleomycin, vinca alkaloids, mitomycin, etc.)
- Paroxysmal nocturnal hemoglobinuria
- Age

Undetermined
- Elevated factor XI levels and VIII levels

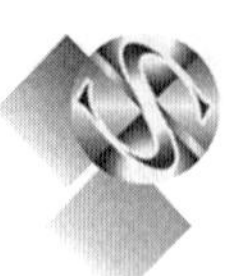

levels of these factors. Hormone replacement therapy and pregnancy are also implicated in raised levels of these factors. Patients on HRT or OC and with elevated factor VIII levels have a 10-fold increased risk of VTE compared to those without these risk factors.

Acquired

The most common cause in this group of conditions is the antiphospholipid antibody (APA) syndrome (Fligelstone et al., 1995). These antibodies bind to plasma proteins that have a high affinity for phospholipid surfaces. The most common of these proteins are the lupus anticoagulant (LA), anticardiolipin (ACL) antibodies, and anti-β_2-glycoprotein-1 antibodies (B_2G). These are usually acquired. Lupus anticoagulant can be suspected if there is an elevated PTT, and ACL and B_2G are detected only by immunoassays. These conditions can be primary, that is, not associated with other autoimmune conditions. They can present with VTE or arterial thrombosis as well as fetal demise. Antiphospholipid antibodies may be associated with infections, cancer, and even certain drugs and hemodialysis, but these are usually IgM as opposed to IgG antibodies and are present in low levels. They do not seem to be associated with thrombotic events.

The overall incidence is 1% to 5% of the normal population. The incidence increases with age and coexisting chronic disease. The incidence in patients with SLE is 12% to 30% for ACL and 15% to 34% for LA. The risk of thrombosis in patients found to have these autoantibodies is unclear but seems to be increased in those with a history of previous thrombosis, with LA and with increased IgG ACL—each of which increases the risk of thrombosis fivefold. The persistent presence of APA also increases the risk of thrombosis. These patients have a high proportion of pregnancy losses as well as an increased incidence of premature births. These patients are best treated with ASA plus heparin to achieve live births.

Interestingly, not all arterial episodes of ischemia or infarction are due to primary thrombosis. Up to 63% of patients with APA syndrome have coexisting valve abnormalities on echocardiography and 4% have vegetations of the mitral or aortic valve. These patients may also be thrombocytopenic (as many as 40–50%)

and may have hemolytic anemia (14–23%) and livedo reticularis (11–22%). Renal involvement may occur, and when it does it usually results in hypertension.

Catastrophic APA syndrome is acute, and multiple simultaneous vascular thrombotic events can occur throughout the body. Small vessels of multiple organs are often affected. The syndrome may result in death. In 78% of these patients the kidneys are involved, followed by the lungs in 66%, the central nervous system in 56%, the heart in 50%, and the skin in 50%. Disseminated intravascular coagulation is a component of this event in 25% of patients. The mortality rate is 50%, usually due to multisystem organ failure. The optimal treatment is not well defined but includes, in various combinations of anticoagulation, steroids and either plasmapheresis or intravenous immune globulin. The condition can be precipitated by surgery, infection, withdrawal of anticoagulation therapy, and drugs, including oral contraceptives.

Heparin-induced thrombocytopenia (HIT) also warrants some discussion. The entity was first described by Towne in 1979 as the white clot syndrome and occurs in 1% to 30% of patients on heparin. Heparin-induced thrombocytopenia is diagnosed by one or more HIT-associated clinical events, such as thrombosis of a graft, and the presence of heparin antibodies. Various tests (Table 5.8) are now available to help in making the diagnosis (Warkentin and Greinacher, 2004). The problem is that the onset of HIT is often delayed or seen after multiple exposures to heparin, where the first few exposures resulted in minimal or no decrease in platelets. Additionally, the delayed onset may be seen only after the offending heparin has been removed. The initial exposure can be as inconsequential as heparin lock flushes to maintain the patency of intravenous lines or standard subcutaneous heparin prophylaxis. Treatment includes stopping the heparin. Coumadin alone is *not* a good treatment due to the hypercoagulable period before anticoagulation is achieved, leading to potential skin necrosis. Additional therapy is switching to hirudin (Refludan), argatroban (Novastartan), or danaparnol (Organan). Additionally, some of the GIIb-IIIa inhibitors have been successfully employed in this situation. Newer agents are under investigation including a recently Food

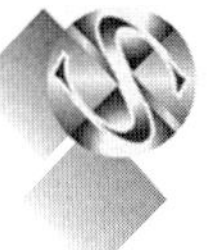

Table 5.8. Testing for heparin-induced thrombocytopenia

	Sensitivity (%)	Specificity (%)	Positive predictive value (%)	Negative predictive value (%)
PF4 + heparin coated plate: anti IgG, IgA, and IgM	97	86	93	91
Serotonin release	88	100	100	81
Platelet aggregation	91	77	89	81

Ig, immunoglobulin; PF4, platelet factor 4.

and Drug Administration (FDA)-approved oral anti–factor Xa agent.

Most malignancies can be associated with a higher incidence of thromboembolic events, in particular, adenocarcinoma and myeloproliferative disorders.

Conclusion

Bleeding and clotting disorders are encountered sufficiently frequently in vascular surgical practice to encourage an awareness of the range of disorders and of the different available therapeutic modalities. A high index of suspicion, a comprehensive medical history, and judicious employment of investigations help guide the experienced clinician to a correct diagnosis. The bleeding disorders are varied, and each requires specific management. The majority of thrombophilic tendencies may simply be treated with appropriate anticoagulation with the exception of catastrophic amyotrophic lateral sclerosis (ALS). The cumulative risks of different inherited and acquired thrombophilic factors have appreciable significance. Individual personalized risk profiles for thrombotic events may have a role to play for patients in the future. An awareness of the broad extent of these conditions helps vascular surgeons provide optimal management for their patients.

References

Donaldson MC, Weinberg DS, Belkin M, Whittemore AD, Mannick JA. (1990) J Vasc Surg 11:825–31.
Fligelstone LJ, Cachia PG, Ralis H, et al. (1995) Eur J Vasc Endovasc Surg 9:277–83.
Nehler MR, Taylor LM Jr, Porter JM. (1997) Cardiovasc Surg 5:559–67.
Ouriel K, Green RM, DeWeese JA, Cimino C. (1996) J Vasc Surg 23:46–51, discussion 51–2.
Warkentin TE, Greinacher A. (2004) Chest 126:311S–337S.

6

Medical Management of Peripheral Arterial Disease

Jill J.F. Belch and Andrew H. Muir

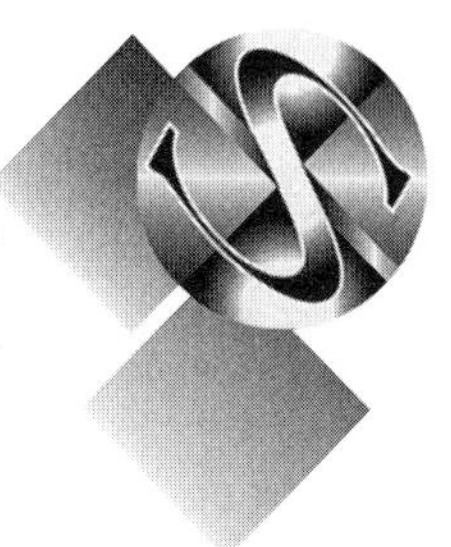

Atherosclerosis

Peripheral arterial disease (PAD) is a marker for multisystem vascular disease. Workers in this field recognized this over 150 years ago, noting the similarity between claudication symptoms and angina. Since then, published work has supported this view, but the commonality of the link between PAD and coronary artery disease (CAD) has only now been fully recognized. Myocardial infarction (MI) and stroke are the biggest risks to life and health for the PAD patient rather than amputation or critical limb ischemia (CLI). The natural history of intermittent claudication (IC), the usual symptom of lower limb atherosclerosis, is often benign. Most patients improve or their disease remains stable. Less than 5% of patients require amputation. In contrast, however, the death rate in these patients is three to four times higher than in patients of similar age without IC (Fig. 6.1). This mortality occurs due to atherosclerosis at other sites within the body. Only one quarter of the mortality of these patients is from nonvascular events. One half die from CAD, 15% as a result of stroke, and 10% from vascular pathology within the abdomen such as ruptured aortic aneurysm. The association between PAD and generalized vascular mortality is so strong that even in asymptomatic PAD [detected by a decrease in the ankle-brachial index (ABI)] the patient's relative risk of a cardiac or cerebrovascular event is very much higher.

Thus we now recognize that atherosclerosis is a systemic disorder affecting the entire vascular tree. Extracranial carotid disease can lead to stroke, CAD to myocardial ischemia/infarction, renovascular disease to hypertension, and aortoiliac and infrainguinal arterial disease to IC or limb-threatening ischemia. The mainstay of the medical management of vascular disease is to understand that it is a systemic disorder and must be managed as such. Thus the medical management of PAD is a complex area that includes strategies for vascular risk reduction, lifestyle advice, and direct pharmacotherapy for the vascular disease. Its implementation requires a multidisciplinary team, which includes not only vascular physicians, vascular surgeons, and interventional radiologists but also many of the professions allied to medicine and, importantly, our primary care colleagues. Areas of focus for such a vascular team are outlined in Table 6.1.

Vascular Risk Factor Modification in Peripheral Arterial Disease

The medical management of vascular disease must focus on modification of the following specific risk factors that promote the progression of the disease: (1) platelet aggregation, (2) smoking, (3) obesity, (4) diabetes, (5) dyslipi-

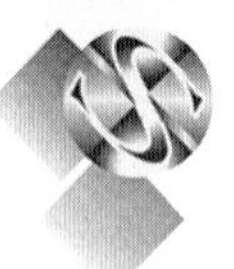

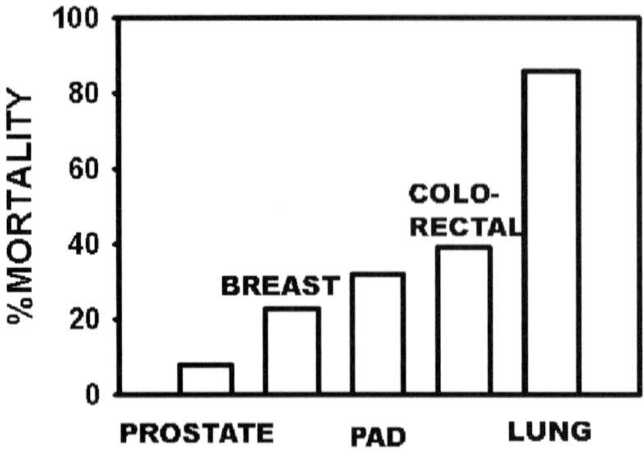

Figure 6.1. Mortality of peripheral arterial disease (PAD). The 5-year mortality of PAD is relatively equivalent to numerous cancers (prostate, breast, colorectal, and lung).

demia, (6) hypertension, (7) sedentary lifestyle, and (8) type A personality or stress.

The literature suggests that cigarette smoking, hypertension, dyslipidemia, and diabetes mellitus are important factors in the development of PAD, and these will be addressed in turn (Table 6.2). A key risk factor for PAD is platelet aggregation along with other hemorheological factors such as increased plasma fibrinogen and decreased fibrinolysis. Currently an area of interest that is being explored is that of the contribution of inflammation to PAD. The high white blood count (WBC) contributes vascular risk to the patient with PAD (Belch et al., 1999) as does increased oxidative stress. Of the above, however, platelet activation and release in the patient with PAD has been well documented and has led to the evidence-based use of antiplatelet agents in PAD.

Platelet Aggregation

Platelet aggregation is increased in patients with PAD, and the role of such aggregates in arterial thrombosis has been well documented. Platelet release products also contribute to the underlying pathology. β-Thromboglobulin is one such product that, once released from platelets, contributes to neutrophil activation. Platelet factor 4 neutralizes heparin, and platelet-derived growth factor stimulates proliferation of vascular smooth muscle cells. Some of the release products are vasoactive, and these include thromboxane A_2 and serotonin, both potent vasoconstrictors.

Antiplatelet Agents

Current interest in antiplatelet agents relates to their use as prophylactic treatments against arterial events in other beds and atherosclerosis disease progression.

Aspirin in Peripheral Arterial Disease

Aspirin is the most commonly used antiplatelet agent, reflecting the fact that it is currently the cheapest agent available and one of the best studied agents in clinical trials. Its action includes the irreversible inhibition of the cyclo-

Table 6.1. Medical strategies for the management of peripheral arterial disease

Address vascular risk
Antiplatelet therapy
Cigarette smoking
Dyslipidemia
Hypertension
Diabetes
Obesity
Thrombophilia
Specific therapy for intermittent claudication
Exercise
?Drug therapy
Vasculitides as a cause of symptoms
Connective tissue disease
Raynaud's phenomenon
Vasculitis
Antiphospholipid syndrome
Embolism as a cause of symptoms
Detect and treat arrhythmia and/or cardiac thrombus
Exclude aortic aneurism
Chronic limb symptoms
Control edema
Control infection
Improve cardiac output
Acute critical limb ischemia (CLI)
Thrombolysis
Anticoagulation
Deep vein thrombosis (DVT)
Prophylaxis
Treatment

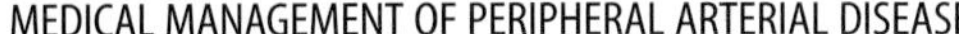

Table 6.2. Risk factors for intermittent claudication

Risk	Management
Other cardiovascular events, e.g., MI, stroke	• Antiplatelet agent Aspirin, clopidogrel, dipyridamole
Smoking	• Cessation program Counseling Nicotine replacement, e.g., patch, gum, spray

Dyslipidemia	• Lipid-lowering therapy
	Diet ± drug
	Target: LDL cholesterol <3.0 mmol/L
	        HDL ≥20%
	        Triglycerides <1.8 mmol/L

Hypertension	• Antihypertensive therapy
	Select: ACE inhibitor
	        Calcium channel blockade
	        Diuretic
	Avoid beta-blockade (unless vasodilatory)
	Target BP <140/85 (in diabetes <140/80)
	(Note: 25% will have renal artery stenosis; watch renal function)

Diabetes	• Check for hyperglycemia
	Fasting glucose ≥ 7.8 mmol/L
	If borderline glucose (random or fasting), glucose tolerance test with fasting and 2-hour sample
	2-hour sample: <7.8 mmol/L normal
	        ≥7.8–11.0 impaired
	        ≥11.1 diabetic

Obesity	• Check for obesity Body mass index ≥30 Low-fat, high-fiber diet, healthy eating Calorie control

Thrombophilia	• Consider referral for thrombophilia screen (inherited or acquired)
	Suspect if:
	    Young (<50 years of age)
	    Connective tissue disease, e.g., SLE
	    Additional history of unexplained venous thrombosis
	    Previous failed vascular reconstruction
	    Strong family history of thrombosis

SLE, systemic lupus erythematosus.

oxygenase enzyme. Platelet aggregation is therefore decreased.

Primary Prevention of Peripheral Arterial Disease

As yet there is no published evidence to suggest that aspirin prevents the primary development of PAD in a normal population. Such a study would require a huge population base. One method of decreasing the numbers required to be studied would be to increase the risk of the population enrolled in the trial. Two such studies are currently under way. In both these studies aspirin is being evaluated in subjects with decreased ABIs but who are currently asymptomatic in terms of PAD. One of the studies is a population-based study and the other is a study of patients with diabetes mellitus. This latter study, Prevention of Progression of Arterial Disease in Diabetes (POPADAD) has recruited 1250 patients with decreased ABI, and aspirin versus placebo is one of the arms of this study, which has a composite end point of vascular events and mortality. This is a Scotland-wide study and results should be available soon.

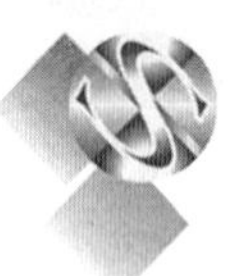

Primary Prevention of Vascular Surgery

Aspirin has been evaluated in the primary prevention of requirement for peripheral vascular surgery in the U.S. Physicians' Health Study. In the aspirin group the risk of undergoing surgery for PAD was decreased by 46% ($p = .03$). Aspirin did not, however, affect the likelihood of developing claudication de novo during the trial period.

Aspirin in the Prevention of Coronary and Cerebrovascular Events in Peripheral Arterial Disease

The Antiplatelet Trialists Collaboration, now called the Antithrombotic Trialists Collaboration, has provided the most convincing data supporting the use of aspirin in PAD. In a meta-analysis of 174 randomized trials of various antiplatelet agents (mainly aspirin), a decrease in nonfatal MI, nonfatal stroke, and vascular death in patients treated by antiplatelet therapy was detected. Subgroup analysis of high-risk patients was carried out. This included patients with PAD, and the percentage of risk reduction versus placebo were as follows: 46% for non-fatal stroke, 32% for the risk of vascular disease, MI, or stroke, and for nonfatal MI, and 20% for death from vascular causes. The most frequently used dosages of aspirin were between 75 and 325 mg per day. Subsequent work has confirmed that there is no evidence that the higher doses are more effective than the lower ones (i.e., >75 mg per day), although bleeding risk is dose dependent.

Clopidogrel

Clopidogrel irreversibly blocks the binding of adenosine diphosphate (ADP) and thus its activation of platelets. The Clopidogrel versus Aspirin in Patients at Risk of Ischemic Events (CAPRIE) study evaluated the risk of vascular death, MI, and stroke in patients with vascular disease receiving either clopidogrel or aspirin. Clopidogrel reduced the event rate by 5.32% per annum versus 5.83% with aspirin ($p = .043$). These figures reflect a relative rate reduction of 8.7% in favor of clopidogrel. No major differences in safety issues between the two drugs was detected. An ad hoc subgroup analysis in patients with PAD suggested greater benefit to these patients from clopidogrel than in other patient populations. An event rate of 3.1 per annum compared to 4.86 per annum in the aspirin group gave a relative risk reduction of 23.8% [95% confidence interval (CI) 8.9–36.2] in favor of clopidogrel ($p = .0028$). A reasonable strategy, therefore, in the 30% of all patients who developed gastrointestinal (GI) side effects from aspirin is to combine the aspirin initially with the gastric protectant, and if this fails, change to clopidogrel. This drug provides an improvement to our therapeutic resources in terms of tolerated antiplatelet drugs.

Dipyridamole

Dipyridamole is an antiplatelet agent that is thought to work through a number of mechanisms including increasing the effect of prostacyclin (PGI_2), and inhibiting the cellular uptake of adenosine and platelet phosphodiesterase, thus enhancing further the effects of PGI_2. The use of dipyridamole itself or in combination with aspirin has produced much controversy. Three decades ago there was excitement about the potential benefits of combining aspirin and dipyridamole, but by the 1980s aspirin alone became the favorite choice. Evidence that the combination treatment is effective has been forthcoming in one of the large stroke studies (Diener et al., 1996), and certainly the combination has been found to be more effective in the prevention of peripheral graft failure in one study. It is our current practice to use both aspirin and dipyridamole in patients with stroke or transient ischemic attack (TIA) but to use aspirin or clopidogrel alone in patients with PAD. In stable PAD we usually reserve dipyridamole for the aspirin-intolerant patient, although clopidogrel is now our first choice for this indication.

Conclusion

There is convincing evidence that antiplatelet agents such as aspirin and clopidogrel are effective in preventing cardiac and stroke events in patients with PAD. It is therefore recommended that an antiplatelet drug should be prescribed for these patients unless there is a clear contraindication to such therapy.

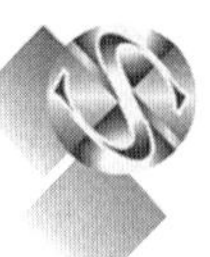

Smoking

Both the risk of PAD and its progression is significantly increased by the smoking of tobacco. Patients who smoke have a significantly increased risk of atherosclerosis and of another tobacco-related peripheral vascular disease, thromboangiitis obliterans (Buerger's disease). Of all the risk factors discussed here, the use of tobacco contributes most to the development of PAD. A number of studies have linked tobacco smoking and the development of IC. In the Framingham study smokers were twice as likely to develop IC. The progression to critical limb ischemia is more likely in smokers, as is amputation. The effect of cigarette smoking on vascular graft patency is well recognized. In one study the 5-year cumulative patency rate for grafts was between 80% and 90% for nonsmokers, with the corresponding patency rates being between 30% and 45% for those who smoked more than five cigarettes a day.

Smoking cessation slows the progression of peripheral arterial disease to critical limb ischemia and lowers the risk of MI and death. The nicotine present in tobacco products is highly addictive; hence, smoking cessation is a very difficult process for patients, and the recidivism rate is high. The key feature in the approach to smoking cessation is for the physician to positively encourage the patient to stop smoking. Without a clear message from the physician that smoking is an underlying cause of atherosclerosis and promotes the progression of atherosclerosis, patients will continue to smoke. Thus, the first step is to clearly tell patients that it is medically indicated that they stop smoking.

Although the majority of smokers would like to quit, 90% are physically addicted to nicotine and at least 75% have tried to stop smoking more than once. Three quarters of those who do stop restart within 3 months, and it is clear that the issue of nicotine dependence must be addressed. During the early stages of quitting, smokers experience both behavioral and physical withdrawal symptoms. It is crucial to explain to the patient that the chemical withdrawal symptoms are short lived as they can exert strong pressure on the smoker's will to stop. This also underlines the fact that we must provide support to these patients. After receiving only medical advice, only 5% of PAD patients stop smoking. Improved cessation rates, however, can be achieved through increasing support through counseling or the provision of judicious nicotine replacement therapy. There are numerous smoking cessation programs and pharmacological aids available for patients. Smoking cessation aids such as nicotine patches and nicotine gum work best in the setting of a specific smoking cessation program. Nicotine chewing gum was the first type of nicotine replacement therapy (NRT) to become widely available, with subsequent development of transdermal patches, intranasal sprays, and inhalers. These latter forms of therapy may attenuate some problems with the gum such as transfer of dependency. A meta-analysis of 53 trials of NRT (42 gum, nine patch, one spray, and one inhaler) (Silagy et al., 1994) showed that NRT increased the odds ratio for abstinence: 1.61 for gum, 2.07 for patch, 2.92 for nasal spray, and 3.05 for inhaled nicotine. Nicotine replacement therapy can be an effective aid to smoking cessation. However, it is contraindicated in acute MI, unstable angina, and in patients with cardiac arrhythmias. Thus, it is important to work with patients to engage them in a specific program.

Finally, because the recidivism rate is high, it is important to be encouraging at follow-up visits once a patient has stopped smoking. Physician encouragement throughout the process of smoking cessation and remaining tobacco free is essential.

Conclusion

Smoking causes PAD. Its cessation is difficult without support. Nicotine replacement and other aids to cessation should be made available to PAD patients.

Obesity

Obesity has reached epidemic proportions in developed countries. Obesity contributes to numerous medical problems including atherosclerosis. It is important to recognize if patients are overweight and to obtain the appropriate dietary consultation to assist patients with weight loss. Most weight-loss programs are not successful unless they include lifestyle modification and a specific exercise program.

Conclusion

Obesity contributes to the development of type 2 diabetes, hypertension, and dyslipidemia, all known to be associated with PAD. Appropriate weight-reduction programs should be recommended. It should be noted that smoking cessation promotes weight gain, and that in a patient with PAD smoking cessation is the most important element in risk reduction. A level of weight gain therefore should be tolerated, at least in the short term.

Diabetes Mellitus

Peripheral arterial disease and diabetes mellitus frequently occur together. Probably half of all patients with diabetes mellitus have evidence of PAD 10 to 15 years after diabetes onset. Furthermore, glucose intolerance correlates with angiographic disease extent. Diabetic patients account for one third of below-knee amputations and 50% of amputations when distal amputations are included. The pathology of the diabetic limb is multifactorial, including contributions from both micro- and macrovascular disease. Asymptomatic PAD occurs in 20% of all diabetic patients with no other evidence of vascular disease (POPADAD screening of 8000 patients). Thus the occurrence of overt diabetes and PAD is well documented. We are less expert at detecting early diabetes in our patients with PAD, however. Distal disease on angiography or increased ABI (due to vessel stiffening) can lead to the retrospective diagnosis of diabetes mellitus, but this still underestimates the figure. Of 100 consecutive patients presenting at our vascular surgery clinic, 40% had abnormal glucose tolerance tests. The majority of these patients had normal random or fasting sugars and were diagnosed only on the basis of this glucose tolerance test. Currently we do not give a glucose tolerance test to all PAD patients but do use this form of diagnosis for patients who have raised ABI in the presence of symptomatic IC, in those in whom the distal distribution of the PAD would arouse a suspicion of diabetes, and in those with a "diabetic" lipid profile where both cholesterol and fasting triglyceride levels are elevated and high-density lipoprotein (HDL) levels are low. Detection of asymptomatic diabetes mellitus in the PAD patient is a major part of the medical management of these patients. It is consistently underdiagnosed in PAD and this can have serious consequences.

Diabetes contributes to atherosclerosis, and studies have indicated that tight glucose control limits the progression of end-organ damage due to diabetes, including atherosclerosis. Physicians involved in the care of diabetic patients with atherosclerosis must work closely, as a team, with other caregivers involved in the management of diabetes to ensure tight glucose control.

Conclusion

It should be remembered that all risk factors are synergistic in terms of vascular disease, not merely additive, and the failure to diagnose underlying diabetes in a PAD patient who smokes will have serious consequences for that patient.

Dyslipidemia

Abnormal lipid profiles are well recognized in patients with atherosclerosis. The relationship between cholesterol level and CAD risk is continuous, with no obvious "safe" cut-off point. Patients with PAD are likely to be identical. A number of studies investigated cholesterol in PAD and found it to be a significant, though weak, risk factor for claudication, and above the age of 55 years to correlate with ABI. Reduced HDL is associated with increased PAD severity,[6] with strong inverse relationships between HDL cholesterol and PAD that persist after adjustment for other risk factors. Furthermore, elevated serum triglyceride levels have been reported in both cross section and longitudinal studies. It has been suggested that the link between increased triglyceride level in patients with PAD and the development of the disease might be explained by the increase in low-density lipoprotein (LDL) providing the enhanced vascular risk.

Despite the links between abnormal lipid profiles and PAD, there have been no clinical studies with the PAD patient as primary end point. The situation has now been overtaken by the Heart Protection Study (2002) and various guidelines with recommendations for lipid-lowering therapy if there is a >3% chance of a vascular event per annum. Such a risk clearly occurs in patients with PAD.

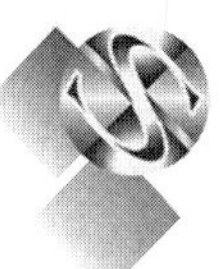

All of the major trials in the field of lipid lowering that have been reported over the past decade have showed variously a decrease in CAD mortality, major coronary events, and the need for coronary revascularization. Together the data suggest that four out of nine deaths occurring in a group of subjects with cholesterol >5.5 mmol/L will be prevented by treatment.

More recently, the Heart Protection Study (HPS) demonstrated for the first time a benefit from statin therapy for prevention of vascular events in patients with PAD (HPS Collaborative Group, 2002). This largest-ever trial of cholesterol-lowering therapy enrolled more than 20,000 high-risk patients, of whom 2700 had symptomatic PAD but no prior CAD. Treatment with simvastatin 40 mg/day reduced major vascular events (coronary events, stroke, and revascularization) by 20% in patients with PAD, a similar reduction to that observed in the study overall. Moreover, the benefits observed in the HPS were not influenced by baseline levels of blood lipids. The findings of the HPS, therefore, strongly suggest that statin therapy should be considered on the basis of high risk rather than high cholesterol, a category into which patients with PAD undoubtedly fall.

Conclusion

Elevated cholesterol and triglycerides contribute to the development and progression of atherosclerosis. Thus, it is important to obtain a lipid profile on any patient with atherosclerosis. Management of dyslipidemia initially involves dietary change followed by specific medical management if necessary. The goal of lipid-lowering therapy is to achieve a serum LDL cholesterol concentration less than 100 mg/dL or 3 mmol/L and a serum triglyceride less than 150 mg/dL.

The first choice for pharmacological therapy is a statin.

Hypertension

Although it has been suggested that raised systolic and raised diastolic blood pressure (BP) are linked to PAD development, results from prospective studies are less convincing. Target levels of blood pressure have been clearly defined in a number of guidelines, For example

the Scottish Intercollegiate Guidelines Network (SIGN) guideline on the management of hypertension and the British Hypertension Society guidelines have given clear guidance in terms of acceptable BP levels. Therapy should be started in all PAD patients with sustained systolic BP elevations recorded above 140 mm Hg or diastolic BP above 90 mm Hg. The optimum target blood pressure is a systolic BP of <135 mm Hg and a diastolic of <85 mm Hg. A more stringent target is required for those patients with diabetes and this is important, as many PAD patients have diabetes mellitus where a target of ≤130/80 mm Hg is recommended. Three long-term double-blind studies (Materson et al., 1993) have compared all the major classes of antihypertensive drug therapy and overall showed no consistent or important differences in terms of efficacy of BP control, side effects from the drugs, or quality of life. It has been suggested that hypertensive patients whose BP is controlled by thiazides or beta-blockers may continue to experience the excess risk of coronary death. These two drug classes change glucose intolerance and lipid profiles in a dose-dependent fashion, and it may be that the lower doses of thiazides currently employed do not show this effect. Although β-adrenergic antagonist drugs have been previously reported to enhance PAD symptoms through their vasoconstrictor effects, more recently it has been suggested that this is not so. It is of interest that the new vasodilating beta-blockers do not even have this theoretical contraindication and might be used safely in patients with PAD. The use of angiotensin-converting enzyme inhibitors in patients with PAD may confer protection against future atherosclerotic events. However care must be taken in the presence of renal artery stenosis, another common finding in patients with PAD.

Care must be taken when treating hypertension in the patient with CLI, as limb perfusion might only be maintained through the elevated BP. Too profound or rapid a decrease in BP may worsen the symptoms, and care must be taken with CLI in the same way as with patients with severe carotid disease.

Conclusion

Hypertension has been implicated in the etiology of PAD and contributes to its vascular comorbidity. Blood pressure should be controlled to levels consistent with local guidelines. Polypharmacy is likely to be required. Caution is advised when high BP is diagnosed in a patient with CLI, as too rapid a decrease in pressure may worsen the limb ischemia.

Sedentary Lifestyle/ Exercise Therapy

Intermittent claudication is a symptom of lower limb peripheral arterial disease. It arises when the blood flow is insufficient to meet the metabolic demands of the leg muscles in ambulating patients. Intermittent claudication is a "leveraged" disability, as pain increases with walking, patients walk shorter distances, muscle strength erodes, and walking distances continue to decrease. This leads to other negative consequences such as weight gain, hypertension, and diabetes. Overall, patients with claudication have a 60% lower functional capacity than age-matched individuals without the disease (Eldridge and Hossack, 1987).

Intermittent claudication is a symptom of systemic atherosclerosis. At least 60% of patients with claudication have significant disease of the cerebral or cardiac circulation. Mortality rates for patients with claudication are very high, with 30% to 50% of patients dying from cardiovascular causes within 5 years of the initial diagnosis. A meta-analysis of 21 studies on the effects of exercise on patients with claudication suggested that the average improvement in walking distance was 122% (Gardner and Poehlman, 1995) and the benefits have been shown to be as high as 180% (Fig. 6.2). The programs with the greatest benefit were those in which patients exercised for 30 minutes at least three times a week for 6 months. However, supervised exercise programs are not currently covered by most medical insurance policies.

There are numerous salutary effects of exercise that contribute to the reduction of cardiovascular events. Exercise is associated with beneficial changes in body fat percentage, lipoprotein profile, carbohydrate tolerance and insulin sensitivity, neurohormonal release, and blood pressure. There is substantial evidence that regular aerobic exercise can even alter

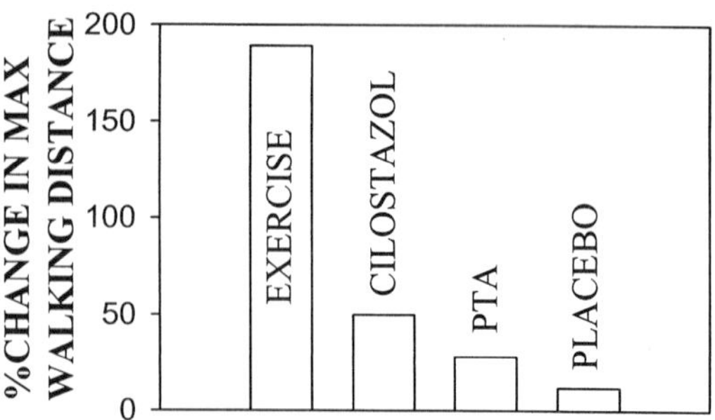

Figure 6.2. Walking distance. The improvement in walking distance is much greater for a graded exercise program compared to the best medical management (cilostazol), percutaneous transluminal angioplasty (PTA), or placebo.

vessel structure. The progression of coronary lesions can be inhibited in those patients who modify risk factors and engage in regular exercise. Numerous studies have demonstrated a significant correlation between exercise and an increase in vessel diameter. Exercise may also induce changes in the lumen diameter in patients after coronary angioplasty. Patients randomized to a 12-week intervention program consisting of daily exercise after balloon angioplasty of the coronary vasculature had a significantly lower rate of re-stenosis than patients in the control group. However, the major benefit of exercise is likely due to the training response.

Thrombophilia

Patients under the age of 50 with manifestations of vascular disease have an increased risk of a defined hypercoagulable disorder. Thus, some believe that these patients should be screened for hypercoagulable disorders. In contrast, most hematology societies indicate that screening for thrombophilia in arterial disease does not yet have an evidence base.

There are two general categories used to describe the hypercoagulable or prothrombotic state: hereditary and acquired. The former is often referred to as inherited thrombophilia disease. *Acquired thrombophilia* is a term reserved for well-defined syndromes such as the antiphospholipid syndrome (APS). This was

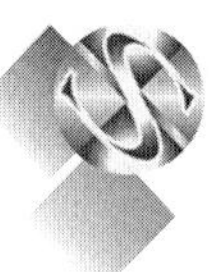

previously termed the lupus anticoagulant. However, the name was changed for two very good reasons. First, the anticoagulant referred to in this latter term reflects the behavior of the blood in the test tube, and in fact a pro-thrombotic effect is observed in vivo. Second, although it can be associated with the connective tissue disease systemic lupus erythematosus, this is by no means necessary and we are increasingly recognizing APS occurring in isolation.

Although the inherited thrombophilic disorders are historically linked to venous thrombosis, there is some evidence suggesting that they may contribute to arterial thrombosis and in particular in patients with PAD. It has been recorded that inherited thrombophilias link to failure of vascular grafting following surgery. In a prospective study hypercoagulability occurs in between 10% and 25% of patients, increasing to about 50% in the presence of clinical markers for thrombophilia. Preoperative identification of such patients is important, as the short- and medium-term failure rates of the graft are reported to be approximately 50% in such patients. Furthermore, such patients are at increased risk of deep vein thrombosis during the operative procedure (see Chapter 5 for the evaluation of these patients).

Conclusion

As the inherited hypercoagulable states such as protein C, protein S, antithrombin II deficiencies, and factor V Leiden occur only infrequently in this patient group, it is not possible to make a formal recommendation for screening of PAD patients. Probably a selective approach is warranted, reserving screening to those patients with bypass failure, a history of thrombotic events, or atherosclerosis at an early age.

Homocystinemia

The clinical features of homocystinemia include the development of premature atherosclerosis, along with manifestations of arterial and venous thrombosis. Disease severity leads to early diagnosis in homozygous patients, but patients with heterozygous disease present merely with premature atherosclerosis; 20%

to 40% of patients presenting with premature PAD have been found to have heterozygous homocystinemia. Pyridoxine supplementation reduces the thrombotic events in homozygous patients. However, it is not known whether this or other vitamins such as folate affect the course of the premature atherosclerosis in the heterozygous sufferers.

Vascular Risk Factor Management in Patients with Peripheral Arterial Disease

The presentation of a patient with PAD to a provider of medical care presents an ideal opportunity for the critical assessment of vascular risk factors. Intervention at this time both decreases the risk of coronary and cerebral events and is likely to limit progression of the arterial disease in the periphery, although the latter is theoretical rather than evidence-based as yet. Thus the modification of vascular risk is of crucial importance in the patient with PAD and is likely to become an even more important area in the future for clinicians involved with the care of these patients.

Drug Treatment of Intermittent Claudication

It is a poor reflection on us, as clinicians involved in the care of the PAD patient, that angina of the legs is addressed far less aggressively than symptoms of claudication in the heart! Part of the problem reflects the concern about the effectiveness of the drug treatment for the symptoms of intermittent claudication and the consequent unease over the use of financial resources to purchase these compounds. Guidelines have been developed for prescribing. There are four oral drug therapies that have a license for use as a treatment for IC in the United Kingdom and two in the United States: Naftidrofuryl (Praxilene, not available in the U.S.), oxpentifylline (Trental), cilostazol (Pletal), and inositol nicotinate (Hexopal). These drugs have been evaluated in clinical

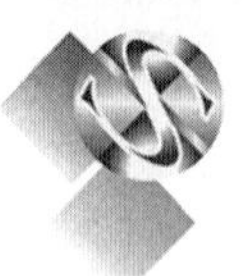

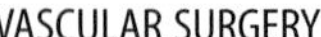

trials in terms of their effectiveness for alleviating the symptoms of leg pain associated with walking (IC).

Naftidrofuryl

Naftidrofuryl is thought to mediate its benefits through vasoactivity (vasodilatation) and via a local anesthetic action. Studies have documented increased tissue oxygenation, increased ADP levels, and reduced lactic acid. The recommended maximum dose is 200 mg three times a day.

A number of double-blind, placebo-controlled studies in this area tend to show a significant placebo response in walking distance approximately 25% improvement in walking distance with placebo. With Naftidrofuryl a further 30% improvement can be expected. These estimates are supported by two meta-analyses.

Pentoxifylline/Oxpentifylline

This is a rheological agent that has been approved for the treatment of intermittent claudication. Only two of the double-blind, placebo-controlled studies of oxpentifylline that measured walking distance using treadmills showed any statistical improvement in such walking distance by patients on oxpentifylline. Furthermore, one of these was a retrospective subanalysis of short-distance claudicants, patients who could only walk short distances before claudication ocurred already included in another study. A meta-analysis of ten randomized, double-blind, controlled studies concluded that the limited amount and quality of data for this drug precluded an overall reliable estimate of its efficacy. We recommend, in the absence of any consistent clinical trial evidence, that oxpentifylline should not be prescribed for use in this indication.

Cilostazol

Cilostazol has recently been approved for the treatment of intermittent claudication. It is a phosphodiesterase inhibitor that has been shown in randomized placebo-controlled trials to improve walking distance by approximately 50%. However, the improvement remains modest compared to exercise programs (180% to 200% improvement). Cilostazol is contraindicated in patients with a history of congestive heart failure.

Inositol Nicotinate (Hexopal)

Inositol nicotinate is licensed for use in the United Kingdom for patients with intermittent claudication. However, the evidence base for this compound is weak. Of the four double-blind, randomized, placebo-controlled trials, three were primary care based and used subjective or questionable objective criteria for assessment of IC without treadmill use. None showed clear evidence of improvement in symptoms with drug use. We suggest, therefore, that the drug may not be of value for patients with IC.

Conclusion

Some patients with IC merit drug treatment due to the severity of their symptoms. It is reasonable to consider Naftidrofuryl or cilostazol for the symptomatic relief of moderate disease. The patients, however, should be reviewed 6 to 12 months after drug commencement to assess its efficacy and the need for continuation. Neither oxpentifylline nor inositol nicotinate can be recommended for the treatment of symptomatic IC.

Summary

Peripheral arterial disease is a marker of systemic atherosclerosis. Patients with PAD are at high risk for MI and stroke. Thus, an integrative approach to risk factor modification and the prevention of the sequelae of atherosclerosis is the mainstay of therapy. Patients must be advised to "stop smoking and keep walking." In addition, however, antiplatelet therapy (e.g., aspirin) is indicated in all patients with peripheral arterial disease in whom there is no contraindication. Hypertension must be appropriately treated and diabetes mellitus detected and managed optimally. The medical management of the symptoms of intermittent claudication should also be addressed if these are significantly impairing the patient's lifestyle.

The key feature, however, in managing these patients is to assess their overall vascular risk and treat accordingly.

References

Belch JJ, Sohngen M, Robb R, Voleske P, Sohngen W. (1999) Int Angiol 18:140–4.

Diener HC, Cunha L, Forbes C, Sivenius J, Smets P, Lowenthal A. (1996) J Neurol Sci 143:1–13.
Eldridge JE, Hossack KF. (1987) Cardiology 74:236–40.
Gardner AW, Poehlman ET. (1995) JAMA 274:975–80.
Materson BJ, Reda DJ, Cushman WC, et al. (1993) N Engl J Med 328:914–21.
Silagy C, Mant D, Fowler G, Lodge M. (1994) Lancet 343: 139–42.

7

Anesthesia for Vascular Surgery

Jamal J. Hoballah and Farid Moulla

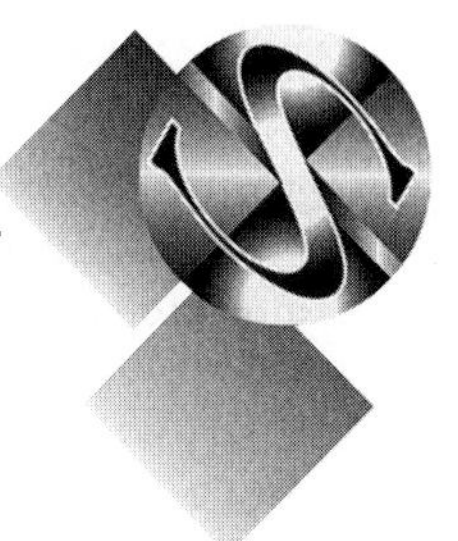

Surgery of the peripheral vascular system requires technical precision and perioperative vigilance. The outcome of vascular procedures depends on various factors. These factors include patient selection, the procedure performed, the surgeon's skills, and the perioperative care. The importance of the perioperative care cannot be underestimated. Patients presenting with a vascular pathology often have comorbidities. The incidence of coronary artery disease (CAD) in patients with carotid disease is estimated at 50%.

Patients with operative lower extremity peripheral vascular disease (PVD) have an even higher incidence of CAD. Hypertension, diabetes, and renal insufficiency are all more frequent in patients with PVD compared to the general population. Following aortic surgery, carotid endarterectomy, and lower extremity revascularization procedures, the most common major complication is a cardiac event. Anesthesia is a risk factor contributing to the perioperative morbidity and mortality of the vascular patient. The preoperative preparation and the intraoperative management can predict and influence the postoperative course. This chapter provides an overview of the various anesthetic techniques that can be used in patients presenting for vascular procedures.

Anesthesia Risks

Depending on the complexity of the vascular pathology, a vascular procedure can be performed under local, regional, or general anesthesia, or a combination of these techniques. Minimally invasive approaches to vascular reconstructions are continuing to be developed, allowing for more localized anesthesia. Often it is assumed that performing a procedure under local or regional anesthesia results in lower mortality and morbidity and allows earlier recovery. Certain trends are apparent in the literature, although not without controversy, comparing these anesthetic techniques and can be outlined as follows:

- While laboratory and monitoring techniques are improving, historically many perioperative cardiac events are "silent" (Steen et al., 1978; Von Knorring and Lepantalo et al., 1986).
- There does not appear to be a discernible difference between regional and general anesthesia with regard to cardiac risk or mortality within the field of vascular surgery. There is a large amount of recent controversy, practice variability, and research related to this point (Bode et al., 1996;

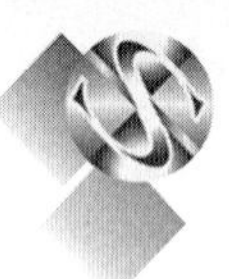

Christopherson et al., 1993; Rigg et al., 2002; Rivers et al., 1991; Rodgers et al., 2000).

- Regional and general anesthesia offer different advantages and disadvantages, but both are safe and appropriate for carotid endarterectomy (Rockman et al., 1996).
- Combinations of anesthetic techniques may offer advantages over single-mode therapy.
- There is a trend toward less need for (immediate postoperative) reoperation for thrombosis when regional anesthesia is employed in lower extremity revascularizations (Christopherson et al., 1993).
- Minimally invasive techniques warrant equally minimally insulting anesthetic techniques, contributing to improved outcomes over standard surgical intervention.

Because of the relative equity of major anesthetic risk between regional and general anesthesia, the site and probable duration of the procedure itself are often the main determinants of anesthetic technique. Lower extremity revascularizations typically last from 2 to 6 hours with significant variability. A single administration of spinal anesthesia offers no ability to redose if the initial infiltration wears off. Epidural anesthesia can be continuously infused both for long procedures and for postoperative pain management. However, it does little to treat the musculoskeletal complaints of an awake patient prostrate for several hours. Conversely, general anesthesia does not allow for patient interaction and requires prophylactic measures to avoid the complications of pressure and immobility. It also has the disadvantage of requiring mechanical ventilation with its potential respiratory complications and possible hemodynamic stresses with induction or extubation. In most cases, regional and general anesthesias are both acceptable alternatives for the common vascular surgeries. Some issues to remember when deciding on anesthetic techniques are as follows:

- Open abdominal vascular surgery such as for an abdominal aortic aneurysm (AAA) is theoretically possible with a celiac axis block or regional anesthesia, but in practice, warrants general anesthesia.
- Epidural anesthesia for supplementation of general anesthesia, as well as for postoperative pain management in major abdominal surgery, is becoming the standard of care as it gains a wealth of supporting literature.
- The need for postoperative full anticoagulation with (or the use of even prophylactic subcutaneous doses of) low-molecular-weight heparin usually precludes epidural catheter use for fear of developing an epidural hematoma upon the removal of the catheter.
- Both prophylactic and therapeutic unfractionated heparin therapy have to be interrupted to allow for normalization of coagulation prior to removing the epidural catheter to avoid a potentially devastating complication.
- Upper extremity vascular procedures can be approached with general, regional, local, or epidural anesthesia. Axillofemoral bypass is a relative contraindication to regional anesthesia as is harvesting of arm veins, although on occasions the vein may be harvested using infiltration of local anesthetics.
- The most common vascular surgery, carotid endarterectomy, has been studied extensively, with ongoing debate regarding the effectiveness of intraoperative monitoring techniques and regional versus general anesthesia.

The following sections review the various anesthetic techniques available for commonly performed vascular procedures.

Anesthesia for Endovascular Interventions

Endovascular procedures vary in complexity and include diagnostic angiograms, balloon angioplasty and stenting, endovascular aortic aneurysm treatment with endografts, and varicose vein treatment by radiofrequency or laser ablation. There is a paucity of studies on the anesthetic requirements of vascular patients treated by endovascular techniques. In general, percutaneous angiography, balloon angioplasty, and stenting are typically performed under local anesthesia. Infiltration of the skin with 1% lidocaine or bupivacaine can provide ample control of pain at the puncture site. It is preferable to premedicate the patient prior to the pro-

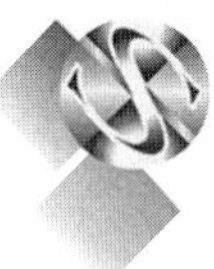

cedure and to augment sedation at the onset of the intervention. Premedication with 25 to 50 mg of diphenhydramine and 5 mg of diazepam given orally 1 hour prior to the procedure relieves many patients of the anxiety and anticipation of the intervention. Once the patient is on the catheterization table, sedation with 1 to 2 mg of lorazepam in addition to 50 μg of fentanyl provides further sedation and excellent pain control. The skin at the puncture site is infiltrated with the chosen local anesthetic and the potential track of the puncture needle is also infiltrated. If during the arterial puncture the patient complains of pain, additional local anesthetic can be infiltrated in the area directly through the Seldinger needle prior to arterial puncture.

Endovascular Aortic Aneurysm Repair

With respect to aortic aneurysm endovascular treatment, most of the procedures were originally done under general anesthesia. As the comfort level of the surgeons with the procedure increased, epidural and local anesthesia started to be used and were noted to be a reasonable alternative to general anesthesia. The idea of being able to treat an abdominal aortic aneurysm under local anesthesia is very exciting and appealing. The question of need for general anesthesia to treat AAA with endovascular technology has been examined (Henretta et al., 1999). In 47 patients treated with local anesthesia and intravenous sedation without intubation, only one required conversion to general anesthesia. The conversion was needed to repair an injury to the external iliac artery. In the remaining 46, there were lower rates of cardiac complications (zero) and shorter hospital stay when compared to those reported with the open technique. Although this study did not compare the results of endovascular AAA treatment under general anesthesia versus local or epidural anesthesia, it clearly proved the feasibility and efficacy of local anesthesia with sedation as an anesthetic technique for endovascular AAA treatment. At the University of Iowa, epidural anesthesia is our preferred technique for endovascular AAA treatment. However, patients' wishes and preferences often play a decisive role in the selection of the anesthetic technique used. The require-

ments for anesthesia are likely to change as rapidly as the endovascular techniques and devices employed.

Lower Extremity Vein Therapy

Radiofrequency or laser ablation of the greater saphenous vein (GSV) is gaining popularity as an alternative, less invasive method for GSV stripping in the treatment of varicose veins. This transforms varicose vein treatment into an office practice and limits the anesthesia needs to infiltration of local anesthetics. The skin is typically infiltrated at the site of insertion of the sheath through which the laser or radioablation catheter is introduced. Because of the heat generated with the venous ablation, additional anesthesia is needed along the course of the GSV. Tumescent anesthesia is used for this purpose. Tumescent anesthesia is prepared by the following concentration:

> 500 cc of normal saline in IV bag
>
> 16 cc of 8.4% sodium bicarbonate solution
>
> 50 cc of 1% lidocaine with epinephrine 1:100,000

It is infiltrated along the course of the GSV using a long spinal needle. In addition to providing anesthesia to the infiltrated area, tumescent anesthesia provides a protective layer between the vein and the dermis to avoid thermal skin injury during the laser or radiofrequency ablation. This tumescent anesthesia is also used during stab avulsion of branch varicosities. In addition to providing pain control, it is useful in minimizing subcutaneous bleeding from the ends of the avulsed veins.

Anesthesia for Open Aortic Surgery

Physiological and Mechanical Considerations

Open aortic procedures are typically performed under general anesthesia. The anesthesia issues in open aortic surgery depend on the level of aortic clamping and the extent of the surgical incision. These issues include the need for cardiopulmonary arrest, spinal cord protection, renal protection, and management of the hemodynamic changes associated with clamping and unclamping of the aorta. Other issues include the need for single-lung ventilation, intraoperative hemodynamic monitoring, and the use of combined epidural and general anesthesia. Although aortic valve, ascending aortic, and arch vessel surgery often require cardiopulmonary bypass, debate still exists regarding descending thoracic and suprarenal aortic surgery. For descending thoracic and suprarenal aortic surgery, the approaches include the clamp and sew technique versus the use of an adjunctive atriofemoral bypass, aortofemoral bypass, or temporary axillofemoral bypass.

In patients requiring a thoracoabdominal incision, the placement of a double-lumen or balloon excluder endotracheal tube is essential to deflate the left lung when needed and maintain the patient on single-lung ventilation. Such a maneuver facilitates better exposure to the thoracic aorta. With respect to spinal cord protection, maintaining distal and pelvic perfusion, reimplantation of intercostals vessels, and control of spinal fluid pressure have been described as essential to minimizing spinal cord ischemia during thoracoabdominal aortic surgery. Although debatable, a spinal catheter is usually inserted prior to induction of general anesthesia, and the spinal pressure is monitored intraoperatively and for 2 to 3 days after the procedure. Spinal fluid is drained to keep the spinal pressure below 10 mm Hg or 14 cm H_2O. Reversal of spinal cord ischemia has been observed in situations where neurological symptoms have developed in the postoperative period in association with elevated spinal fluid pressure. Debate still exists with respect to hemodynamic goals and monitoring, visceral organ protection, and control of cardiac responses to clamp stresses.

Aortic cross-clamping leads to an increase in cardiac afterload. This acute increase in afterload is both measurable and manipulable, directly and indirectly. Uncontrolled hypertension, although tolerated by the healthy heart, can lead to systolic or diastolic dysfunction and cardiac decompensation. Blood pressure is often viewed as dependent on circulating blood volume, cardiac preload and afterload, and cardiac function. All of these factors are influenced by, and essentially precluded by, the ability of the heart to withstand the stress of any acute physiologic change. The effects of aortic cross-clamping are initially mechanical due to abrupt change of afterload. The rough percentage of cardiac output blocked by clamping at various levels is as follows: infrarenal, 10% to 15%; suprarenal, 15% to 25%; and supraceliac, 55%. The precise percentage varies with certain disease states, such as aortic occlusive disease and collateralization. Typically, the surgeon works in concert with the anesthesiologist to decrease the afterload (lower the blood pressure) prior to applying a clamp on the aorta. In thoracoabdominal procedures where an aortofemoral or axillofemoral bypass is being used, the increase in afterload with cross-clamping is less pronounced. The use of the cardiopulmonary pump in these procedures facilitates easier manipulation and removal of circulating blood volume to treat hypertension. The importance of continuous communication between the surgeon and the anesthesia team cannot be overemphasized. Cross-clamping or unclamping of the aorta should not be performed before the anesthesia team has made all the necessary interventions needed to address the hemodynamic changes expected with the aortic clamp application or removal.

Pharmacological Considerations

Although mechanical intervention related to circulating blood volumes are undertaken routinely, so too is pharmacological control of the vascular system. Nitroprusside and nitroglycerine titrations are often employed to decrease afterload and preload, respectively. The advantages of nitroprusside include its effectiveness in peripheral arteriolodilatation and titratability. Furthermore, the vasodilatation of the vascular beds causes decreased oxygen extraction ratio and decreased cardiac work. Nitroprusside effects cardiac preload to a lesser extent, but it can possibly decrease the perfusion pressure to infra-clamp tissues provided by collateral arterial supply due to arteriolar dilatation. A common side effect is pulmonary vasoconstriction, arteriovenous shunting, and resultant desaturation of blood. Furthermore, prolonged use of nitroprusside can result in systemic cyanide toxicity. Nitroglycerine decreases cardiac preload and is titratable. It vasodilates coronary circulation and indirectly decreases cardiac work. It does not effect infra-clamp organ perfusion and has less systemic toxicity, seen as methemoglobinemia; however, it is not as potent as nitroprusside. Other factors for visceral protection include the use of mannitol 12.5 g intravenously a few minutes prior to suprarenal cross-clamping in an attempt to decrease renal reperfusion injury.

Anesthesia in Carotid Surgery

General anesthesia is the traditional anesthetic technique for carotid endarterectomy (CEA). In 1962 Spencer and Eiseman described a local anesthetic technique for CEA. A "cervical block" is regional anesthesia consisting of infiltration of the paravertebral nerve roots at C2–C4 with one or a mix of local agents. General anesthesia and regional anesthesia are equally acceptable approaches to anesthesia for a patient undergoing a carotid endarterectomy and depend on the experience of the operative team.

Pros and Cons of Regional Anesthesia and General Anesthesia for Carotid Endarterectomy

The advantage of general anesthesia goes beyond keeping the patient motionless. The brain's metabolic demand is usually reduced with general anesthesia, and thus acts as a protective mechanism against ischemia. The disadvantages of general anesthesia in carotid surgery include the need to routinely place a shunt or the use of EEG or stump pressure monitoring to selectively shunt. The decision to shunt is sometimes determined preoperatively in cases of contralateral occlusion, history of ipsilateral stroke, or known lack of collateral circulation (from cerebral angiogram). In these cases, many surgeons would routinely shunt during general anesthesia.

The advantages of regional anesthesia are more often seen in a different patient population than with that of general anesthesia. Published selective shunt rates in regional anesthesia are in the range of 15%, which is a lower rate of shunting than techniques that involve monitoring. Regional anesthesia has been shown to invoke less postoperative hypertension and hypotension and reduced postoperative intensive care unit and hospital stay.

"Cerebral protection" in CEA refers to protection of the brain from ischemia induced by blood flow changes at the time of CEA. Cerebral protection can be obtained from a shunt, or monitoring for its need. The placement of a shunt from the common carotid artery to the internal carotid artery is the standard way to maintain intracerebral blood flow during CEA. The disadvantages of shunting include potential injury to the proximal and distal ends of the shunted vessel (intimal flaps), increased blood loss, the rare potential for embolism through the shunt, and the technical aspects of performing the endarterectomy around the shunt device. It is for these reasons that selective shunting is advocated by some. Monitoring for significant cerebral effects of carotid cross-clamping has been shown to decrease the need for shunting, and thus allows for use of a selective shunt only if brain tissue is thought to be compromised. Electroencephalography, transcranial Doppler, and ipsilateral stump pressure measurement are techniques most often employed.

Cerebral perfusion pressure (CPP) is equal to the mean arterial pressure (MAP) minus the intracranial pressure (ICP). Thus, an additional approach to cerebral protection is to maintain an elevated MAP during CEA. One approach is to maintain the patient's blood pressure at the same level or within 20 mm Hg higher than the patient's baseline blood pressure. Again, this requires a coordinated effort between the surgeon and anesthesiologist.

Regional Anesthesia Techniques for Carotid Endarterectomy

The dermatomal distribution of the neck innervation is in cervical nerves 2 through 4. Regional block anesthesia is targeted at these nerves in a paravertebral location. The cervical plexus is comprised of the anterior divisions of cervical nerves 1 through 4. The plexus sits anterior to the median scalene and levator scapulae, and behind the sternocleidomastoid muscles. The cervical plexus divides into superficial and deep branches. It is the deep branches that innervate the deep structures of the neck including the muscles via an internal and an external series of nerves. The internal series consists of the following nerves: communicating branches, mus-

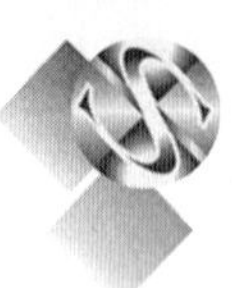

cular branches, communicantes cervicales, and phrenic. The external series includes the communicating and the muscular nerves. The superficial branches of the cervical plexus become the following sensory nerves: smaller occipital, great auricular, cutaneous cervical, and supraclaviculars. A deep cervical plexus block is a paravertebral block targeted to C2 through C4. Due to its proximal location, an effective block involves the superficial and deep branches. A superficial cervical block has the advantage of not involving any nerves that innervate muscle including the phrenic, and the disadvantage of not involving the deeper sensory nerves that the deep branches of the plexus innervate.

Deep Cervical Plexus Block: Selected Division Blockade Technique

After placing the patient in a neutral supine position, and appropriately prepping the skin for aseptic technique, a 4- or 5-cm 22-gauge needle with a short bevel is used to instill local anesthetic. An example of local anesthetic that could be used is a half-and-half mix of 1% lidocaine and 0.5% bupivacaine. A total of about 3 or 4 cc of local anesthetic should be used at each level. To find the proper position for needle placement at all levels, an imaginary line can be drawn between the tip of the mastoid process and Chassaignac's tubercle of C6, which is palpable at the level of, and posterior to, the cricoid cartilage. The C2 injection is performed about 1 to 1.5 cm below the mastoid process on this line, just posterior to the sternocleidomastoid. Moving about 1.5 cm caudad from the C2 site along the same line can place injections at C3 and C4. A horizontal line from the ramus of the mandible posterior can be a guide to the level of the C4 injection site as well. A slight caudal angle of the needle can prevent the needle from tracking to the intervertebral space, and thus avoiding peridural or spinal anesthesia. If the transverse process is hit with the tip of the needle, paresthesias result. This indicates that the needle tip is in the proper vicinity and the injection can be performed.

The complications of this approach to deep cervical block include intravertebral artery injection causing convulsions, unconsciousness, or temporary blindness. The nerve block can also spread to prevertebral (superficial) fascia and the cervical sympathetic chain, causing Horner's syndrome or hoarseness secondary to recurrent laryngeal nerve involvement.

Deep Cervical Plexus Block: Interscalene Technique

This technique utilizes the proximity of the cervical plexus branches' proximity to each other to administer a single dose of anesthetic. Using the same needle as the selective approach but a larger syringe to inject 10 yo 12 cc of an equivalent anesthetic, a single bolus of local is injected in an "interscalene" location as follows: Palpate the interscalene groove separating the anterior and middle scalenes at a level of the cricoid again using Chassaignac's tubercle of C6. At this location, enter using a caudal and slightly posterior angle. A C5-6 dermatomal paresthesia is elicited, and 10 to 40 cc of local is injected while holding caudal pressure. A 40-cc injection without caudal pressure also involves the brachial plexus. Regardless of the amount or pressure used, the ipsilateral phrenic nerve is blocked by this procedure, an effect that is usually well tolerated.

The complications of this approach of deep cervical blockage include phrenic nerve involvement and the same complications as for the selective technique; however, there is a lower chance of inadvertently puncturing the vertebral artery.

Superficial Cervical Plexus Block

Using a 22-gauge, 4-cm needle, local is injected just posterior to the midpoint of the posterior border of the sternocleidomastoid muscle. The injection should be angled to attempt infiltration of the posterior and medial aspects of the muscle. As it only affects the cutaneous nerves, the complications of this approach are minimal.

Anesthesia for Vascular Surgery of the Lower Extremity

Transfemoral thromboembolectomy, focal vein bypass revisions, and even femorofemoral bypasses can be effectively performed under

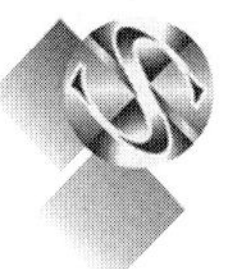

local anesthesia. In most other procedures where long skin incisions, long segments of vein harvesting, deep exposures, and tunneling are required, the options include regional or general anesthesia. Regional anesthesia appears to avoid the hypercoagulability noted with general anesthesia and appears to provide an early patency advantage with infrainguinal bypass procedures (Christopherson et al., 1993). However, in prolonged procedures, the patient may become restless and uncomfortable due to prolonged immobility.

Conditions that suggests avoiding regional anesthesia include tremor at rest, inability to follow commands (the level of cooperation of the patient), peripheral neuropathy limiting the sensation of pain of the distal lower extremities, and a history of lower back surgery or pain. In the presence of severe heart failure or diastolic dysfunction, general and regional anesthesia have been shown to be similar in overall outcome. In these high-risk patients, local anesthesia with monitored anesthesia care is the best option if the surgical procedure is appropriate for such anesthesia.

In the presence of significant pulmonary disease [forced expiratory volume in 1 second (FEV_1) <1.0], the risk of prolonged intubation or pulmonary infection after endotracheal intubation would indicate regional anesthesia. However, some patients with significant pulmonary disease are unable to maintain a supine position for prolonged periods.

Significant coagulopathy precludes spinal and epidural anesthesia due to the risk of epidural hematoma and subsequent paralysis. Furthermore, an infection either in the region of placement of a regional anesthetic or causing systemic sepsis usually precludes regional anesthesia due to the risk of seeding the paraspinal space.

During procedures involving the foot such as toe or forefoot amputations, an ankle block can be an ideal regional anesthesia. The technique for ankle block involves infiltrating the ankle circumferentially with a local anesthetic just at the level of the medial malleolus. Further infiltration of the posterior tibial nerve is usually needed to achieve adequate anesthesia. The neuropathy associated with diabetes can lead to a nearly anesthetic foot, and procedures can be performed with minimal anesthesia.

Anesthesia for Vascular Surgery of the Upper Extremity

In general, most vascular procedures in the upper extremity can be managed by local or regional anesthesia. In spite of the lack of evidence of the benefit of regional anesthesia versus general anesthesia in randomized studies in terms of morbidity and mortality, there is enough proven or anecdotal benefit in terms of pain relief, cost-efficiency, and time to discharge. These benefits of regional anesthesia are particularly valued in outpatient surgery and should therefore encourage its use.

Regional Anesthesia Techniques for the Upper Extremity

The brachial plexus supplies all of the motor, and most of the sensory, innervation to the upper extremity. It is important to remember that the medial aspect of the upper arm to near the elbow is enervated by the medial cutaneous and intercostobrachial nerves and not the brachial plexus. Similarly, the skin on the shoulder is supplied by the "caudal" branches of the cervical plexus supply. The common regional anesthesia techniques of the upper extremity are categorized based on location of surgical dissection.

Axillary Artery/Vein Dissection

Axillary artery and vein exposure including axillofemoral bypass proximal dissection can be performed under local anesthesia, or with an intrascalene approach to block the brachial and cervical plexus. Applying inferior pressure on the interscalene groove can guide the infiltration of local anesthesia superiorly along the scalene muscles to effect a predominantly cervical plexus block. Using less pressure inferiorly can result in a predominantly brachial plexus block.

Brachial Artery/Vein

This is the "gray zone" of brachial plexus blocks, as the skin overlying the brachial vessels is often at least partially innervated by the medial cutaneous and intercostobrachial nerves. However, if local anesthesia is used in combination with the brachial plexus block, adequate and safe anesthesia can result.

Radial, Ulnar, and Antecubital Regional Anesthesia

The region from the elbow to the wrist is ideal for a brachial plexus block. The techniques include an intrascalene approach, as mentioned above, and a subclavian approach. The intrascalene approach, as mentioned in the discussion of cervical plexus block, above, often involves the ipsilateral phrenic nerve and possibly some cranial nerves. The subclavian approach has less phrenic nerve involvement (50%) and requires smaller volumes of anesthetic, but can lead to pneumothorax.

Distal Ulnar and Radial Artery, and Hand Surgery

Local anesthesia is the best option in the compliant patient. Axillary blockade is another option for distal arm/hand surgery and is relatively easy and safe. However, axillary blockade effects only the forearm, requires arm abduction, and can lead to hematoma.

Conclusion

Numerous approaches to vascular anesthesia are available. The approach must be tailored to the patient and the procedure. It is important that the operative team, surgeons and anesthetists, work in concert throughout any vascular procedure.

References

Bode Jr RH, Lewis KP, Zarich SW, et al. (1996) Cardiac outcome after peripheral vascular surgery: comparison of general and regional anesthesia. Anesthesiology 84:3–13.

Christopherson R, Beattie C, Frank SM, et al. (1993) Perioperative morbidity in patients randomized to epidural or general anesthesia for lower extremity vascular surgery. Anesthesiology 79:422–34.

Henretta JP, Hodgson KJ, Mattos MA, et al. (1999) Feasibility of endovascular repair of abdominal aortic aneurysms with local anesthesia with intravenous sedation. J Vasc Surg.

Rigg JRA, Jamrozik K, Myles PS, et al. (2002) Epidural anaesthesia and analgesia and outcome of major surgery: a randomized trial. Lancet 359:1276–82.

Rivers SP, Scher LA, Sheehan E, Veith FJ. (1991) Epidural versus general anesthesia for infrainguinal arterial reconstruction. J Vasc Surg 14:765–70.

Rockman CB, Riles TS, Gold M, Lamparello PJ, Giangola G, Adelman MA. (1996) A comparison of regional and general anesthesia in patients undergoing carotid endarterectomy. J Vasc Surg 24:946–56.

Rodgers A, Walker N, Schug S, et al. (2000) Reduction of postoperative mortality and morbidity with epidural or spinal anaesthesia: results from overview of randomized trials. BMJ 321:1493–7.

Steen PA, Tinker JH, Tarhan S. (1978) Myocardial reinfarction after anesthesia and surgery. JAMA 239:2566.

Von Knorring J, Lepantalo M. (1986) Reduction of perioperative cardiac complications by electrocardiographic monitoring during treadmill exercise testing before peripheral vascular surgery. Surgery 99:610.

8

Nonatherosclerotic Vascular Disease

Jonathan R.B. Hutt and Alun H. Davies

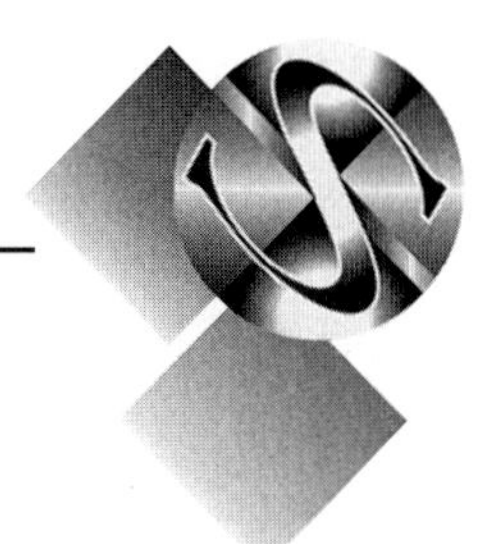

Vasospastic Disorders

Raynaud's Phenomenon

In 1862 Maurice Raynaud first described the problem of an asphyxia and symmetrical gangrene of the extremities. Raynaud's phenomenon is now defined as episodic vasospasm of arterioles in the extremities. It is classified as either an idiopathic form, known as primary Raynaud's or Raynaud's disease, or as secondary Raynaud's or Raynaud's syndrome, where it occurs in the presence of an underlying cause (Table 8.1).

Raynaud's has an incidence of up to 5%. It is found worldwide, but due to the common precipitant factor of cold extremities, it appears to have a higher incidence in countries with a low ambient temperature. It affects women far more than men at a ratio of 9:1. In the case of primary Raynaud's, there is evidence of a genetic predisposition, as 25% of sufferers have a first-degree relative who is affected.

The underlying pathophysiology of Raynaud's presents a complicated picture. The overall effect is due to vasospasm of small muscular arteries and arterioles. Many factors and mechanisms have been implicated in this process, and it is occasionally unclear whether they are causal as part of the primary pathology or consequential as a result of it. That there are many causes of secondary Raynaud's is testament to the fact that there may be subtly differ-

ent underlying mechanisms with a similar final end point. In a similar vein, although some factors may not be primary instigators of the problem, their activation and subsequent action may contribute to the severity of the pathology and thus provide therapeutic targets in certain situations. The increasing number of implicated mechanisms may also indicate the future potential for further delineation of the spectrum of disorders associated with Raynaud's into more distinct pathological mechanisms.

Broadly speaking, the etiological factors that have so far been implicated in the development of Raynaud's can be divided into local factors present at the immediate neurovascular level, and more general humoral factors (Fig. 8.1).

The Local Microvascular Unit

Neurogenic Mechanisms

Vasoconstriction of the cutaneous vessels when induced by cold is regulated by α_2 receptors. This mechanism is open to derangement in the pathology of Raynaud's. It has been shown that sufferers have a reduced basal blood flow, which would obviously be further decreased in the setting of sympathetic-induced vasoconstriction. Notably, it also appears that baseline cutaneous blood flow is decreased in healthy women compared with men, which may provide an insight into the condition's preference for the female sex. Although there is no increase in background catecholamine circulation detected in affected patients, dermal arteriolar

Table 8.1. Secondary causes of Raynaud's phenomenon

Mechanical
Frostbite
Vibration

Rheumatological disease
Scleroderma
Systemic lupus erythematosus
Dermatomyositis
Polymyositis
Rheumatoid arthritis
Sjögren's syndrome
Takayasu's arteritis
Giant cell arteritis

Arterial disease
Brachiocephalic atherosclerosis
Buerger's disease
Thoracic outlet syndrome

Vasospastic disorders
Migraine
Prinzmetal's angina

Endocrine disorders
Carcinoid syndrome
Hypothyroidism

Blood dyscrasias
Cryoglobulinemia
Paraproteinemia
Polycythemia

Infective causes
Parvovirus B19
Helicobacter pylori

Drugs
Vinblastine
Bleomycin
Methysergide
Ergot alkaloids
Beta blockers

samples from Raynaud's patients show an exaggerated response to α_2-stimulating agents. The use of sympathectomy as a therapy and the documented benefits from the α_2-blocking agent Prazosin also support a place for abnormal sympathetic activity in Raynaud's pathophysiology.

Another neurological factor is calcitonin gene-related peptide, a powerful vasodilator found in cutaneous nerve endings. Response to this mediator is unaffected in diseased tissue, but immunocytochemistry demonstrates a decrease in calcitonin gene-related peptide levels in the local digital neurons of people with primary and secondary Raynaud's. Intravenous infusion of calcitonin gene-related peptide has also been shown to increase blood flow in the hands and may also help digital ulceration in more severe cases.

Endothelial Mechanisms

At the level of the endothelium, there are a number of mechanisms which may have been implicated in the pathophysiology of Raynaud's. Endothelin-1 is a vasoconstrictor derived from vascular endothelial cells. Increased levels of this mediator have been described in patients presenting with Raynaud's. Similarly, nitric oxide, an endogenous vasodilator, appears to be present at reduced levels. It appears, however, that these findings may be more consequential than causal. Reports on patients with primary Raynaud's have not shown increased levels of endothelin-1, and it is accepted that endothelial damage is more a feature of secondary disease. Moreover, endothelin-1 levels correlate with severity of disease and are also shown to decrease in patients with systemic sclerosis as digital ulcers undergo healing. Administration of L-arginine, a precursor of nitric oxide synthesis, has no benefit, and samples from

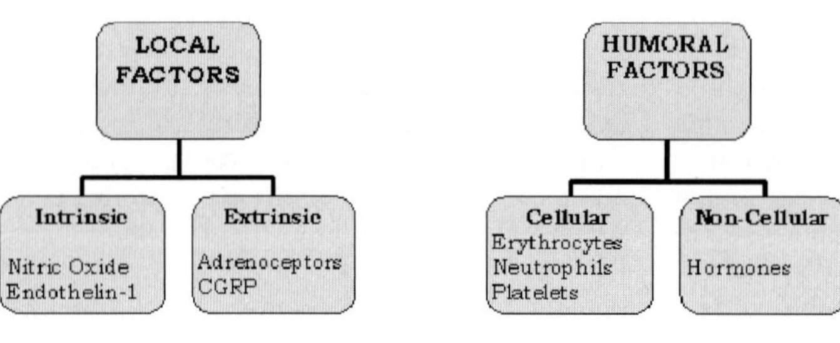

Figure 8.1. Etiological mechanisms in Raynaud's phenomenon. Both local and humoral factors have been implicated. CGPR, calcitonin gene-related peptide.

nonaffected arterioles from patients with systemic sclerosis show normal endothelium-mediated vasodilatory responses. This suggests that this mechanism is unlikely to be a primary causative one.

Humoral Factors

Cellular

Platelets

The potential for platelets to act as a significant pathological factor is high. Activated platelets have the ability to aggregate and cause mechanical blockage, or release mediators that are both prothrombotic and stimulate vasoconstriction. Similar to the effects seen on endothelial cells, increased expression of α_2 receptors on platelets in Raynaud's patients may provide a lower threshold for activation in the presence of sympathetic stimulation. Platelets from Raynaud's patients also appear to be hypersensitive to 5-hydroxytryptamine (5-HT) (serotonin) stimulation. An increase in activation of platelets is seen in Raynaud's, with augmented release of the mediators thromboxane A_2 and serotonin. Similar to endothelin-1, thromboxane A_2 is related to disease severity, primarily in secondary disease. Administration of antagonists to this substance, however, does not appear to have a marked effect on disease expression or progression.

The potential for platelets to be primary etiological agents is also called into question with the interesting observation that sufferers of Glanzmann's thrombasthenia, who display a complete lack of platelet aggregation, may still suffer attacks of Raynaud's syndrome.

Neutrophils

Although they are unlikely to be causative factors, circulating neutrophils may certainly have a propensity for causing damage. Trapping and activation in the setting of occluded vessels followed by ischemia and reperfusion lead to an escalation of the reactive response in the local vicinity of the arterioles. However, in primary Raynaud's, endothelial damage is not really a feature. In light of this fact, this mechanism may simply represent an augmenting effect.

Erythrocytes

Abnormalities of erythrocyte aggregation and deformability have been described in Raynaud's patients.

Hormonal

Estrogen

Certainly the large predilection for the female sex that Raynaud's displays is cause enough to consider an underlying hormonal basis. Different phases of the menstrual cycle are associated with varying responses of digital blood flow to cold stimuli, which certainly suggests that female sex hormones may have an etiological role.

Clinical Factors

Raynaud's is characterized classically by the following symptoms:

- Initial pallor due to vasoconstriction
- Cyanosis due to sluggish blood flow
- Redness due to hyperemia

This gives the classical picture of white, blue, and then red discoloration described by sufferers. This picture usually occurs in the presence of cold or emotional stress. It may be accompanied by numbness and burning pain, which may be severe as the blood flow returns. The most common site to be affected is the fingers, with the toes involved to a lesser extent. More rarely, other extremities such as the nose, ears, tongue, or nipple may be affected. The attacks range from mild, with an asymptomatic picture when seen by the clinician, to more severe effects with necrosis and gangrene of peripheral tissues. In extreme cases, this may progress from superficial to deep structures and require amputation.

In the setting of the presentation of Raynaud's as a primary complaint rather than on the background of known disease, investigation into underlying causes is required. Up to 5% of patients presenting with primary Raynaud's ultimately develop a connective tissue disorder. It does appear that there are notable differences in the demographics and presentation between primary and secondary disease, as outlined in Table 8.2.

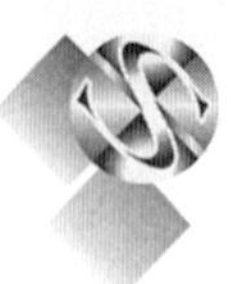

Table 8.2. Clinical differences between primary and secondary Raynaud's

Feature	Primary	Secondary
Age at onset	≤30	≥30
Digital gangrene	Rare, superficial	Common
Nail fold capillaries	Normal	Large and tortuous
Auto antibodies	Negative or low titer	Frequent

History and examination should be directed at the exclusion of secondary causes of Raynaud's phenomenon. History should include questioning on symptoms of connective tissue diseases as well as details of drugs and exposure to toxic agents. A history of vibrating tool use, trauma, or positional triggering consistent with thoracic outlet syndrome is also helpful. Routine examination should not omit careful examination of the peripheral pulses and blood pressure (BP) in both arms, along with neck examination for the presence of a cervical rib.

A further test that can be performed at the consultation is capillaroscopy of the nail fold, where capillary loops lie horizontal to the surface (Box 8.1). Other techniques for the measurement of peripheral blood flow such as analysis of digital systolic pressure during cooling or red blood cell velocity in nail fold capillaries have yet to find their way into clinical practice.

A chest radiograph shows a cervical rib if it is present, and may also show changes consistent with connective tissue disease. Blood testing for autoantibodies or prothrombotic states can provide good indicators for the presence of underlying disease. Further tests such as Doppler imaging or angiography of vessels as well as further blood tests, should be instigated on the basis of previous indications. A potential pathway for diagnosis in Raynaud's is shown in Figure 8.2.

As an idiopathic cause, primary Raynaud's should be considered a diagnosis of exclusion, to coincide with the following criteria:

- Symmetrical vasospastic attacks
- Absence of necrosis or gangrene
- History and physical findings not indicative of secondary cause
- Normal capillaroscopy of nail bed
- Normal erythrocyte sedimentation rate (ESR) and negative serology for autoantibodies

A follow-up period of 2 years is likely to be sufficient to pick up any underlying pathology of what initially appears to be Raynaud's disease. The most likely culprits by far that may reveal themselves are the connective tissue diseases.

Treatment

Acute Ischemia

In the setting of acute tissue-threatening ischemia, instigation of vasodilatation is the key treatment. Intravenous prostaglandin analogues such as iloprost are effective. In the absence of the availability of such therapy, a short-acting calcium channel blocker such as nifedipine can be given, along with aspirin as antiplatelet therapy. A digital or wrist block with local anesthesia without adrenaline may be beneficial both for pain relief and for the underlying pathology, as it effectively provides a localized chemical sympathectomy.

In persistent cases, a prolonged infusion of IV heparin may be required, and in intractable cases, surgical intervention with localized digital sympathectomy is indicated.

In the absence of tissue-threatening complications, disease therapy is best approached in a stepwise manner. Increasing levels of intervention can then be introduced if the disease proves refractory to a particular level of therapy. A potential pathway for the treatment of Raynaud's disease is shown in Figure 8.3.

Box 8.1. Capillaroscopy

The nail-fold capillaries can be visualized through immersion oil placed on the finger. Although best seen with a microscope, they can also be viewed using an ophthalmoscope set at a diopter of 10–40. In the presence of connective tissue disease, the nail-fold vessels are tortuous and dilated.

Figure 8.2. Algorithm for the diagnosis of Raynaud's phenomenon.

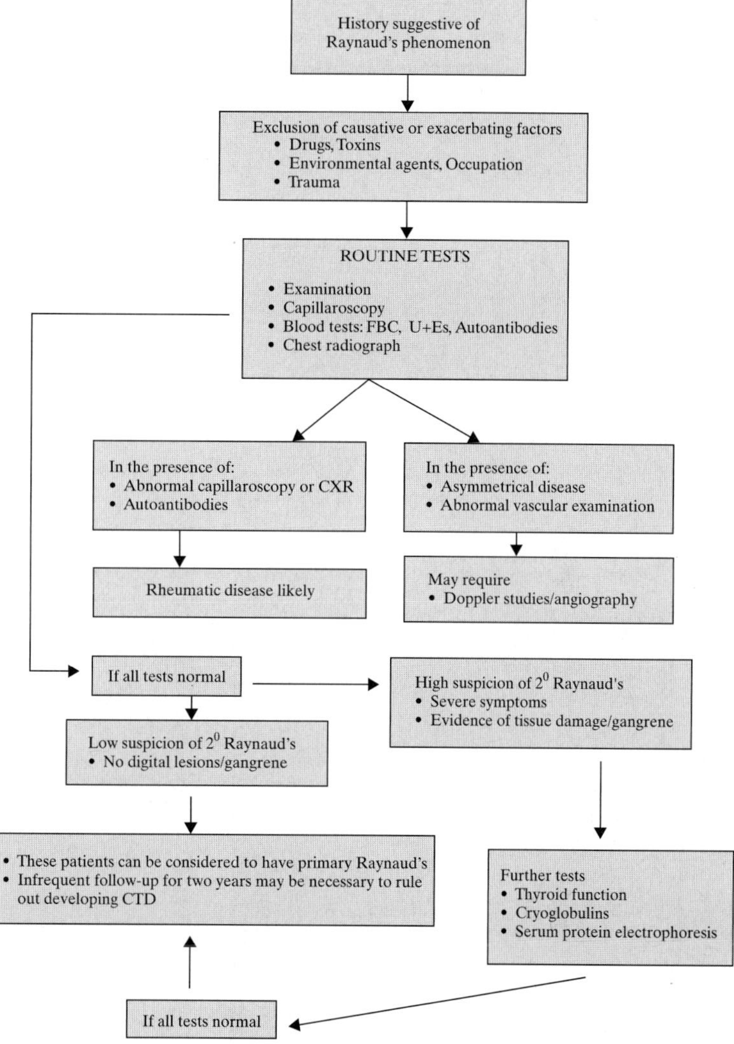

Nonpharmacological Therapy

Initial treatment is based on the avoidance of precipitants, such as cold and emotional stress. Prevention of exposure to cold is best based on a total body approach, rather than just localized to fingers and toes, and may include specifically designed clothing such as heated gloves. The cessation of contributing factors is also involved at this step. This includes lifestyle modifications regarding smoking and caffeine intake, plus other vasoconstricting substances such as cocaine and amphetamines. Any medical therapies that may be contributing to the disease should be stopped or modified to other, less harmful agents. Use of vibration-proof impact tools or in certain cases a change of job may prevent the progression of secondary Raynaud's associated with hand–arm vibration syndrome.

Pharmacological Therapy

There are a multitude of putative pharmacological therapies for Raynaud's, some of which have a more solid evidence base than others:

Ca$^+$ channel blockers: These have been the mainstay of treatment for some time. The best agents are those based on dihydropyridines, due to their decreased action on

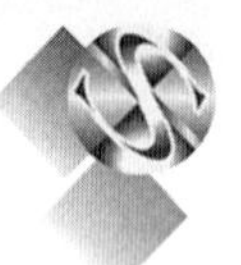

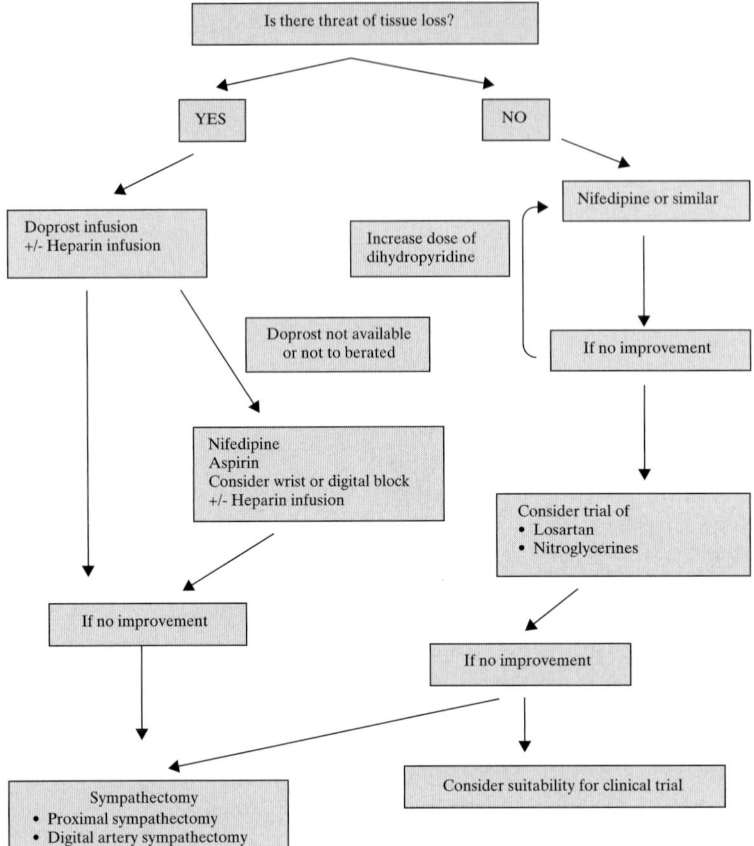

Figure 8.3. Algorithm for the treatment of Raynaud's disease.

cardiac muscle and relative selectivity for vascular smooth muscle. Classically, nifedipine is the drug of choice, but newer dihydropyridines such as amlodipine and felodipine are also effective. These are usually started at a low dose with gradual escalation as required.

Angiotensin II receptor antagonists: Trials with losartan show a good efficacy compared with nifedipine in reduction of quantity and severity of attacks (Dziadzio et al., 1999).

Serotonin modulation: The serotonin antagonist Ketanserin has been used in treatment, particularly in the setting of scleroderma, although its evidence base may be questionable. There is also some evidence that selective serotonin reuptake inhibitors (SSRIs) such as fluoxetine may have a beneficial effect.

Nitroglycerines: The use of topical nitrates may aid in symptomatic relief and in the reduction of the number of attacks, although side effects may limit their usefulness.

Prostaglandins: There is good evidence that an intravenous infusion of iloprost, a synthetic prostacyclin analogue, is efficacious in Raynaud's, certainly in severe disease. The key to its widespread use in less acute settings lies in the production of an effective oral preparation. However, attempts to date to produce a similar effect to that seen with intravenous administration have proved equivocal and have been troubled by a high incidence of side effects.

Future possibilities: Further medical treatments are likely to continue to appear, in the light of the large quantity of mooted causative factors. Initial trials with calci-

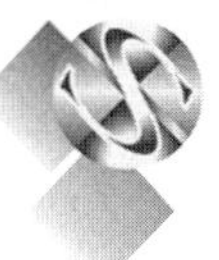

tonin gene-related peptide certainly indicate potential for development. Further delineation of the genomics behind primary Raynaud's may show the road to more interventional possibilities in the setting of gene therapy.

Surgical Therapy

Due to its invasive nature as well as its inherent complications, surgery for Raynaud's is usually reserved for cases that are refractory to medical therapy. The main surgical option is sympathectomy, which may be performed as a proximal procedure, or as a microsurgical localized operation:

Upper limb: This involves destruction of the second and third thoracic ganglia and their interconnections, which may be performed through a number of surgical approaches. Results are disappointing in terms of relapse rate, although it may still have a role in severe cases.

Lower Limb: This involves destruction of the second, third and sometimes fourth lumbar sympathetic ganglia plus interconnections. It appears to be a more effective therapy than the similar procedure in the upper limb.

Another option, this one microsurgical, is digital artery sympathectomy, a more effective procedure than proximal sympathectomy. Although effective, its place probably lies in treatment of tissue-threatening disease or in cases refractory to medical therapy.

Other Vasospastic Disorders

Erythromelalgia

This is a rare condition characterized by vasodilation associated with erythema and increased temperature of the extremities along with a burning pain. Similarly to Raynaud's phenomenon, it may occur in an idiopathic form or secondary to other disease. Associated pathology includes hypertension, myeloproliferative disorders, diabetes, rheumatic disease such as rheumatoid arthritis or systemic lupus erythematosus (SLE), gout, spinal cord disease, and multiple sclerosis.

The clinical picture varies in severity. Therapy with aspirin and vasoconstrictive agents can be helpful, and treatment of the underlying disease may aid symptoms in secondary disease.

Acrocyanosis

This presents as a symmetric cyanosis of the hands or less commonly of the feet, which is both persistent and painless. Affected body parts show decreased temperature and blue discoloration, and they may be swollen and sweaty. Examination of peripheral pulses is normal. Generally, it is not a harbinger of underlying or threatening pathology, and supportive treatment with reassurance and advice about avoiding the cold is usually sufficient.

Vasculitis

Vasculitis is broadly defined as inflammation of the vessel wall. It covers a wide range of clinical and pathological entities, which have both confusing similarities and yet important distinctions, most notably in their treatment and prognosis.

Classification of these diseases is complicated, as there is considerable overlap both in clinical presentation and histological appearance. The most common approach used is to classify them by consideration of the size of the vessels that the disease affects (Table 8.3). Vasculitis that affects the smaller arteries can be further classified according to whether or not antineutrophil cytoplasmic antibodies (ANCAs) are found. Such a distinction is possible at a histological level, as only those associated with ANCAs affect the small arteries, with the others affecting arterioles, venules, and capillaries.

The underlying pathophysiology of many of the noninfective vasculitides appears to have an immunological basis. This is clear not only from the temporal associations of some of the conditions with certain viral infection, but also from the fact that the majority are treated with various combinations of immunosuppressants.

Their clinical presentation arises from the consequences of vessel wall inflammation. These include thrombosis and subsequent ischemia or infarction, aneurysm formation, and hemorrhage. The extremely broad range of clinical phenomena and affected target vessels

Table 8.3. Classification of the vasculitides

Large-vessel vasculitis
Giant cell arteritis
Takayasu's arteritis
Medium-vessel vasculitis
Kawasaki's disease
Polyarteritis nodosa
Small-vessel vasculitis
ANCA associated
Wegener's granulomatosis
Churg-Strauss syndrome
Microscopic polyangiitis
Not ANCA associated
Henoch-Schönlein purpura
Cryoglobulinemic vasculitis
Cutaneous leukocytoclastic angiitis

ANCA, antineutrophil cytoplasmic antibody.

means that the vasculitides present to a myriad of clinicians: dermatologists, rheumatologists, and gastrointestinal(GI) and vascular surgeons.

Large-Vessel Vasculitis

Giant Cell Arteritis

This is a granulomatous inflammatory disease of the aorta and its branches. It has a tendency to affect the extracranial branches of the carotid artery, hence its other name of temporal arteritis. It was first described by Sir Jonathan Hutchinson in 1890, who noticed it in a retired hospital porter who was unable to wear his hat due to tender and inflamed temporal arteries. It is a disease that is predominantly seen in Europeans over 50 years old, and has a slightly higher incidence in women, with a male to female ratio of 1:2. Incidence can be up to 25/100,000 in the older age groups. Although the actual cause remains a mystery, it has a strong association with polymyalgia rheumatica, which is present in up to 50% of cases. Both these conditions share genetic risk factors and geographical populations.

At a microscopic level, there is intimal thickening and edema. A chronic inflammatory picture is seen with giant cell and granuloma formation.

The usual clinical presentation is with severe unilateral occipital or temporal headaches. There is scalp tenderness, which classically becomes evident on brushing or combing hair.

Features of vascular insufficiency may also be present, such as jaw claudication, or, more rarely, tongue or limb claudication. These symptoms may be accompanied by systemic symptoms of fever, malaise, fatigue, and a sore throat.

The most feared complication is involvement of the ophthalmic artery. This leads to ischemia of the optic nerve and sudden painless visual loss, which can be temporary or may be permanent.

On examination, there may be swelling and tenderness of affected superficial arteries, which will be pulseless. The most notable finding on simple blood tests is a significantly raised ESR and C-reactive protein (CRP).

The key to diagnosis of this condition is obtaining histology from an arterial biopsy, which is usually taken from the temporal arteries. Due to the nature of the disease, which occurs as skip lesions, it is important to take a multiple sections, each of an amount of at least 3 to 5 cm.

The most effective treatment is corticosteroids, and if a diagnosis of giant cell arteritis (GCA) is suspected, immediate initiation of steroid therapy is required to prevent the onset of blindness. A prompt biopsy should then be organized, preferably within 7 days of starting the steroid course. This reduces the possibility of a negative biopsy in an affected patient, avoiding the clinical conundrum that follows of a patient on long-term steroids without a definitive diagnosis.

In 75% of patients, the disease settles within a period of 3 years, but in others it proves refractory to treatment. As in all diseases treated with long-term steroids, the side effects of the treatment itself can lead to difficulties. Currently, however, it appears that no steroid-sparing agent has emerged as a suitable alternative or adjunct.

Takayasu's Arteritis

In 1908 Mikito Takayasu, a Japanese ophthalmologist, described the association of retinal arteriovenous anastomoses and absent upper extremity pulses. Takayasu's arteritis is a rare granulomatous arteritis of the aorta and its major branches. It has a predilection for females, and tends to affect people in their second and third decades, although it has been reported in patients as young as 6 months and in adults at every age. Although it is encountered worldwide, it is especially prevalent in people of Asian descent.

Pathologically, Takayasu's arteritis somewhat resembles giant cell arteritis, displaying severe necrotizing inflammation that leads to marked intimal thickening. This causes eventual narrowing and occlusion of the lumen. It can also weaken the vessel wall, providing a predisposition to aneurysm formation.

Clinically, patients suffer from systemic symptoms such as fever, malaise, weight loss, arthralgia or myalgia, and night sweats. More specific symptoms are related to the affected arterial system and related end-organ ischemia, (Table 8.4). Clinical presentation can vary from incidental discovery in the asymptomatic patient to a catastrophic event.

Physical examination may reveal bruits or decreased pulses (Takayasu's is also known as pulseless arteritis). Blood pressure may be elevated, and also asymmetrical due to subclavian stenosis. There may be valvular regurgitation and arterial tenderness. This latter sign may be especially noticeable over the carotids.

Investigation is primarily by arteriography. Neither the level of symptoms nor other indicators of disease such as the ESR provide a clear indication of disease extent or severity. As a rule, these indicators are thus not a good guide to management.

Table 8.4. Site-dependent presentation of Takayasu's arteritis

Clinical presentation and severity depend on:	
Site	
Degree of stenosis	
Availability of collateral blood supply	
Subclavian:	Arm claudication, Raynaud's
Carotids:	Visual changes, syncope, TIAs/ stroke
Vertebrals:	Visual changes, dizziness
Aortic arch:	Aortic insufficiency, CHF
Aorta (includes main enteric branches):	
	Abdominal pain, nausea, vomiting
Renal arteries:	Hypertension/renal failure
Iliac arteries:	Leg claudication
Pulmonary arteries:	Atypical chest pain, dyspnea
Coronary arteries:	Chest pain/MI

CHF, chronic heart failure; MI, myocardial infarction; TIA, transient ischemic attack.

Treatment

Some patients demonstrate a self-limiting disease that requires minimal intervention, whereas others require more intensive therapy.

Medical

In the first instance, treatment is with glucocorticoids. If the disease proves refractory to steroid therapy, or if the patient is unable to be weaned off their long-term use, further treatment with cytotoxic agents is indicated. Adjunct therapy with methotrexate is effective in increasing progression to remission as well a having steroid-sparing effects. Cyclophosphamide has similar properties, but due to its significant toxicity is probably best used as a third-line treatment in those who are intolerant of or nonresponsive to methotrexate.

Surgical

There is a place for open vascular surgery and endovascular options in the cure of fixed vascular lesions producing significant ischemia. Indications include cerebral hypoperfusion, hypertension due to renovascular disease, and aneurysms or valvular insufficiency. Clinically significant improvement of symptoms is usually possible with surgery, although restenosis is common.

Prognosis

Takayasu's is a chronic disease with a 45% relapse rate, although 23% of patients never reach a state of remission. Following diagnosis, survival rates are greater than 80%. However, the disease still carries a significant morbidity.

Cogan's Syndrome

This rare disorder of young adults of either sex warrants a mention at this point primarily due to the vessel it affects. It is an inflammatory process that leads to interstitial keratitis and may lead to permanent hearing damage or effects on the vestibuloauditory system, although these effects appear unrelated to the vasculitic phenomena. From a vascular point of view, patients may suffer aortitis or other large-vessel inflammation. The primary source of morbidity is cardiovascular involvement and auditory problems.

Treatment is with prednisolone, and is indicated for severe ocular or auditory disease and vasculitis. Prompt treatment at the first sign of hearing damage improves the prognosis for overall hearing loss and return of function.

Medium-Vessel Vasculitis

Kawasaki's Disease

Kawasaki's disease was first identified in 1967 by Tomisahu Kawasaki, a Japanese pediatrician, and is also called mucocutaneous lymph node syndrome. Although it is seen in adults, this is primarily a disease of childhood, and the major cause of acquired heart disease in children in the United States and Japan. Despite the original demographical description, it is a disease that is found worldwide. In the United Kingdom the incidence is less than 5/100,000 in children less than 5 years old; 80% of sufferers are in this age bracket, and males are affected with slightly greater frequency than females at a ratio of 2:1.

Clinical Factors

The condition begins with an acute febrile illness. This is followed by a polymorphic rash that may affect any part of the body, congestion of the conjunctivae, dryness and erythema of the oral mucosa, cervical lymphadenopathy, and erythematous edema of the palms and soles. These features are the criteria for the diagnosis of Kawasaki disease (Table 8.5). Other clinical features are outlined in Table 8.6.

The major cause of morbidity and mortality in the disease arises from the cardiovascular complications, including pancarditis, but more specifically the vasculitic changes in the coronary arteries may lead to the formation of

Table 8.5. Diagnostic criteria for Kawasaki's disease

Fever plus:
Rash
Conjunctival injection
Oral mucosal changes
Brawny induration of extremities
Cervical lymphadenopathy

Table 8.6. Other clinical features of Kawasaki's disease

System	Feature
Cardiovascular	Pancarditis
Gastrointestinal	Diarrhea
Genitourinary	Albuminuria
Neurological	Aseptic meningitis
Joints	Arthralgia
Blood	Leukocytosis, thrombocytosis, raised C-reactive protein

aneurysms. These occur 1 to 4 weeks after the onset of fever, and are seen in up to 25% of untreated cases. Thus, monitoring of the disease is usually structured with an electrocardiogram (ECG) performed in the first week of illness, with an echocardiogram both initially at diagnosis and repeated 2 to 4 weeks later.

Treatment is twofold. High-dose IV immunoglobulin is given as a single infusion. This prevents the formation of coronary aneurysms but also decreases fever and inflammation in the myocardium. Patients are also given aspirin as an antithrombotic measure. In certain cases, long-term follow-up and anticoagulation may be required.

Polyarteritis Nodosa

Polyarteritis nodosa (PAN) was the name eventually given to the disease process in the first definitive report of a patient with necrotizing arteritis, which was written in 1866. For some time, before it was clear that there were further underlying pathological mechanisms, all patients presenting with necrotizing arteritis were given a diagnosis of PAN. In truth, it is an uncommon disorder. Unlike other vasculitic disorders, PAN is most frequently observed in middle-aged men. It often leads to severe systemic complications affecting many of the organ systems. The underlying pathology of PAN is one of florid acute inflammatory changes seen in a pattern of fibrinoid necrosis. This is similar to what is seen in models of immune complex vasculitis, and there is some evidence that certain viruses have associations with the development of PAN. These include the hepatitis B and C viruses and HIV. Clinically, the patient may present with a number of complaints, due to the widespread nature of the disease (Table 8.7).

Table 8.7. Clinical manifestations of polyarteritis nodosa

System	Manifestation
Cardiovascular	Coronary arteritis may lead to MI or HF
Respiratory	Asthmatic symptoms + hemoptysis, (rare)
Gastrointestinal	Hemorrhage and mucosal ulceration Presentation may mimic the acute abdomen
Genitourinary	Hematuria
Neurological	Mononeuritis multiplex (involvement of vasa nervorum)
Joints	Subcutaneous nodules,* hemorrhage, and gangrene Livedo reticularis, (seen if chronic)
Blood	Leukocytosis, thrombocytosis, raised CRP

* These occur due to the involvement of subcutaneous arteries and, although uncommon, they are part of the reason why the disease was originally named.

CRP, C-reactive protein; HF, heart failure; MI, myocardial infarction; TIA, transient ischemic attack.

Blood tests in PAN reveal anemia, leukocytosis, and a raised ESR; ANCA is rarely positive in classic PAN. Diagnosis is primarily by two methods. Histologically, biopsied lesions show a classical pattern of necrotizing arteritis, whereas angiography reveals microaneurysms, which may be found in hepatic, intestinal, or renal vessels.

Treatment of the condition is primarily with immunosuppressants. Therapy is initially with corticosteroids, but further agents such as azathioprine or cyclophosphamide may be indicated in life-threatening disease.

In cases where the vasculitis occurs in a picture of viral infection, control of the inflammation with immunosuppression may be necessary before effective antiviral therapy can be considered. However, combination antiviral therapy may prevent the problems of conventional treatment, which may enhance viral replication, increasing the chance of progression to chronic infection. In viral-associated vasculitis, plasma exchanges may also be considered, as they are effective in reducing the amount of circulating immune complexes.

The prognosis, perhaps unsurprisingly, is worse in those patients who suffer multisystem involvement. Five-year survival with treatment is 80%, and it is a disease that relapses only infrequently.

Small-Vessel Vasculitis

Estimates of incidence of the small-vessel vasculitides vary, most likely due to variations in the diagnosis. They share similar nonspecific systemic features such as fever, malaise, weight loss, arthralgia, and myalgia. Investigation of these patients should include screening for antineutrophil cytoplasmic antibodies (Box 8.2).

Broadly speaking, the vasculitides of the small vessels can be divided into those in which the ANCAs are positive or negative (Table 8.8).

Wegener's Granulomatosis

In Wegener's (named for Friedrich Wegener, a German pathologist, 1907–1990), the small arteries are predominantly affected above all others. It may occur at any age, and appears to show no predilection for either sex (Hoffman et al., 1992).

Pathologically, it has a pattern of necrotizing granulomatous vasculitis and is typically characterized by lesions that involve three main

Box 8.2. Antineutrophil cytoplasmic antibodies

Antineutrophil cytoplasmic antibodies (ANCA)

There are two primary types of ANCA, differentiated on the basis of their pattern of immunofluorescence on ethanol-fixed neutrophils.

cANCA

Antibodies directed against serine protease proteinase 3 (PR3).

These give a cytoplasmic pattern.

pANCA

Antibodies directed against the enzyme myeloperoxidase (MPO).

These give a perinuclear pattern.

The ANCA typing can be combined with antigen-specific testing for PR3 and MPO to increase specificity.

Table 8.8. Distribution of ANCA among the small vessel vasculitides

ANCA positive	ANCA negative
Wegener's granulomatosis	Henoch-Schönlein purpura
Churg-Strauss syndrome	Cutaneous leukoclastic angiitis
Microscopic polyangiitis	Cryoglobulinemic vasculitis

ANCA, antineutrophil cytoplasmic antibody.

organ systems: the upper respiratory tract, the lungs, and the kidneys. Greater than 90% of patients seek help for symptoms related to the respiratory tract.

Patients suffer initially from severe rhinorrhea. This is followed by nasal and sinus inflammation, which eventually leads to cartilaginous ischemia, the sequelae of which are perforation of the nasal septum and saddlenose deformity of the nasal bridge. Tracheal inflammation and sclerosis lead to stridor and potentially dangerous airway stenosis. This particular complication is more common in children who are affected. Disease activity in the lower respiratory tract leads to cough, hemoptysis, and pleuritic pain. Renal tract disease manifests as glomerulonephritis. This is present in only 20% of patients at the time of diagnosis, but appears overall in 80% eventually.

A chest radiograph may show nodular masses, which can be multiple. There may also be ground-glass infiltration and cavitation. Over time, the lesions show a migratory pattern, disappearing in one area only for new lesions to appear in others.

The typical histology of Wegener's is best seen in the kidney. A renal biopsy demonstrates necrotizing microvascular glomerulonephritis. However, diagnosis is often by nonrenal biopsy, which demonstrates the granulomatous necrotizing inflammation with neutrophil aggregation and vasculitis. The site of biopsy is important. An upper airway biopsy, although easy to perform, demonstrates diagnostic changes in only 20% of cases. A more invasive biopsy of the lung parenchyma shows the diagnosis in 90%.

Before treatment became available, patients suffering from Wegener's granulomatosis would have a mean survival time of only 5 months before succumbing to pulmonary or renal failure. Even with treatment, relapse is seen in around 50% of cases. The presence of lung or kidney involvement at diagnosis is a poor prognostic indicator. Wegener's also has an especially mutilating form, known as midline granuloma, which carries a particularly poor outlook.

Therapy is with a combination of glucocorticoids and other immunosuppressants. Treatment with prednisolone alone is ineffective, and the decision on which further agent to use is based on a number of factors. In active Wegener's where the disease is life threatening, treatment with prednisolone is combined with cyclophosphamide. This leads to a 90% improvement rate, achieving complete remission in around 75% and giving a survival rate of 80%. The main drawback with this regimen is the significant toxicity associated with cyclophosphamide use. To avoid it, a progressive approach may be needed, using cyclophosphamide until the disease is in remission, then changing to another agent such as methotrexate or azathioprine, which can then be tapered out. In active disease that is not life threatening, combination treatment with prednisolone and methotrexate is equally as good at maintaining remission compared with a cyclophosphamide, and a similar regimen may also be used in those patients who are intolerant of cyclophosphamide.

Churg-Strauss Syndrome

Churg-Strauss syndrome, named for Jakob Churg, a Polish-American pathologist (1910–1966) and Lotte Strauss, an American pathologist (1913–1985), has an incidence of about 3 per million. The typical patient is usually male and in the fifth decade of life. Classically the syndrome is a triad of rhinitis and asthma, eosinophilia, and systemic vasculitis. Because of its makeup, there are a number of theories about the underlying pathophysiology. It may be a progression of an allergic phenomenon, or a primary vasculitis that has an asthmatic component due to the involvement of eosinophils.

Pathologically, the picture is one of eosinophilic infiltration, which typically affects the lung, peripheral nerves, and the skin. Histologically, a necrotizing vasculitis of the small

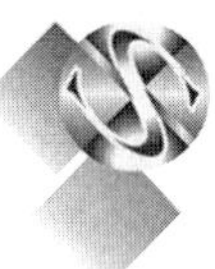

arteries is seen along with extravascular, allergic granulomas.

Although initially presenting as above, the syndrome has a progressive nature, which is eventually vasculitic and involves the lungs, nerves, heart, and the GI and renal tracts. A complete blood count shows a high eosinophil count.

Treatment is primarily with corticosteroids alone, although in life-threatening cases cyclophosphamide can be added. Due to its association, it may be difficult to taper prednisolone treatment when the vasculitic parts of the disease are in remission, as this may lead to asthmatic exacerbations.

Microscopic Polyangiitis

Another vasculitis that primarily affects the small vessels, microscopic polyangiitis has only recently been distinguished from PAN, and for this reason there is a relative dearth of data about the disease. Pathological distinction from PAN is accepted to be on the basis that microscopic polyangiitis leads to vasculitis in vessels smaller than arteries, whereas PAN can be diagnosed if these vessels are not involved. Histologically, it represents a necrotizing vasculitis, with few immune deposits and no granuloma formation.

Clinically, microscopic polyangiitis mainly affects the kidney, presenting with glomerulonephritis and hemoptysis. It may also be associated with mononeuritis multiplex and fever. Diagnosis is usually based on clinical features, testing for ANCAs, and renal biopsy. It can be severe, and survival rates at 5 years may be as low as 74%. In disease that is potentially life threatening, treatment is with prednisolone and cyclophosphamide.

Non–Antineutrophil Cytoplasmic Antibody–Associated Small-Vessel Vasculitis

Henoch-Schönlein Purpura

This is the most common systemic vasculitis in children. It is named for Edouard Henoch, a German pediatrician (1820–1910), and Johann Schönlein, a German physician (1793–1864). The peak incidence is at 5 years. Pathologically,

it is characterized by the deposition in vascular structures of immunoglobulin A (IgA)-containing immune complexes. It has a preference for venules, capillaries, and arterioles. The common clinical presentation is usually with arthralgia, colicky abdominal pain, and a purpuric rash; 50% of sufferers have hematuria or proteinuria. However, this compromises renal function in only 15%.

It is important to distinguish Henoch-Schönlein as a distinct pathological entity from other small-vessel vasculitides. It has an excellent prognosis, and supportive care is usually sufficient for most patients, in contrast to the life-threatening disease that can be caused by the other inflammatory disorders. End-stage renal failure occurs in less than 5% of patients.

Cutaneous Leukocytoclastic Angiitis

This is the most common cutaneous vasculitic lesion. It is an acute purpuric skin lesion, underlying which is an inflammation of the dermal postcapillary venules. Although primarily affecting the skin, it may also be associated with an arthralgia or glomerulonephritis. Etiologically, there is some indication that viral agents such as hepatitis C virus may play a part. It can also result from drug therapy with certain agents such as sulfonamides or penicillin.

Most patients suffer a single episode, with resolution occurring over a few months. About 10% suffer recurrent disease at varying intervals. Symptomatic relief from cutaneous irritation and associated arthralgia and myalgia is possible with antihistamines and nonsteroidal antiinflammatory drugs. Treatment of severe cutaneous disease is with corticosteroids.

Cryoglobulinemic Vasculitis

Cryoglobulins are cold-precipitable immunoglobulins that may be monoclonal or polyclonal. They are encountered in myriad disease pictures including lymphoid and plasma cell neoplasms and chronic infective and inflammatory processes. Essential mixed cryoglobulinemia describes the presence of cryoglobulins in the absence of any precipitating underlying pathology. Although this has been described historically, it appears that most of these cases are related to infection with hepatitis C virus (HCV).

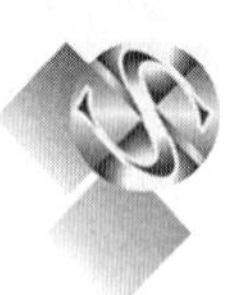

Vasculitis occurring in association with cryoglobulins affects people at about 50 years of age. A clinical picture of palpable purpuric lesions, arthritis, weakness, neuropathy, and glomerulonephritis is seen. The latter complication has an association with a poor prognosis, if not always a progression to end-stage renal failure. A useful diagnostic test is to look at complement levels. A distinctive picture of low levels of C4 with normal or slightly low C3 is seen. Renal biopsy shows an endothelial membranoproliferative glomerulonephritis with intraglomerular deposits.

Mild disease can be approached symptomatically. Antiviral therapy that produces a sustained response appears to be the most effective way of treating HCV-associated cryoglobulinemic vasculitis. In severe disease, the use of immunosuppressants has been advocated, although as expected, these agents may lead to an increase in HCV viremia.

Miscellaneous Disorders

Buerger's Disease

This eponymous disease, named for Leo Buerger, an Austrian-born American physician and urologist (1879–1943), is also known by the more descriptive term *thromboangiitis obliterans*. It is an occlusive disease of the small and medium-size arteries of the extremities, which it affects in a segmental fashion. It primarily affects young people, with a median age of 34 years. Initial descriptions by Buerger noted a strong predilection of the disease for men, affecting 2 of 500 cases that he reported. More recent studies report a male to female ratio of up to 5:1. The disease also has a somewhat unusual geographical distribution. It has a low incidence in people of European descent, but is high in India, Japan, Korea, and the Middle East, especially among Jews of Ashkenazi descent. In fact, in this latter micropopulation, Buerger's disease accounts for up to 80% of cases of peripheral vascular disease.

The primary causative factor associated with Buerger's disease is tobacco usage. Although this usually manifests as smoking, it has also been observed in patients who chew tobacco. Tobacco use holds the key not only to causation but also to persistence, progression, and recurrence. This much is clear from observations of the patient base, although interestingly the actual underlying mechanism has proved elusive. The indications appear to be that of an immune-mediated pathology, and a high prevalence has been associated with certain tobacco types in India and Bangladesh. Histologically, the disease manifests as an intense endarteritis with cellular infiltration, giant cell foci, and the presence of cell rich thrombi, which may show recanalization. Other immunological markers have also been demonstrated within the intima of the vessels. The internal elastic lamina and overall vascular wall architecture are well preserved.

Clinically, there is a picture of ischemia of the distal extremities with rest pain, ulceration, and gangrene (Ohta and Shionoya, 1988). Both upper limb and lower limb disease is seen in 40% of cases. In 10% there is only upper limb involvement, and in 50% only the lower limb is affected. Claudication is a rare symptom due to the distal nature of the diseases, and if present occurs most notably on the instep.

Diagnosis is based both on typical clinical features as well as the exclusion of other causes, as outlined in Table 8.9.

The investigations are thus directed initially at ruling out other conditions. The next step is to image the affected vessels. Arteriograms of the upper limb often show occluded radial and ulnar arteries that have become tortuous where they have recanalized. There may also be "pruning" of the digital arteries. In the lower limb, the vessels are often normal down to the popliteal trifurcation. Distal to this, segmental occlusive disease is seen. This frequently affects the tibial branches more than the popliteal. None of these changes, however, is pathognomonic.

Although the treatment of infected lesions with antibiotics and debridement where necessary is similar to that of other ischemic disease, the mainstay of therapy in Buerger's disease is the cessation of smoking. Recurrence is almost always associated with resumption of tobacco usage, and new ischemic lesions are rare without reexposure. Conversely, persistent abstinence from tobacco results in quiescence of the disease process. As the lesions in Buerger's disease appear to have healing potential, this intervention can have a significant clinical effect.

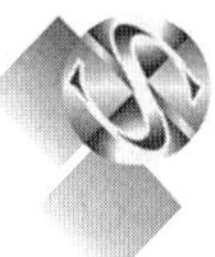

Table 8.9. Features of Buerger's disease

1. Distal extremity ischaemic symptoms
2. Exclusion of other causes
   - Proximal embolic source
   - Localised lesion (popliteal entrapment, cystic disease
   - Vasculitis
   - Drugs—ergot
   - Hypercoagulable states
   - Trauma
3. Onset at <45 yrs
4. Tobacco usage
5. Supporting features
   - Migratory superficial phlebitis
   - Raynaud's phenomenon
   - Upper limb involvement

Distal extremity ischemic symptoms
Exclusion of other causes
   Proximal embolic source
   Localized lesion (popliteal entrapment, cystic disease)
   Vasculitis
   Drugs: ergot
   Hypercoagulable states
   Trauma

Onset at <45 years of age
Tobacco usage
Supporting features
   Migratory superficial phlebitis
   Raynaud's phenomenon
   Upper limb involvement

Other options are used in refractory progressive disease. Sympathectomy has been advocated, and surgical bypass may occasionally be attempted. This latter treatment, however, has a poor rate of success. The results are affected not only due to the segmental, distal nature of the disease, but also because the associated phlebitis makes the veins poor conduits.

A number of new treatments are being evaluated, including implantation of spinal cord stimulators and intramuscular injections of vascular endothelial growth factor. The use of iloprost has also been advocated, although a significant clinical effect seems to be absent.

The final surgical option is amputation. It should be noted that healing of surgical amputation is much improved when patients are free from tobacco usage.

Compared with other necrotizing arteritides, Buerger's disease has a worse prognosis with regard to limb loss. Some form of amputation, ranging from digital to major lower limb removal, is required in up to 20% of patients. The extreme importance of smoking is again evident here. In one study, 94% of patients who quit smoking remained amputation free, whereas 43% of those who continued eventually required at least one amputation. Interestingly, and perhaps due to the distal nature of the vasculature affected, the long-term survival of patients with Buerger's disease is affected only very slightly, with life expectancies approaching that of the normal population.

Fibromuscular Dysplasia

This is a noninflammatory, nonatherosclerotic vascular disease affecting arteries of small and medium size. It appears in a variety of histological manifestations depending on the arterial wall layer that is most significantly involved (Table 8.10). Although different types show a slight variation epidemiologically, the commonest form has a predilection for females in their second to fourth decades. Disease has been noted in patients as young as 2 months old.

The etiology of fibromuscular dysplasia (FMD) is still unclear, but it appears to be multifactorial. Suggested factors include localized ischemia due to poor perfusion from the vasa vasorum, sequelae of mechanical damage, and there is evidence for a familial link. There are also many documented associations, both with diseases such as pheochromocytoma, neurofibromatosis, Ehlers-Danlos, Alport's, Rubella syndrome, and heterozygous α_1-antitrypsin deficiency as well as other factors such as ergotamine and methysergide.

Symptomatic disease from FMD may result from vessel stenosis, dissection, embolization, thrombosis, or rupture of associated aneurysms. Disease and thus symptoms have been recorded across the whole spectrum of the

Table 8.10. Histological classification of fibromuscular dysplasia

Classification	Frequency (%)
Intimal fibroplasia	5
Medial fibroplasias	1–2
Medial hyperplasia	80–90
Perimedial fibroplasia	10–15

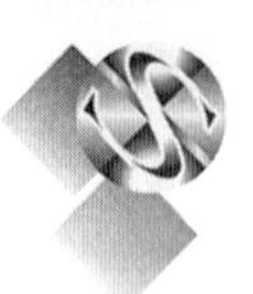

vascular bed, and it is likely that there will be subclinical disease present in other areas in most patients. The most common manifestations are hypertension from renovascular disease and stroke from carotid disease. In terms of the kidney, a significant proportion of renovascular disease arises on a background of FMD, the primary result of which is hypertension. However, as renovascular disease is a relatively uncommon cause of hypertension in itself, FMD is not a major contributing factor to adult hypertension. When it affects the cerebrovascular system, it is predominantly seen in the internal carotid artery, and frequently is seen bilaterally. Vertebral artery involvement also occurs, although rarely in isolation from carotid disease. There is also a reported association between cerebrovascular FMD and intracranial "berry" aneurysms of an order of around 7%. The symptoms of cerebrovascular disease depend on the location and severity of the lesions.

Where visceral vessels are affected, symptoms are usually due to ischemia. Infarction is rare due to the collateral arterial supply. In the peripheral vascular tree, lesions at all levels have been identified. The commonest sites are the subclavian artery in the upper limb and the external iliac artery in the lower limb.

Investigations are directed at ruling out other causes of disease, but ultimately are based on imaging of the affected arterial system. As a noninflammatory process, FMD is not associated with any of the acute-phase changes seen in the vasculitides, which can be detected by simple blood tests.

Imaging can be either by noninvasive methods such as duplex scanning or magnetic resonance angiography (MRA), or by angiography. The angiographic appearance of the most common histological type of FMD is of a string of beads. If duplex scanning is used to image the carotid system, it is important to image as distally as possible in order not to miss FMD, which in contrast to atherosclerotic lesions is not commonly seen around the carotid bifurcation.

Therapeutic intervention in FMD should be considered on an individual basis and depend on the individual as well as the location and severity of the disease. In renovascular disease, initial medical therapy for hypertension is usually indicated. It should be remembered that as with other reno-occlusive disease angiotensin-converting enzyme (ACE) inhibitors should be avoided. If pharmacological treatment fails, there are a number of options. Percutaneous transluminal angioplasty (PTA) is an effective intervention, and although it is associated with up to a one in five re-stenosis rate, the rate of reappearance of hypertension is lower. Given the success in actually curing hypertension, PTA should probably be considered earlier in younger patients to avoid unnecessarily long courses of medical therapy along with progressive deterioration of renal function. There are also a number of surgical options, which carry a higher morbidity and mortality. However, if considered in the appropriate setting both in terms of patient suitability and available expertise, they can be very effective.

Management of cerebrovascular FMD depends on the presence or absence of symptoms to a certain extent. However, there is not a great deal of information on the progression of the disease with which to make this judgment. In the asymptomatic setting, medical therapy is appropriate. In the presence of symptoms, intra-operative or percutaneous dilatation of lesions can be considered.

Where the visceral vessels are affected, surgical treatment may be indicated when medical therapy fails. Treatment of peripheral disease can broadly be considered as medical therapy, dilation therapy, either percutaneously or by open technique, and surgical bypass or reconstruction.

Cystic Adventitial Disease

This is a rare, nonatherosclerotic cause of limb claudication. Since being first reported in 1947, there have been less than 350 documented cases. It affects people mostly in the fourth and fifth decades, with a male to female ratio of 5:1.

Pathologically, it is defined by synovial-like cysts in the adventitial layer of the arterial wall. These contain a mucinous gel that contains various proportions of mucoproteins, mucopolysaccharides, hyaluronic acid, and hydroxyproline. Although the exact underlying etiology is unclear, a number of mechanisms have been proposed. It has been suggested that the fluid may come from the reactivation of mesenchymal cells trapped in developing

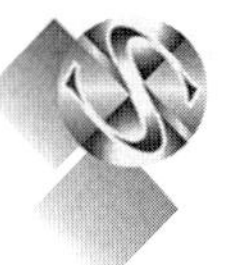

vessels during embryological vessels. Another, more widely supported hypothesis is that the cysts develop from a herniation of adjacent synovium. This latter theory is backed up by imaging results and by the late age of onset of disease.

From the reported cases, cystic adventitial disease has a predilection for the popliteal artery above all others, but has also been described in the external iliac, axillary, and distal brachial, radial, and ulnar arteries. In the acute setting the picture is of sudden onset and progressive claudication. Physical examination may reveal a mass. Indeed, some of the cases are discovered in patients referred for investigations of a soft tissue mass, before the emergence of significant vascular symptoms.

The mainstay of investigation is imaging. Although the main accepted method is angiography, good diagnostic results can also be obtained from less invasive techniques. Duplex ultrasonography can reveal the cystic disease itself, which appears as anechoic or hypoechoic masses in the external wall. It also has the advantage of providing information as to the degree of vascular impairment. Magnetic resonance imaging also produces characteristic images, demonstrating multiple intramural cystic masses oriented along the long axis of the vessel.

There are numerous therapeutic options. Spontaneous resolution of symptoms with conservative management has been documented. The cysts can also be drained percutaneously under computed tomography or ultrasound guidance. Surgical intervention consists of either excision of the cysts and diseased wall with preservation of the artery or use of an interposition graft. Both of these techniques have good initial results, although long-term follow-up data are lacking.

Given the paucity of cases on which to base interventional judgment, the decision is probably best made by considering the clinical urgency and available expertise.

References

Dziadzio M, Denton CP, Smith R, et al. (1999) Arthritis Rheum 42:2646–55.
Hoffman GS, Kerr GS, Leavitt RY, et al. (1992) Ann Intern Med 116:488–98.
Ohta T, Shionoya S. (1988) Br J Surg 75:259–62.

9

Lower Limb Ischemia

Rajabrata Sarkar and Alun H. Davies

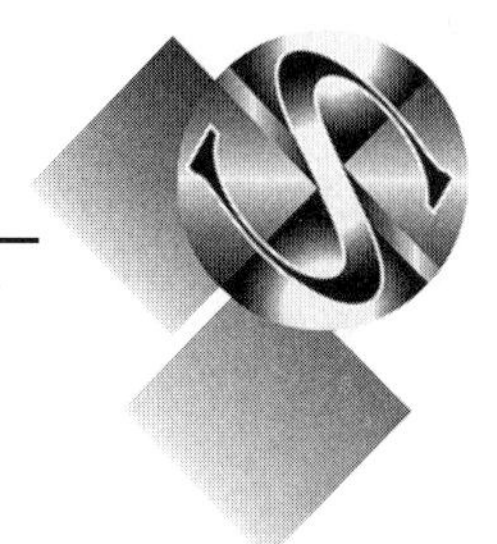

Lower limb ischemia is an increasingly prevalent disorder that has a wide range of clinical presentations and variable consequences for the patient. Although atherosclerosis is by far the most common cause of lower extremity ischemia, a variety of other conditions can cause either acute or chronic lower extremity ischemia. Three major factors are contributing to an increase in both the prevalence and incidence of lower extremity ischemia. The first is the general aging of the population in developed countries, with its attendant increase in the prevalence of atherosclerosis, peripheral aneurysms, and other vascular lesions associated with advanced age. The second factor is the alarming increase in the incidence of diabetes, particularly among adolescents and younger adults. As diabetes accelerates the progression of atherosclerosis and lower extremity ischemia, we can anticipate further increases in the number of patients presenting at a younger age with lower extremity ischemia. The third factor is the increasing numbers of patients who have undergone prior peripheral arterial bypass surgery and are potentially at risk for either graft occlusion or progression of disease. At many major medical centers the majority of patients presenting with acute limb ischemia are those with thrombosis of a prior lower extremity arterial reconstruction. This chapter reviews the causes, clinical presentations, diagnostic approach, treatment options, and outcomes of chronic and acute lower extremity ischemia.

Etiology and Presentation

Peripheral arterial occlusive disease due to atherosclerosis is the most common cause of lower extremity ischemia in developed countries, with 3% to 6% of the population over the age of 65 suffering from symptomatic disease. The clinical presentation of long-standing ischemia can be variable, with symptoms ranging from intermittent claudication to rest pain, arterial ulcers, and frank gangrene. The classic progression of symptoms in atherosclerotic lower extremity ischemia is (1) decreased pulses without any symptoms, (2) intermittent claudication, (3) rest pain, and (4) arterial ulceration or gangrene (Fig. 9.1). Patients with limited ambulation due to other causes (e.g., stroke, musculoskeletal disorders) or diabetic neuropathy may present initially with evidence of advanced ischemia such as arterial ulceration or frank gangrene. Limb ischemia should always be considered in the evaluation of the older patient who presents with a nonhealing ulcer of the lower extremities, or with an extensive or persistent skin or soft tissue infection of the foot.

Other causes of limb ischemia include embolic or thrombotic sequelae of aortic or peripheral aneurysms, embolization from the heart or proximal arterial sources, and arterial dissection (usually aortic). More unusual causes include popliteal entrapment syndrome, adventitial cystic disease, and Buerger's disease (thromboarteritis obliterans). Some of these etiologies such as embolization or thrombosis of

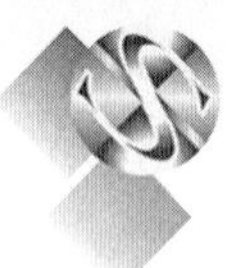

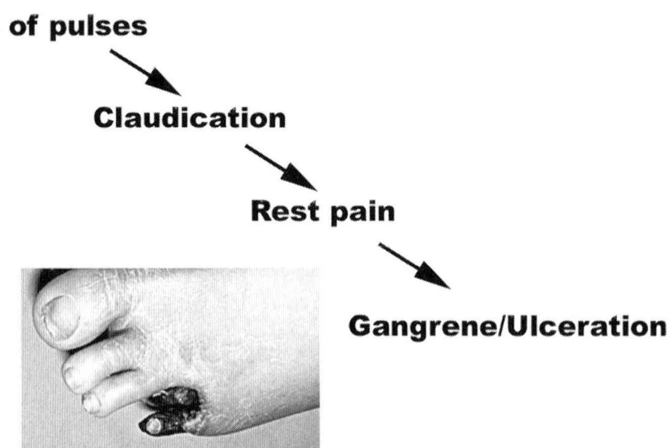

Figure 9.1. Chronic limb ischemia, progression of disease. Atherosclerosis leads to arterial occlusion, resulting in loss of pulses followed by claudication. In patients with mild peripheral arterial disease, the best treatment option is risk factor modification and exercise. In more severe cases there is rest pain, which usually occurs at night followed by gangrene (photo insert) or ulceration. Rest pain and gangrene/ulceration are considered limb threatening ischemia and the surgical options are amputation or revascularization. Aggressive attempts at revascularization are usually undertaken in ambulatory patients.

an aneurysm present as acute limb ischemia, which is characterized by the 5 P's: pulselessness, paralysis, paresthesia, poikilothermia (coolness), and pallor.

Chronic Ischemia

Patient History

Patients are often referred for vascular evaluation if they have reproducible pain in the lower extremities with walking. Although many disorders can cause these symptoms, several basic questions can be asked to ascertain a vascular etiology. Patients with vascular claudication always have pain when they walk a relatively constant distance on level ground; they do not have variable days when they can walk for considerably greater distances without pain. Often patients know exactly how far or for how long they can walk before the symptoms occur. This is in contrast to patients with neurogenic claudication or musculoskeletal causes of lower extremity pain, where the symptoms occasionally occur at rest or at with highly variable walking distances. Stopping results in resolution of vascular claudication within a few minutes, and this resolution occurs if the patient simply stops and stands in place. Patients with neurogenic claudication usually have to sit down to relieve their pain. Neurogenic claudication and musculoskeletal pain are often induced by standing in one place for prolonged periods (waiting in line at the bank or washing dishes). This is not the case with vascular claudication, where lower extremity muscular oxygen demands are not as greatly increased by standing as they are by prolonged walking. Neurogenic claudication is relieved by leaning forward, so patients with this disorder often note that they can lean forward onto a grocery cart or lawn mower and go substantially further than they can walk unaided. Similarly, the patient with neurogenic claudication often can walk further on an incline, whereas vascular claudication is marked worsened if the patient is on an incline. Patients with musculoskeletal disorders often have pain that is present at rest, or worsened by standing or sitting in certain positions. The pain in neurogenic claudication often is described as originating in the thigh and then extending down the leg, which is quite different from the focal posterior calf pain usually noted in vascular claudication. Together, these aspects of the history of the patient's

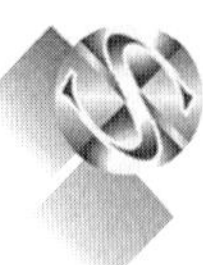

symptoms help differentiate vascular from neurogenic claudication.

More pronounced ischemia results in pain at rest, which also has specific features that distinguish it from the many other causes of lower extremity pain. Ischemic rest pain occurs when the blood flow to the foot is decreased to the point where ischemia of the sensory nerves occurs, hence the burning causalgia-like quality of the pain. Cardiac output decreases with sleep, and most patients describe symptoms that are initially present only at night. As the ischemia becomes advanced, the pain is present constantly. The more distal aspects of the lower limb are the most ischemic, and rest pain is most commonly described as occurring across the metatarsal heads of the affected foot. Ischemic pain awakens the patient from sleep and is relieved by dangling the affected limb over the edge of the bed, which patients quickly learn will allow uninterrupted sleep. Alternatively patients awakened by the pain find that rubbing the foot or walking to stimulate circulation relieves the pain. Dangling (or standing) causes the perfusion pressure of the foot to be augmented by the hydraulic pressure due to the gravity component of the height of the calf. This is approximately 40 cm of water pressure (length of the calf), which equals a 29 mm Hg augmentation of foot perfusion pressure. This increase is enough to overcome the critical closing pressure (CCP) of the precapillary sphincter in the vascular bed and restore flow to the ischemic regions of the foot. With progression of disease and more pronounced ischemia, this maneuver no longer provides relief as the net pressure falls below the CCP and capillary perfusion ceases. Several other disorders cause lower extremity pain at night and can be confused with ischemic rest pain. Diabetic leg cramps are quite common and occur at night, but the site of pain is variable and the pain often migrates up or down the leg. Musculoskeletal pain rarely occurs in the midfoot at night, and is usually localized to the joint in question (commonly the ankle or knee). Musculoskeletal causes of foot pain are usually exacerbated by walking or standing and relieved by rest, in contrast to ischemic pain. Infections in the foot, particularly osteomyelitis, can cause constant pain at rest but are often easily recognized due to other signs and symptoms.

History-taking in the patient with lower extremity ischemia should also focus on symptoms of atherosclerosis in other vascular beds, particularly the cerebral and coronary circulation. Patients with symptomatic lower extremity ischemia have a 20% to 60% incidence of significant coronary artery disease, and the coexistence of cerebrovascular and lower extremity arterial occlusive disease is also well established. Symptoms of angina, congestive heart failure, and transient ischemic attacks or strokes should be diligently investigated as many patients may ascribe these symptoms to a nonvascular cause and may not volunteer this important information. The history should also include any prior events, such as blue or painful toes, which may be suggestive of an embolic cause of the ischemia.

Physical Examination

The physical examination should be complete and focused on the detection of occlusive and aneurysmal disease throughout the peripheral circulation. The presence (or absence) of carotid bruits, cardiac arrhythmias, peripheral pulses, and bruits should be documented, and any prior scars consistent with arterial bypass surgery or vein harvest should be noted. This is of particular importance when planning reoperative infrainguinal bypass surgery, which may involve harvesting autogenous vein from multiple sites and limbs. The stigmata of chronic occlusive or embolic disease should be diligently sought, including muscle atrophy, loss of secondary skin structures such as hair and nails, dependent rubor, splinter hemorrhages, and embolic skin lesions or dusky toes. Nonpalpable pulses should be interrogated with a handheld Doppler, and a bedside ankle—brachial index (ABI) determined with an inflatable blood pressure cuff placed above the site of the Doppler signal and then at the wrist. Peripheral and aortic aneurysms may be difficult to detect on physical examination, particularly in the obese patient. A wide or easily palpable popliteal pulse is suspicious for a popliteal aneurysm, and evaluation with ultrasound or computed tomography (CT) scanning is indicated to determine the true diameter of the vessel.

More advanced limb ischemia may be associated with arterial ulcers or frank gangrene.

their ability to exercise or perform job-related tasks. The role of revascularization, whether catheter-based or surgical, in patients with claudication remains controversial. Factors that should be considered include ongoing cigarette use, the patient's commitment to exercise and physical activity, and the anatomical level of occlusive disease that requires correction. Aortoiliac occlusive disease, as judged by physical examination and noninvasive studies, can be treated well by angioplasty and stenting with minimal risk to the patient. More extensive disease, particularly involving either the infrarenal aorta or the external iliac arteries, is better treated with aortobifemoral bypass grafting. The long-term results of aortobifemoral bypass grafting are excellent, with patencies exceeding 90% at 5 years. Although aortoiliac endarterectomy was the first procedure developed for the treatment of occlusive disease of these vessels, it has largely been replaced by bypass grafting. Extensive unilateral disease, particularly occlusion of the external iliac artery, can often be treated with femoral–femoral bypass grafting. This is a procedure of substantially smaller magnitude than an aortobifemoral bypass, and is often the procedure of choice in patients with coexisting cardiac and pulmonary disease. Femoral–femoral bypass requires normal flow in the contralateral ileofemoral system, and mild to moderate disease of the contralateral artery can be treated with angioplasty and stenting to obtain sufficient inflow to support the femoral–femoral bypass graft. Although some centers have advocated axillofemoral bypass grafts for mild to moderate limb ischemia and claudication, our policy is to reserve this form of extensive extraanatomical bypass for poor-risk patients with limb-threatening ischemia or when revascularization is required after removal of infected aortic grafts.

Occlusive disease of the distal superficial femoral artery, another common site in mild to moderate limb ischemia, generally requires bypass with either prosthetic or autologous grafts (Table 9.1). Femoral-popliteal bypass grafting is often performed with excellent results in patients with disabling claudication. A randomized prospective trial of prosthetic versus greater saphenous vein bypass grafts in the femoral to above-knee popliteal artery did not demonstrate a difference in long-term

Table 9.1. Conduits for revascularization

Axillofemoral, aortofemoral, femoral–femoral	Dacron or ePTFE
Femoral: above the knee	Autologous vein, Dacron, or PTFE
Femoral: below the knee	Autologous vein

PTFE, polytetrafluoroethylene; ePTFE, expanded PTFE.

patency (Veith et al., 1986). A randomized multicenter trial demonstrated an improved graft patency and decreased risk of subsequent amputation with heparin-bonded Dacron grafts in comparison to polytetrafluoroethylene (PTFE) grafts (Devine et al., 2001), and represents the first major advance in synthetic vascular grafts that has been shown to improve clinical results relative to standard materials. Self-expanding and balloon-expandable stents in conjunction with balloon angioplasty are being applied to stenoses and occlusions of the distal superficial femoral artery with improving results, and are extending the ability to provide percutaneous revascularization of moderate lower limb ischemia.

Occlusive disease of the popliteal artery or more distal vessels, although uncommon in the nondiabetic patient with claudication, requires bypass with autogenous vein to the distal popliteal artery or tibial vessels. These procedures are generally reserved for more severe ischemia where salvage of the extremity is in question. If there is calf claudication with extensive occlusive disease of the proximal aspects of the tibial arteries, a femoral-tibial bypass to a distal vessel may result in excellent perfusion of the foot with minimal relief of claudication. This is due to the lack of retrograde perfusion to the geniculate arteries that supply the major muscles of the upper calf.

More advanced ischemia of the lower limb generally requires a more aggressive approach to revascularization if long-term viability of the limb is to be preserved. The need for revascularization needs to be combined with a complete evaluation of the medical and functional status of the patient. Patients with critical limb ischemia, which presents with rest pain, arterial ulcers, or frank gangrene, commonly have multilevel occlusive disease, which usually requires

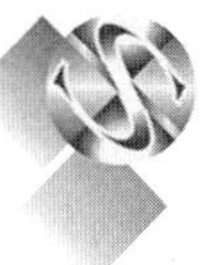

major surgical revascularization to achieve long-term limb salvage. They also have correspondingly more advanced atherosclerosis in their coronary and cerebrovascular circulation, and their perioperative morbidity and mortality is higher than for patients with claudication. The incidence of renal insufficiency or chronic failure as well as diabetes is higher in patients who present with signs of critical limb ischemia, and these medical factors have been noted in several multivariate analyses to be independent predictors of poor outcomes and higher mortality after arterial reconstruction.

Revascularization in patients with critical limb ischemia often requires correction of both aortoiliac and infrainguinal (femoral-popliteal-tibial) occlusive disease. In patients who present with advanced tissue loss or gangrene and multilevel occlusive disease, restoration of in-line arterial flow to the foot is required to heal the large tissue defects. A combination of percutaneous treatment of the aortoiliac disease (if anatomically suitable) with femoral-popliteal or femoral-tibial bypass can be used to rapidly restore foot perfusion in these cases. If the presenting ischemic symptoms are rest pain or small arterial ulcers, then correction of one level of occlusive disease (usually the aortoiliac) with angioplasty/stenting or surgical bypass relieves the symptoms.

The conduit of choice for femoral-tibial bypass, or femoral-popliteal bypass with poor runoff is the greater saphenous vein (Table 9.1). Prospective studies comparing reversed versus in situ saphenous vein grafts have not demonstrated a difference in patency or limb salvage rates between the two techniques (Harris et al., 1987). In many patients with critical limb ischemia, the ipsilateral greater saphenous vein is not available for use as a conduit due to prior harvest or vein stripping. If the contralateral greater saphenous vein is not available, then secondary sources of autogenous vein such as the lesser saphenous vein or arm veins should be preoperatively mapped by duplex scanning and utilized. The use of spliced segments of autologous vein was recently compared to PTFE grafts with vein cuffs in a randomized prospective trial of patients without an available greater saphenous vein (Kreienberg et al., 2002). Patency was greater in the spliced arm vein group (87% vs. 59% at 2 years) with similar rates of limb salvage (94% and 85%). Alternative choices for conduit include cryopreserved cadaver saphenous vein, umbilical vein grafts, conventional prosthetic grafts (PTFE and Dacron), and heparin-bonded Dacron. These have variable patency rates, all of which are inferior to saphenous vein or spliced autologous veins when utilized for femoral-tibial bypass.

A useful technique in patients with limited amounts of available vein is to originate the graft from a more distal site than the common femoral artery, thus requiring shorter segment of vein conduit. Long-term patency is not compromised by originating the graft from the deep femoral artery, the superficial femoral artery, or the popliteal artery provided that there is not significant occlusive disease above the inflow site (Wengerter et al., 1992). Autogenous vein grafts should be studied postoperatively along their entire length periodically with duplex ultrasound to identify potential areas of midgraft stenosis, which should be corrected with either balloon angioplasty or surgical repair before graft thrombosis occurs.

Many patients with critical limb ischemia are bedridden or do not ambulate because of neurological or musculoskeletal problems. In these patients, primary amputation is a safer and more expeditious means of dealing with foot gangrene than surgery for revascularization. The level of amputation, which is always of great patient concern even when ambulation is not an issue, is determined by the ambulation potential of the patient and the degree of perfusion required to heal the amputation. Although there are numerous guidelines and means of measuring skin perfusion to determine the appropriate level of amputation, clinical judgment remains the final factor. Enthusiasm for various quantitative means of measuring limb and skin blood flow has been tempered by prospective studies of these various techniques, which have failed to identify one quantitative test that preoperatively estimates probability of healing with sufficient positive and negative predictive value. Transcutaneous oxygen testing ($TcPO_2$) is the most readily available of these sophisticated blood flow measurements, which include radiolabeled xenon washout, laser Doppler velocimetry, and photoplethysmography perfusion studies. A $TcPO_2$ of greater than 40 mm Hg at the level of proposed amputation is predictive of healing, and a $TcPO_2$ of less than 20 mm Hg is indicative

of a high likelihood of failure to heal. Unfortunately, many patients with lower extremity ischemia fall into the range of 20 to 40 mm Hg, where clinical judgment must be used to decide on the level of amputation.

We recommend attempting a below-knee amputation in any ambulatory patient with reasonable rehabilitation potential in whom there is detectable popliteal artery Doppler signal. This approach is based on the known benefits with preservation of the knee joint for ambulation, and will predictably result in a small number of failures that require revision as a cost of salvaging as many below-knee amputations as possible. In the nonambulatory patient with advanced ischemia, a primary above-knee operation is performed if perfusion at the level of the popliteal artery is poor or nondetectable. Although there is some benefit to preservation of the knee joint even in the nonambulatory patient for aid in transferring from bed, major amputations in this population carry at least a 10% to 15% mortality per procedure and it is recommended to perform a single definitive above-knee procedure if there is questionable perfusion in a nonambulatory patient.

Outcomes

There has been a steady improvement in limb salvage rates due to refinements in both percutaneous and surgical revascularization for chronic limb ischemia. In particular, the widespread application of femoral-tibial bypass has led to revascularization of limbs that until recently would have been deemed inoperable. Awareness of limb ischemia as a cause of nonhealing ulcers and patient and practitioner education are responsible for earlier evaluation and referral of patients for revascularization. The success of aortoiliac angioplasty and stenting has led to relief of claudication in patients without the morbidity and length of hospital stay previously associated with aortofemoral bypass.

Despite the advances in percutaneous and surgical revascularization, a large number of patients with critical limb ischemia will eventually undergo an amputation (>50,000 cases per year in the United States). Many patients are not candidates for standard revascularization techniques because of anatomical or medical factors. The discovery that endogenous peptides can induce growth of new blood vessels (angio-genesis) has spurred interest in applying angiogenic therapy to patients with limb ischemia. Preliminary results with growth factors such as fibroblast growth factor are encouraging (Lederman et al., 2002), and further studies are needed to define the optimal growth factor, route of delivery, and duration of therapy. Similarly, the finding that circulating bone marrow—derived stem cells contribute to the angiogenesis and spontaneous revascularization seen in experimental hindlimb ischemia has led to trials of stem cell therapy for the treatment of chronic limb ischemia in humans, with promising preliminary results (Tateishi-Yuyama et al., 2002). These areas of investigation should lead to therapies for critical limb ischemia that will complement surgical revascularization and extend our ability to provide limb salvage.

Acute Ischemia

Patient History

The most important determination in the evaluation of acute limb ischemia is whether the ischemia is due to an arterial embolus or thrombosis of a chronically diseased artery. Two aspects of the patient's history contribute to this decision. The first is the onset of symptoms. Embolic occlusion of a normal arterial bed results in sudden onset of symptoms, and the patient can often recollect the exact moment of onset of the ischemia. In contrast, thrombotic occlusion of a diseased native artery occurs more gradually, with symptoms often worsening over several days. The second important aspect of the history is the presence or absence of chronic peripheral arterial occlusive disease, which is more frequently associated with thrombosis rather than embolism. Thus the presence of previous symptoms such as claudication or rest pain, or a history of prior interventions for peripheral arterial occlusive disease, strongly suggests that the acute ischemia is secondary to thrombosis of a diseased vessel or bypass graft. Many of these patients have an antecedent history of acute dehydration from gastrointestinal causes or poor perfusion, from acute cardiac dysfunction. Conversely a lack of prior claudication coupled with the presence of risk factors for arterial embolization (atrial fibrillation, a recent

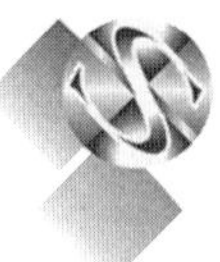

myocardial infarction, dilated cardiomyopathy, or prior embolic event) is more consistent with either arterial embolization or another unusual nonatherosclerotic cause of acute ischemia such as dissection or thrombosis of a peripheral aneurysm. Unfortunately, this maxim cannot always be relied on, as up to 25% of patients with embolism as a cause of acute limb ischemia have long-standing signs and symptoms of prior peripheral arterial occlusive disease.

Physical Examination

Acute limb ischemia is characterized by the five P's: pulselessness, paralysis, paresthesia, pain, and pallor. The level of arterial occlusion is generally one anatomical level higher that the clinical manifestation of the ischemia. Thus patients with an embolus lodged in the proximal superficial femoral artery present with an ischemic calf. The severity of the ischemia can be determined from the physical findings, with pain and pallor occurring early and paresthesia and paralysis being later findings. Paresthesia is due to direct ischemia of the sensory nerves within the extremity and is often reversed with prompt revascularization. Paralysis can be due to either ischemia of the motor neurons or muscle death. Muscle death can be determined on examination by rigidity of the ischemic muscle to palpation (rigor) and corresponding difficulty moving the joints with passive motion. If skeletal muscle death has occurred, there is little to no chance for meaningful limb salvage.

A major problem with diagnosis of acute limb ischemia remains the failure to consider ischemia as a cause of acute symptoms in the limb, leading to delays in treatment that can lead to limb loss. These delays are usually seen in patients without known prior peripheral vascular disease, such as those with undiagnosed popliteal aneurysms, aortic dissection, or (most commonly) arterial embolism. The most common misdiagnosis is a primary neurological problem, such as spinal cord impairment or stroke, to which the paresthesia and paralysis of ischemia is attributed.

Diagnostic Studies

The history and physical examination in acute limb ischemia are focused on the critical issue of whether the occlusion is due to embolism or thrombosis of a diseased artery, as this distinction leads to either immediate surgical embolectomy or preoperative angiography to delineate the cause of ischemia. The arteries of the lower extremity have tremendous capacity for collateral flow, and thus thrombosis of a native artery occurs only when atherosclerotic lesions are very advanced. Such advanced atherosclerosis is usually symmetrical, and the contralateral limb does not have a normal pulse exam. The presence of normal pulses in the contralateral limb is highly suggestive of an embolism as a cause of acute ischemia, and warrants operative embolectomy without the delay associated with preoperative angiography. Unfortunately, the converse is not always true, as signs and symptoms of prior peripheral arterial occlusive disease do not guarantee that the acute ischemia is due to thrombosis rather than embolism. Thus the presence of significant peripheral arterial occlusive disease (defined by both prior symptoms or physical findings in the contralateral limb) in patients with acute limb ischemia is an indication for angiography. Angiography definitively identifies the cause of the acute ischemia and delineates the proximal and distal arterial anatomy should a bypass be required either immediately or subsequently to relieve ischemia. Nonembolic causes of acute ischemia include thrombosis of a chronically diseased vessel, thrombosis of a previous bypass graft, thrombosis of a peripheral aneurysm (particularly a popliteal aneurysm), and proximal arterial dissection (usually aortic). The treatment of these conditions is quite varied, and immediate surgical exploration without angiography is often unsuccessful in restoring flow. In many cases, angiography is not only diagnostic but is therapeutic in terms of initiating thrombolytic therapy for occlusion of bypass grafts or thrombosed popliteal artery aneurysms. Aside from assessment of limb perfusion by Doppler examination, immediate angiography is the only diagnostic study utilized in the evaluation of acute limb ischemia.

Treatment

For any form of acute limb ischemia, systemic anticoagulation with intravenous unfractionated heparin is immediately instituted while

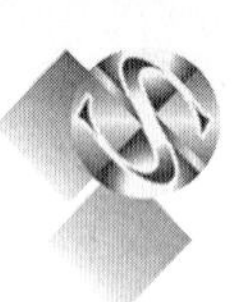

preparations are made for surgery or angiography. Patients with known sensitivity to heparin or a documented history of heparin-induced thrombocytopenia can be treated with direct thrombin inhibitors. Anticoagulation alone usually does not relieve the ischemia, but it helps prevent further propagation of the thrombus and preserve flow in collateral vessels around the occlusive thrombus. The specific treatment of acute limb ischemia rests on preoperative establishment of the cause of the acute ischemia. In a patient with a prior history of peripheral bypass surgery, the most common cause of acute limb ischemia is thrombotic occlusion of the bypass graft. In these patients, as well as patients with preexisting chronic peripheral vascular occlusive disease, preoperative angiography is usually obtained to determine the location of the occlusion and the inflow and outflow sites for bypass grafting. Preoperative angiography is not utilized in those cases of advanced acute ischemia where the location of the problem is clinically obvious, such as a patient with a prior aortobifemoral bypass graft, an absent femoral pulse, and a profoundly ischemic limb. The delay associated with obtaining preoperative angiography is also avoided in patients with suspected arterial embolism, which is treated with emergent catheter embolectomy.

Restoration of a functional and viable intact limb is extremely rare when skeletal muscle death has already occurred. If physical examination suggests that limb paralysis is due to death of the skeletal muscle, then the status of the muscle is determined by operative exploration. The high likelihood of amputation is discussed with the patient and family members prior to surgery, and primary amputation is performed if there is no bleeding from the muscle and no muscle contraction with direct electrical stimulation. Aortoiliac revascularization may be subsequently required to obtain adequate blood flow to allow healing of the definitive amputation site.

Treatment of lower limb ischemia secondary to aortic dissection can be either directed at correcting the dissection or an extra-anatomical bypass to relieve the limb ischemia. Correction of the underlying dissection may require surgical repair of the thoracoabdominal aorta, although these procedures are formidable undertakings in patients who are often critically ill with concurrent renal, mesenteric, or spinal cord ischemia. Mortality rates approaching 40% have been reported from major centers in patients with coexisting cardiac and renal disease. Advances in catheter-directed therapy for acute dissection are allowing rapid restoration of perfusion to the involved branches of the aorta without the physiological stress of operative repair of the thoracoabdominal aorta (Slonim et al., 1996). These procedures include endovascular stenting of dissections within the thoracic aorta and catheter-based percutaneous fenestration to restore perfusion to both false and true aortic lumina.

For limb ischemia secondary to suspected femoral, iliac, or aortic bifurcation emboli, embolectomy is performed via the common femoral artery. For bilateral limb ischemia where the embolus is lodged in the aortic bifurcation, bilateral transfemoral embolectomy is performed. Catheter embolectomy should be performed both proximally and distally from the common femoral artery. This is usually performed through a transverse arteriotomy in the common femoral artery placed opposite the orifice of the deep femoral artery to facilitate passage of the catheter into both the superficial and deep femoral arteries. The first priority should be establishment of adequate inflow to the common femoral artery. This is usually accomplished easily with catheter embolectomy, but occasionally the arterial flow from the external iliac artery may be unsatisfactory even after removal of all possible thrombus. This is usually due to preexisting chronic occlusive disease of the iliac arteries, but can also be caused by dissection of a diseased vessel during the embolectomy. There are two options to manage inadequate inflow after transfemoral embolectomy. The traditional solution is surgical bypass, usually with a femoral–femoral or axillofemoral graft. More recently, intraoperative angioplasty and stenting of the iliac system can be used to treat occlusive disease or dissection of the ipsilateral iliac arteries. This can be performed via either an ipsilateral retrograde approach or the contralateral femoral artery. The use of angioplasty and stenting in this setting can often restore adequate inflow more rapidly than constructing an extra-anatomical bypass, and is the procedure of choice if the appropriate expertise and equipment are available.

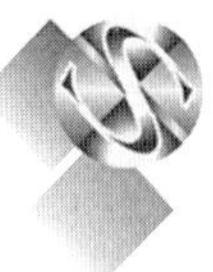

Caution must be taken when restoring blood flow to the severely ischemic limb, as the stagnant and ischemic venous blood contains toxic metabolites from the limb. Sudden return into the systemic circulation can be associated with serious complications including acidosis, cardiac arrhythmias, or arrest and renal damage. Release of the venous return from the ischemic limb to the body is done in close cooperation with the anesthesiologists, and administration of antiarrhythmic agents, sodium bicarbonate, and mannitol may be required. In patients with prolonged ischemia, particularly those with preexisting cardiac dysfunction, consideration is given to draining the initial venous return from the limb to prevent flow of these toxic metabolites back to the circulation of a compromised patient. The common femoral vein is encircled at the level of the inguinal ligament with a Rummel tourniquet and the first 300 to 600 mL of venous blood is exsanguinated via a transverse venotomy at the time that arterial inflow to the limb is restored. Appropriate replacement with banked blood is essential to maintain adequate cardiac output and oxygen delivery, and should be done concurrently with the venous drainage.

Most emboli of cardiac origin lodge in the common femoral or proximal superficial femoral artery. Smaller emboli may lodge in the popliteal artery, and embolic occlusion of individual tibial arteries from a cardiac source is unusual. Once adequate inflow to the common femoral artery is established as described above, the embolectomy catheter is directed distally down the superficial femoral artery to retrieve distal thromboemboli. Restoration of backbleeding from the superficial femoral artery is followed by embolectomy of the profunda femoris artery, which is rarely the site of embolization. Propagation of a secondary thrombus, however, does occur in the proximal aspect of this vessel, although more distal segments remain patent due to collateral circulation via the numerous branches. Transfemoral embolectomy of the distal circulation may sometimes not result in restoration of a satisfactory Doppler signal at the level of the ankle. There may be subsequent propagation of thrombus distally into tibial vessels, or fragments of more proximal emboli may become dislodged into the distal circulation during catheter embolectomy. In this case on-table angiography is performed to determine the location and amount of residual thrombus. If thrombus is found in the proximal aspects of the individual tibial arteries and blood flow to the remains poor, then more distal embolectomy is performed to restore blood flow to the foot. This is usually performed via the infrageniculate popliteal artery, which is exposed via a medial incision down distally to the tibioperoneal trunk in order to allow the passage of the embolectomy catheter into each of the tibial vessels. If the infrageniculate popliteal artery is small or diseased, a longitudinal arteriotomy is closed after embolectomy with a small vein patch; otherwise a transverse arteriotomy can be primarily closed with interrupted sutures.

Irrigation of the distal circulation with heparinized saline containing papaverine helps relieve spasm of the tibial vessels induced by passage of the embolectomy catheter. Intraoperative instillation of thrombolytic therapy, usually urokinase or streptokinase, has been described as a means of treating residual thrombus that cannot be retrieved by catheter embolectomy. Dramatic increases in patency of the distal circulation have been noted after intraoperative thrombolytic therapy, and this technique is particularly useful when there appears to be insufficient runoff to maintain patency of either a distal bypass graft or the native proximal popliteal artery.

Arterial bypass plays an important role in the management of acute limb ischemia, particularly in patients with ischemia secondary to thrombosed popliteal artery aneurysms, arterial dissection of the ileofemoral arteries, or thrombosis of a chronically diseased aortoiliac segment. Bypass operations for acute occlusion of the aortoiliac segment include aortofemoral bypass, femoral–femoral bypass, and axillofemoral bypass. The latter two are less extensive procedures that are particularly useful in the emergent management of acute aortoiliac thrombosis secondary to acute medical illness such as cardiogenic shock. The femoral–femoral bypass is performed for acute unilateral ischemia if embolectomy fails to restore adequate inflow or if the acute ischemia is due to any nonembolic cause. A clinically normal contralateral femoral pulse is a prerequisite for a femoral–femoral bypass graft, and a decreased contralateral pulse would favor the placement of an axillofemoral bypass or aortofemoral bypass in the patient whose medical condition will tolerate it. Emergent axillofemoral bypass and aortofemoral bypass are also used to treat bilateral acute limb ischemia. Axillofemoral bypass is applied in the unstable or critically ill patient in whom the more extensive incisions, prolonged time to revascularization, and greater fluid shifts associated with aortofemoral bypass may be detrimental. Emergent aortofemoral bypass for acute ischemia has the advantage of providing definitive revascularization from the most reliable source of inflow, namely the nondiseased juxtarenal aorta. The disadvantage of urgent or emergent aortofemoral bypass is the substantial magnitude and duration of an aortic procedure in a potentially ill or medically unstable patient with insufficient time for preoperative optimization of associated medical conditions.

Infrainguinal bypass procedures are also commonly used in the management of acute limb ischemia. Thrombosis of a popliteal artery aneurysm or a diseased popliteal artery is a typical indication, as are symptomatic acute thrombosis of the superficial femoral artery and dissections extending more distal to the common femoral artery. Acute thrombosis of a popliteal artery aneurysm or diseased popliteal artery can be successfully treated with popliteal or tibial bypass only if a patent target vessel below the popliteal artery is identified on preoperative angiography. Although some authors have advocated bypass to isolated or "blind" segments of the popliteal or tibial arteries, we prefer to utilize target vessels that flow across the ankle joint to supply the pedal arch, or in the case of the peroneal artery, collateralize via the anterior or posterior branch at the malleolus to provide flow to either the anterior tibial or posterior tibial artery that subsequently supplies the foot. Failure to visualize any target vessel in the calf below the level of acute thrombosis is an indication for intraarterial thrombolytic therapy to improve the outflow and provide a suitable target for a subsequent bypass graft. Neurological changes secondary to acute ischemia are traditionally considered contraindications for thrombolytic therapy due to the time required for effective thrombolysis. However, the results with thrombolytic therapy for moderate to severe acute ischemia (particularly thrombosed popliteal aneurysms) are substantially better than the dismal outcomes

Table 9.2. Controversies in the management of limb ischemia

Primary amputation versus complex bypass for limb salvage in patients with critical limb ischemia and renal failure and diabetes
Thrombolytic therapy versus surgical thrombectomy for aortofemoral graft occlusion.
Thrombolytic therapy versus surgical therapy for primary aortoiliac thrombosis.

of attempted bypass surgery to a distal vessel not angiographically visualized below the level of acute thrombosis. Accordingly, we utilize thrombolytic therapy even in the presence of early neuromuscular changes if there are no vessels visualized initially that are suitable targets for bypass grafting (Table 9.2). Although thrombolytic therapy is usually associated with improvement in the acute ischemia, serial examination of these patients for worsening ischemia is critical to determine if thrombolytic therapy should be terminated and surgical bypass performed.

The conduit of choice for infrainguinal bypass to treat acute limb ischemia is the greater saphenous vein, either from the involved limb or if necessary from the contralateral leg. There is usually insufficient time for preoperative vein mapping in such patients, and the suitability of the saphenous vein is defined by operative exploration if there are no signs of prior harvest. If there is no available saphenous vein, which is often the case in patients with acute ischemia secondary to thrombosis of a prior saphenous vein graft, then a prosthetic (usually PTFE) graft with a vein patch or cuff or a cryopreserved cadaver vein can be used. Both of these options are associated with substantially worse long-term patency than autologous saphenous vein, particularly when used for bypass to the below-knee popliteal artery or tibial arteries.

After revascularization for acute limb ischemia, consideration is given to immediate fasciotomy if the ischemia was severe and of greater than 4 to 6 hours' duration. Immediate prophylactic fasciotomy avoids problems with identifying compartment syndrome subsequently in patients who are receiving pain medication or sedation and already have pain in the limb from the surgical incisions (particularly if the popliteal artery was exposed below the

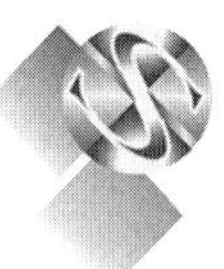

knee). The need for fasciotomy is less common in patients with preexisting arterial insufficiency, as they possess preformed arterial collateral pathways that decrease the degree of acute ischemia induced by the superimposed thrombosis or embolus. Nonetheless, either immediate fasciotomy or careful observation for development of elevated compartment pressures is mandatory following any prolonged period of ischemia of the lower extremity. This is particularly true in patients with thrombosis of an aortobifemoral bypass limb with poor outflow, as profound ischemia is produced when the inflow graft occludes.

The early signs and symptoms of compartment syndrome are the 3 P's: pink, painful, and pulses (present). Before the capillary leak induced by the ischemia-reperfusion causes intracompartment pressures to eventually exceed mean arterial pressure, there is a palpable pulse in the involved limb. The skin appears pink as the dermal plexus of arterioles maintains perfusion despite ischemia of the underlying muscle. The pain induced by compartment syndrome in the conscious patient is initially present only with motion of the muscles in the affected compartment. Thus passive stretching of the first toe is one of the most sensitive tests for compartment syndrome of the anterior compartment of the lower leg. As the ischemia becomes advanced, pain is present at rest and becomes excruciating. Immediate four-compartment fasciotomy is performed via double incisions if there is any clinical suspicion or signs of compartment syndrome after revascularization.

In the intubated or otherwise unresponsive patient where the diagnosis is unclear, measurement of intracompartment pressures with either a Stryker device or an intravenous infusion pump [with pressure sensing capability, i.e., an intravenous accurate control (IVAC) machine] enables the diagnosis of compartment syndrome to be made in the absence of the characteristic signs and symptoms. Pressures greater than 12 to 15 mm Hg are treated with fasciotomy. Fasciotomy of the lower limb is usually performed through two incisions, although a single incision fasciotomy with fibulectomy can enable decompression of all four fascial compartments. The skin incisions can often be closed at the time of fasciotomy, and this allows more rapid healing than the

weeks associated with healing open wounds by secondary intention. If there is a question of whether the edema will compromise skin closure, we place interrupted nylon horizontal mattress sutures in the skin and leave them untied at the time of fasciotomy. Once the edema subsides (usually 1 to 3 days), delayed primary closure is accomplished by tightening and tying these sutures at the bedside under intravenous sedation. The muscle ischemia in compartment syndrome results in myoglobinemia and myoglobinuria, and precautionary measures to protect the kidneys from precipitation of myoglobin within the renal tubules are instituted in all patients with compartment syndrome. Alkalinization of the urine is accomplished by administration of intravenous sodium bicarbonate, and close monitoring of serum electrolytes as well as serum myoglobin and creatine kinase (CK) levels is continued until the syndrome subsides. In patients with documented myoglobinurea, we routinely monitor urine pH to confirm alkalinization of the urine.

Outcomes

The probability of limb salvage in acute lower limb ischemia is dependent on two factors. The first and more important is the duration and degree of ischemia prior to revascularization. In patients with prior peripheral vascular surgery, diagnosis and treatment are usually not delayed, as both the patient and physician are focused on ischemia as a cause of the symptoms in the limb. As discussed above, patients with arterial embolism or aortic dissection can be misdiagnosed as having a primary nonvascular cause of their limb symptoms. The associated delay in treating the ischemia can often contribute to ultimate limb loss. The second factor in determining the outcome in acute limb ischemia is the success of revascularization, which is related to the level of disease responsible for the acute ischemia. More proximal occlusive disease, particularly aortoiliac disease or occlusion, is readily treated with embolectomy or bypass and generally associated with good outcomes. Acute limb ischemia due to failure of a prior infrainguinal bypass graft placed for prior critical limb ischemia, particularly if there have been multiple prior bypass procedures in the involved limb, is associated with worse

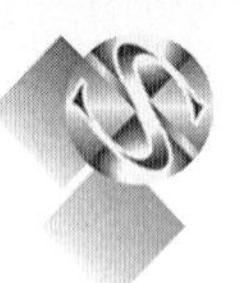

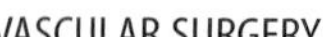

outcomes as the quality of the distal target vessel and available bypass conduit progressively decreases.

Long-term outcomes after arterial embolism are determined by the underlying medical condition of the patient, particularly the cardiac status. Despite long-term anticoagulation, up to 20% of patients with arterial embolism suffer another embolic event. Ischemic neuropathy of either the sensory or motor nerves can persist after revascularization for acute limb ischemia, and can be a source of frustration to both the patient and physician. Newer nonnarcotic modalities for chronic pain and dysesthesia are emerging, including electrical nerve stimulation, use of tricyclic drugs, and other options to treat chronic neuropathy.

Patients who present with acute ischemia secondary to thrombosis of a popliteal aneurysm have a high rate (40% to 50%) of limb loss despite modern advances in thrombolytic therapy and peripheral bypass surgery. These results reinforce the need to aggressively diagnose and treat popliteal aneurysms prior to thrombosis, and the finding that 15% of patients with aortic aneurysms have evidence of an aneurysm in the lower limb when prospectively screened (Diwan et al., 2000) provides a basis for such a strategy.

References

Devine C, Hons B, McCollum C. (2001) J Vasc Surg 33: 533–9.

Diwan A, Sarkar R, Stanley JC, Zelenock GB, Wakefield TW. (2000) J Vasc Surg 31:863–9.

Gardner AW, Poehlman ET. (1995) JAMA 274:975–80.

Harris PL, How TV, Jones DR. (1987) Br J Surg 74:252–5.

Kreienberg PB, Darling RC 3rd, Chang BB, et al. (2002) J Vasc Surg 35:299–306.

Lederman RJ, Mendelsohn FO, Anderson RD, et al. (2002) Lancet 359:2053–8.

Money SR, Herd JA, Isaacsohn JL, et al. (1998) J Vasc Surg 27:267–74; discussion 274–5.

Slonim SM, Nyman U, Semba CP, Miller DC, Mitchell RS, Dake MD. (1996) J Vasc Surg 23:241–51; discussion 251–3.

Tateishi-Yuyama E, Matsubara H, Murohara T, et al. (2002) Lancet 360:427–35.

Veith FJ, Gupta SK, Ascer E, et al. (1986) J Vasc Surg 3:104–14.

Wengerter KR, Yang PM, Veith FJ, Gupta SK, Panetta TF. (1992) J Vasc Surg 15:143–9; discussion 150–1.

10

Chronic Venous Insufficiency, Varicose Veins, Lymphedema, and Arteriovenous Fistulas

Andrew W. Bradbury and Peter J. Pappas

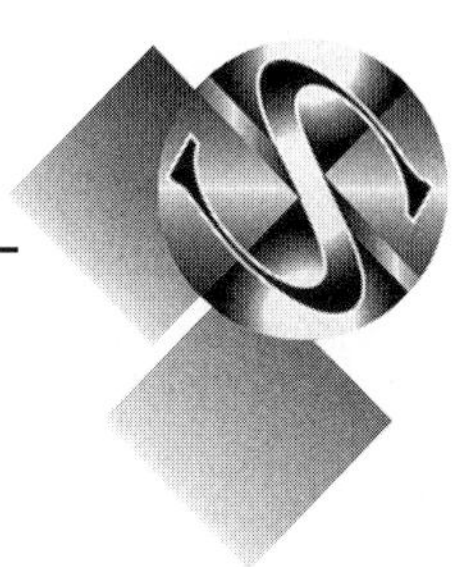

Chronic Venous Insufficiency

Chronic venous insufficiency (CVI) may be defined as symptom or signs of ambulatory venous hypertension. In developed countries, CVI affects up to half of the adult population. Furthermore, the treatment of CVI consumes up to 2% of total health spending and is a major cause of lost economic productivity. These startling data, coupled with the ineffectiveness of current treatment modalities in many of the most severely affected patients, underscore the need for more research.

Classification

Chronic venous insufficiency has proved difficult to classify for the purposes of scientific reporting. This has obfuscated attempts to directly compare the findings of different epidemiological, pathophysiological, and clinical studies. The clinical, etiological, anatomical, and pathophysiological (CEAP) classification, proposed in 1994 by the American Venous Forum, is now the most widely accepted system (Table 10.1).

Epidemiology

In industrialized countries the lifetime risks of developing varicose veins (VVs), skin changes (corona phlebectatica, lipodermatosclerosis, varicose eczema, atrophie blanche), and chronic venous ulceration (CVU) are 30% to 50%, 5% to 10%, and 1% to 2%, respectively. The bulk of advanced disease affects the elderly, with up to 5% of women over the age of 65 years having a history of CVU. However, up to 50% of affected patients, especially men, develop their ulcer before their 50th birthday. Women often relate the development of VVs to pregnancy and childbirth. The increase in female sex hormones and blood volume during the first trimester may be responsible. However, there is little evidence of an association with (multi)parity, and men and women appear to be affected almost equally by CVI. The excess of women observed in clinical practice is mainly due to their longevity and the reluctance of men to seek medical attention. There is no clear evidence that low socioeconomic class predisposes to CVI, although CVU healing and recurrence rates may be worse. Clinical experience suggests that occupations involving prolonged standing are associated with an increased prevalence and severity of CVI, poor ulcer healing, and increased recurrence rates. Data on the relationships between physical activity and CVI are conflicting, but it seems reasonable to assume that an individual with a well-developed calf muscle pump is less likely to develop CVI. Although a consistent relationship between weight and height is lacking, VVs appear to be commoner in tall men and CVU in obese women. Similarly, there is growing evidence of a hereditary predisposition to CVI. For example, patients whose parents both have VVs have a 90% chance of developing

Table 10.1. Clinical, etiological, anatomic, and pathophysiological (CEAP) classification

Clinical[1]	
Class 0	No visible or palpable signs of venous disease
Class 1	Telangiectasia[2] or reticular veins[3]
Class 2	Varicose veins[4]
Class 3	Edema
Class 4	Skin changes (lipodermatosclerosis, atrophie blanche, eczema)
Class 5	Healed ulceration
Class 6	Active ulceration
Etiological	
E_C	Congenital (may be present at birth or recognized later)
E_P	Primary (with undetermined cause)
E_S	Secondary (with known cause): postthrombotic, posttraumatic, other
Anatomical	
A_S	Superficial veins (numbered 1 to 5)[5]
A_D	Deep veins (numbered 6 to 16)[6]
A_P	Perforating veins (numbered 17 and 18)
Pathophysiological	
P_R	Reflux
P_O	Obstruction
$P_{R,O}$	Both

[1] Supplemented with (A) for asymptomatic or (S) for symptomatic, e.g., $C_{6,A}$.

[2] Intradermal venules up to 1 mm in diameter.

[3] Subdermal, nonpalpable venules up to 4 mm.

[4] Palpable subdermal veins usually larger than 4 mm.

[5] Telangiectasia/reticular veins (1); greater (long) saphenous vein above (2) below (3) knee; lesser (short) saphenous vein (4); nonsaphenous (5).

[6] Inferior vena cava (6); common (7), internal (8), external (9) iliac; pelvic (10); common (11), deep (12), superficial (13) femoral; popliteal (14); crural (15); muscular (16).

VVs, and CVU patients have a higher prevalence of inherited thrombophilia (TP). The influence of race and ethnicity is unclear, as there are few reliable data from nonwhite populations.

Normal Venous Function

Venous blood from the lower limbs returns to the right heart against gravity through the deep and superficial venous systems. The deep veins follow the named arteries and are often paired. The superficial system comprises the long saphenous vein (LSV) and short saphenous vein (SSV) and their tributaries. As there are numerous communications between the long and short saphenous systems, and between the superficial and deep systems through junctional and nonjunctional perforators, these three elements are highly interdependent, both anatomically and functionally, in health and in disease. Most of the blood draining into the superficial veins from skin and subcutaneous tissues immediately enters the deep venous system via perforators in the foot, calf, and thigh. In healthy subjects, less that 10% of the total venous return from the lower limb passes through the LSV and SSV to the saphenofemoral junction (SFJ) and saphenopopliteal junction (SPJ), respectively. Blood is forced back up the leg during leg muscle systole, and prevented from flowing back down the leg under the influence of gravity during diastole, through the actions of the muscle pumps and closure of venous valves, respectively. The act of walking sequentially compresses venous sinuses in the sole of the foot, the calf (soleus, gastrocnemius), and to a lesser extent the thigh and buttock. During relaxation these sinuses fill from the deep and superficial venous systems and valves close in the superficial and axial veins to prevent reverse flow (reflux). In both the superficial and deep systems, the density of valves is greatest in the calf and gradually diminishes in the thigh. The iliac veins and inferior vena cava are frequently devoid of valves.

When standing completely motionless, with all the leg muscles relaxed, the venous valve leaflets come to lie in a neutral midposition. As a result, the venous pressure in the dorsal foot veins comes to represent the hydrostatic pressure exerted by the unbroken column of venous blood stretching up from the foot to the right atrium (approximately 90 to 100 mm Hg in a person of average height). Contraction of the leg muscles immediately leads to the compression of deep veins and sinuses and to the movement of venous blood cranially. Retrograde blood flow is terminated by valve closure, and perforators that allow unidirectional flow from the superficial to the deep venous system only. Conventionally, this has also been ascribed to the closure of valves within the perforators. However, several studies have shown that many perforators are devoid of valves. Instead, outward flow through perforators may be

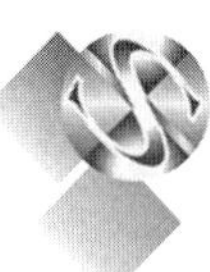

limited by external compression from contracting muscle and a pinch-cock mechanism involving the deep fascia. The importance of these mechanisms is that the very high pressures (up to 200 mm Hg) generated within the calf muscle pump are used exclusively to propel blood back up the leg against gravity, and are not transmitted to the superficial or distal deep systems. When the muscle pump relaxes, the previously expelled venous blood tends to flow caudally under gravity but is prevented from doing so by valve closure. This has the effect of dividing a single long (and heavy) column of blood into a series of shorter columns lying between closed valves. The pressure within each of these segments is low and the ambulatory venous pressure (AVP) in the dorsal foot veins falls typically to <25 mm Hg. During muscle pump diastole, blood in the superficial system flows in to the deep system along a pressure gradient.

Pathophysiology

There are three basic mechanisms that lead to raised AVP and the symptoms and signs of CVI: (1) muscle pump dysfunction, (2) valvular reflux, and (3) venous obstruction.

Aging, general debility, and a wide range of musculoskeletal or neurological lower limb pathologies can impair calf muscle pump function. The "fixed" ankle secondary to arthritis or trauma is a common example. Muscle bulk and tone are also important factors in the maintenance of perforator competence (see above). Failure of perforator competence leads to calf pump inefficiency (akin to mitral regurgitation), as well as the transmission of high pressures directly to the skin of the gaiter area.

Reflux is present in more than 90% of patients with CVI; 5% to 10% have isolated deep, 30% to 50% isolated superficial, and 50% to 60% combined. In general, superficial reflux has a better prognosis than deep reflux (especially when the latter is postphlebitic), and proximal reflux has a better prognosis than distal reflux. Valvular reflux can arise in two ways that are not mutually exclusive in any one patient:

Primary valvular incompetence (PVI): A loss of elastin and collagen in the vein wall around the valve commissures leads to dilatation, separation of the valve leaflets, and reflux. As the vein dilates, the tension in the wall increases according to the law of Laplace, which leads to further dilatation. The end result is an incompetent, elongated and tortuous varicose vein. Primary valvular incompetence may also affect the deep venous system.

Postthrombotic syndrome (PTS): Approximately 25% of CVU patients have a clear history of deep venous thrombosis (DVT), and many more have probably suffered a subclinical or undiagnosed thrombosis. Deep venous thrombosis leads to endothelial hypoxia, valvular destruction, and mural inflammation. Even though most DVTs recanalize, the end result is a thickened, valveless tube that permits gross reflux and poses an anatomical (narrowing, fibrous webs) and functional (lack of compliance) obstruction to venous outflow. Obstruction leads to the formation of collateral pathways. For example, blood may be forced out of the calf via perforators into the superficial venous system and thence up the leg with the formation of secondary VVs. Removal of such VVs increases AVP. Most patients with severe and intractable CVU have PTS.

Clinical Assessment

History

Inquiry should be made as to the duration of the present ulcer as well as the duration of ulcer disease, the number of episodes, and any precipitating factors (Table 10.2). Previous treatment history and contact allergies are recorded. Peripheral artery disease (20%), diabetes mellitus (5%), and rheumatoid arthritis (8%) often coexist. Malignancy must not be overlooked. Many patients with lower limb symptoms, and who coincidentally have VVs, have other pathology to explain their symptoms. Orthopedic, neurological, and arterial causes of leg symptoms must be excluded. Particular attention must be paid to a history of "white leg" of pregnancy, prolonged immobilization, phlebitis, and major lower limb fracture, any of which may suggest previous the PTS. A family history of venous disease, particularly early-onset, recurrent, or unusual thrombotic events, should be sought (Cornu-Thenard, 1994).

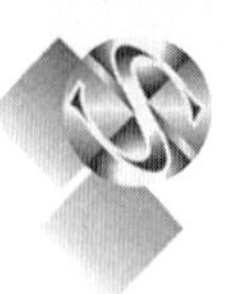

Table 10.2. Distinguishing features of arterial and venous ulcers

Clinical features	Arterial ulcer	Venous ulcer
Gender	Men > women	Women > men
Age	Usually presents >60 years	Typically develops at 40–60 years but patient may not present for medical attention until much older; multiple recurrences are the norm
Risk factors	Smoking, diabetes, hyperlipidemia and hypertension	Previous DVT, thrombophilia, varicose veins
Past medical history	Most have a clear history peripheral, coronary, and cerebrovascular disease	More than 20% have clear history of DVT, many more have a history suggestive of occult DVT, e.g., leg swelling after childbirth, hip/knee replacement or long bone fracture
Symptoms	Severe pain is present unless there is (diabetic) neuropathy, pain may be relieved by dependency	About a third have pain but it is not usually severe and may be relieved on elevation
Site	Normal and abnormal (diabetics) pressure areas (malleoli, heel, metatarsal heads, fifth metatarsal base)	Medial (70%), lateral (20%) or both malleoli and gaiter area
Edge	Regular, punched-out, indolent	Irregular, with neoepithelium (whiter than mature skin)
Base	Deep, green (sloughy) or black (necrotic) with no granulation tissue, may comprise major tendon, bone and joint	Pink and granulating but may be covered in yellow-green slough
Surrounding skin	Features of SLI	LDS, varicose eczema, atrophie blanche
Veins	Empty, guttering on elevation	Full, usually varicose
Swelling	Usually absent	Often present

Symptoms

Localized discomfort in the leg: Usually at the site of the visible VV, particularly after prolonged standing. Prominent varices may be tender, particularly in menstruating women.

Pain: Severe pain is unusual and suggests infection or arterial insufficiency.

Swelling: A feeling of swelling is common.

Venous claudication: This is unusual and due to extensive postthrombotic iliofemoral venous occlusion. There is bursting pain in the calf on walking, which is relieved only by elevating the leg. In addition, patients often complain of heaviness in the calf with ambulation.

Itching: This is common and may lead to scratching, infection, and ulceration.

Physical Examination

Varicose veins: Note the distribution of varices and any surgical scars.

Corona phlebectatica (ankle/malleolar flare): One of the earliest skin manifestations of CVI comprises dilated intra/subdermal veins at or just below the medial malleolus. Overlying skin is thin and fragile leading to a blue-bleb appearance. Trauma frequently leads to hemorrhage and ulceration.

Lipodermatosclerosis: The skin is brown (red or purple) and indurated due to hemosiderin and plasma protein deposition, leading to dermal fibrosis.

Atrophie blanche: Thin and pale skin due to the thrombotic obliteration of papillary capillaries; often at the site of previous ulceration.

Varicose eczema: Scaly dry (or weeping) skin that is often intensely pruritic and can demonstrate blanching erythema (mimicking cellulitis).

Edema: A common presentation in patients with CEAP class 3 or greater CVI. Chronic venous insufficiency may coexist with other diseases that cause edema, such as

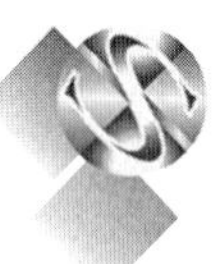

congestive heart failure, and must be considered when evaluating CVI patients (Table 10.3).

Hemorrhage: Can be alarming, even life threatening, may be spontaneous or follow trauma. Direct pressure and elevation always arrest venous hemorrhage. As recurrent bleeding is almost inevitable, the patient should be hospitalized for definitive treatment.

Ulceration: Most CVUs can be easily differentiated from other forms of ulceration.

Arterial circulation: If pedal pulses are impalpable, measure the ankle–brachial index (ABI). An ABI of <0.8 mandates referral to a vascular surgeon. The ABI is unreliable in diabetic patients.

Investigations

Virtually all patients with CVI require further investigation, and duplex ultrasound (DU) has largely replaced all other modalities in routine clinical practice. It allows Doppler velocity information to be color coded and superimposed in real time upon a gray scale (B-mode) image. It determines the location and severity of reflux, the location of the SPJ and nonjunctional perforators, and whether the deep veins are patent. Plethysmography involves the assessment of venous function through the measurement of limb volume and nowadays is primarily a research tool. Photo (PPG) and air (APG) plethysmography are probably the most popular techniques. Ambulatory venous pressure is measured by cannulating and transducing a dorsal foot vein; it remains the research reference standard. Ascending venography determines the presence of residual thrombus, the extent of recanalization, and the distribution of collaterals. Contrast medium is injected into a dorsal foot vein and directed into the deep veins by the placement of an ankle tourniquet. The iliac system and the vena cava may not be visualized, in which case a separate injection can be made in the common femoral vein (CFV) (cavography). Descending venography involves injecting contrast medium into the CFV with the subject positioned at 60 degrees with the head up in order to assess reflux. Venography is largely reserved for patients being considered for deep venous reconstruction because it is superior to DU in determining the presence and extent of the PTS. Ovarian vein reflux and pelvic varices can be visualized by placing a catheter into the ovarian or internal iliac veins via the CFV approach. As well as this imaging being diagnostic, it also enables the ovarian vein to be embolized in women suffering from pelvic congestion syndrome. Ulcers that fail to heal, tend to bleed, or have unusual features should be biopsied at base and margin under local anesthesia.

Table 10.3. Etiological classification of lymphedema

Primary lymphedema	Congenita (onset <2 years old): sporadic
	Congenita (onset <2 years old): familial (Milroy's disease)
	Praecox (onset 2–35 years): sporadic
	Praecox (onset 2–35 years): familial (Meige's disease)
	Tarda (onset after 35 years of age)
Secondary lymphedema	Bacterial infection
	Parasitic infection (filariasis)
	Fungal infection (tinea pedis)
	Exposure to foreign-body material (silica particles)
	Primary lymphatic malignancy
	Metastatic spread to lymph nodes
	Radiotherapy to lymph nodes
	Surgical excision of lymph nodes
	Trauma (particularly degloving injuries)
	Superficial thrombophlebitis
	Deep venous thrombosis

Nonsurgical Management

The mainstay of treatment is compression with or without superficial venous surgery in the great majority of patients who have CVI due to reflux. A small minority of patients who have deep venous obstruction may benefit from surgical or endovascular reconstruction. There is considerable controversy over the role of sclerotherapy.

Dressings

No particular dressing or topical agent has been shown unequivocally to significantly

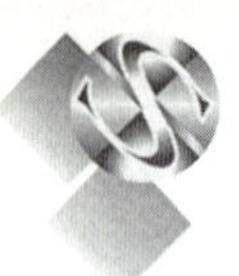

hasten CVU healing. However, they do have different physical properties, and the surgeon needs to have a basic grasp of the underlying science (and art) of wound care. Enzymatic agents (e.g., streptokinase-streptodornase) undoubtedly digest the constituents of slough. However, they are relatively ineffective against deep necrosis or hard eschar. There is evidence that they speed up healing, and may damage the wound environment. Hydrocolloid dressings come in many forms, and are generally impermeable to gases, water vapor, and bacteria. They produce a moist, acidic, low-oxygen tension wound environment that has been shown experimentally to enhance wound healing. Patients like these dressings because they are easy to use, and patients can bathe with the dressing in situ. The dressings absorb exudate (reducing the frequency of dressing changes, smell, risks of cross-infection, and costs) and may provide superior pain relief. However, in randomized controlled trials where both treatment arms have received equal and adequate compression, hydrocolloid dressings have not be shown to improve overall healing compared to any other dressing. Bead dressings (such as cadexomer iodine and dextranomer) comprise hydrophilic, polysaccharide materials that absorb large amounts of fluid and slough. The former also releases iodine in to the wound. Although they may speed up desloughing, they have not been shown to enhance healing. Paste bandages comprise a plain weave cotton fabric impregnated with zinc oxide paste, either alone or with calamine, calamine and clioquinol, coal tar, or ichthammol. These additives are designed to soothe venous eczema but are actually a common cause of contract allergy, and patch testing is recommended. Paste bandages do not retain moisture, and for this reason, and to apply compression, additional layers of bandaging are required. The Unna boot is a paste bandage containing glycerin that hardens into semirigid dressing. In trials where equal amounts of compression are applied, no form of paste bandage has been shown to improve healing over other forms of dressing. Their principal benefit is provision of inelastic compression. Alginate dressings absorb exudate and create a moist wound environment but have not been proved to speed healing. Biological dressings comprising cultured human epithelium or fibroblasts may act as a source of growth factors and act as a scaffold for the patient's own epithelial cells. But they are extremely expensive and as yet unproven.

Topical Agents

Dermatitis is common and may be endogenous (varicose or venous stasis dermatitis) or exogenous due to topically applied substances (contact dermatitis). Dermatitis is extremely morbid, associated with nonhealing, and may be irritant or allergic due to cell-mediated, delayed hypersensitivity. Early patch testing is mandatory. The use of bland paraffin preparations greatly reduces the risks of dermatitis. In patients with marked exudate, zinc oxide paste can be used to protect the surrounding skin. Acute dermatitis must be treated with removal of the offending allergen and topical steroid therapy. Topical antibiotics should be avoided.

Physical Therapy

Prolonged bed rest with leg elevation will heal virtually all CVUs. However, it is logistically impossible, and associated with decubitus complications, and as it does not address the underlying hemodynamic abnormality, recurrence is virtually inevitable. Exercise therapy aimed at improving calf muscle pump function may be of benefit and trials are under way.

Compression Therapy

Compression undoubtedly retards the development and progression of CVI. However, it is still more of an art than a science, and the quality of scientific reporting remains low. Elastic bandaging (the four-layer bandage) is favored in the United Kingdom, whereas in mainland Europe and North America inelastic bandaging (the Unna boot) is preferred. The four-layer bandage comprises orthopedic wool (to protect the bony prominences and to absorb any exudates); crepe bandage (to compress and shape the wool, and to provide a firm base for the compression bandages), elastic bandage (e.g., Elset™, Seton, applied at 50% stretch) and a self-adhesive elasticated bandage (e.g., Coban™, 3M to add to compression and fix the bandaging in place). This bandage typically exerts 40 mm Hg at the ankle and 20 mm Hg just below the knee. Once the ulcer is healed, the patient should be pre-

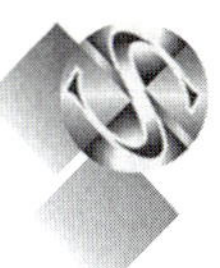

scribed stocking. There is no evidence that extending compression above the knee confers benefit. Compliance is a major problem.

Sclerotherapy

The role of sclerotherapy is controversial, with practitioner's views based largely on professional background and country of origin rather than on clinical comparative studies. Some sclerotherapists believe they can treat all VVs, but most accept the superiority of surgery in the presence of main stem, SFJ, or SPJ incompetence. However, the advent of foam sclerosants may revolutionize the management of such disease. The aim is to place a small volume of sclerosant in the lumen of a vein empty of blood, and then appose the walls of that vein with appropriate compression. The vein then fibroses closed without the formation of clot. Some practitioners use magnifying loupes for smaller veins, and there is increasing interest in injecting larger veins under ultrasound guidance (echosclerotherapy). The vein must be kept empty of blood both during and after the injection to prevent thrombophlebitis. Adequate compression is difficult in the perineum, upper thigh, and popliteal fossa, especially in the obese. Patients should be mobilized immediately afterward. In the U.K., most surgeons use detergents that act by directly damaging the endothelium. In mainland Europe and North America, hypertonic saline is also popular. Err on the side of caution with regard to volume and concentration until the patient's response can be assessed. The complications of injection sclerotherapy include anaphylaxis (<0.1%), allergic reactions (uncommon), ulceration (extravascular injection), arterial injection (rare and serious), pigmentation (extravasation), superficial thrombophlebitis (inadequate compression), and DVT (inadequate mobilization).

Surgical Management

There is growing evidence that saphenous surgery improves the quality of life in patients with VVs, and augments the healing and reduces the recurrence of CVU better than compression alone (Dwerryhouse et al., 1999). For optimal results, it is necessary to define the extent and severity of venous disease, usually by means of DU, prior to surgery. Surgery for CVU is different from that for uncomplicated VVs in a number of important ways. The patients are older and often have multisystem, medical comorbidity; the risks, especially DVT, are higher. Patients may require inpatient optimization of cardiorespiratory function, treatment of dermatitis, edema reduction, and desloughing of the ulcer. The effect of deep venous reflux on the efficacy of superficial venous surgery is controversial and incompletely defined. Deep reflux due to PVI may reverse once superficial reflux has been eradicated. However, most agree that patients with extensive PTS gain less benefit from surgery. Secondary VVs that are acting as collaterals must not be removed. Although postoperative compression therapy has been shown to reduce VVs and CVU recurrence, compliance is poor.

Varicose Vein Surgery

Long Saphenous Surgery

Safe and effective surgery depends on observing a few sound principles. In a patient of normal build the SFJ lies directly beneath the groin crease; in the obese it lies above. An incision made below the crease is likely to be too low. Resist the temptation to operate through an excessively small incision. Do not divide any vein until the SFJ has been unequivocally identified. Unless all tributaries are taken beyond secondary branch points, a network remains of superficial veins connecting the veins of the thigh with those of the perineum, the lower abdominal wall, and the iliac region. These cross-groin connections are a frequent cause of recurrence. Ligate the LSV deep to all tributaries flush with the CFV using nonabsorbable transfixion suture to reduce neovascularization through the stump. Directly ligate, and if large, consider stripping, any high anterolateral or posteromedial or thigh branches to reduce hematoma formation and recurrence. There is evidence to show that stripping the LSV to a hand's breadth below the knee significantly reduces recurrence by disconnecting the thigh perforators and saphenous tributaries and by removing the conduit that will allow neovascularization in the groin to reconnect with the remaining superficial venous system of the thigh and calf. Confining stripping to just below the knee, and to a downward direction, reduces

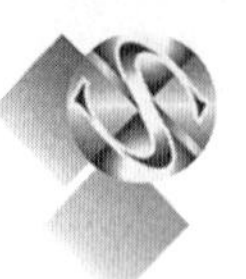
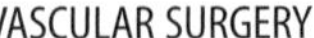

saphenous nerve injury. The theoretical advantages of invagination stripping in terms of reducing blood loss, hematoma, nerve injury, and scars have not been confirmed in trials.

Short Saphenous Surgery

Saphenopopliteal junction ligation can prove to be a challenging procedure, especially when performed for recurrent disease. Always mark the junction preoperatively with DU (some surgeon still prefer venography). The SSV can be found by following the Giacomini vein, which is a superficially placed tributary of the SSV that runs up the thigh to join the LSV. This may be large and confused with the SSV, especially if the SPJ is absent; the importance of this will be apparent on the preoperative DU. Be aware that traction on the SSV can tent up and damage the mobile and thin-walled popliteal vein. Palpation of the artery gives an indication of the depth of dissection. Beware the common peroneal nerve under medial edge of biceps femoris, which is at risk from overzealous lateral retraction as well as from a careless stitch when closing the popliteal fascia. The SSV is often closely associated with sural nerve injury and is also at risk, particular if stripping is undertaken. There are still a number of controversial issues regarding the SSV. Is it always necessary to ligate the SSV flush with the popliteal vein? Experience suggests that this counsel of perfection is hard to achieve in a significant proportion of patients without risk of collateral damage. This raises the question of what should be done with the gastrocnemius and other, often large and refluxing, muscular veins? Should the SSV be stripped or is it permissible just to remove a segment through the popliteal fossa wound? It seems likely, although there is no proof, that SSV stripping, for the same reasons as for the LSV, would reduce recurrence. However, there is concern about sural nerve injury.

Perforator Ligation

Although the advent of DU-guided subfascial endoscopic perforator surgery (SEPS) has rekindled interest in perforator ligation, there is no evidence that it alters the natural history of venous disease. Clearly, the only way to resolve this issue once and for all is to perform a randomized controlled trial of compression vs. compression and saphenous surgery vs. compression, saphenous surgery, and SEPS.

Surgery for Recurrent Veins

Recurrent LSV VVs arise because of inadequate dissection of, or neovascularization at, the SFJ in the presence of a nonstripped or incompletely stripped LSV. Standard teaching is to approach the SFJ through nonoperated tissues (usually from a lateral approach that first exposes the common femoral artery) so that the CFV can be skeletonized of branches using nonabsorbable sutures for 1 to 2 cm above and below the junction. The top of the LSV is dissected from the mass of scar tissue so that it can be stripped. However, this can be a difficult and potentially morbid operation. When the preoperative DU indicates neovascularization as opposed to an intact SFJ, the LSV can be located at the knee, a stripper passed up toward the groin, and the vein stripped without a formal redissection.

Complications

Fortunately, major complications following VV surgery are relatively rare. However, up to 20% of patients may suffer some form of minor morbidity, such as hematoma, lymphatic leak, pain, saphenous neuritis, and venous thrombosis. In the U.K., VV surgery is the commonest cause of litigation against general and vascular surgeons. This not a field for the unsupervised, inexperienced surgeon and it behooves surgeons who undertake VV surgery to carefully audit their management, techniques, and outcomes.

Deep Venous Reconstruction

These procedures have not gained widespread acceptance largely because there is little data to support their efficacy. Several different techniques have been described for suturing the edges of "floppy" valve cusps to the vein wall, rendering the valve competent. Autologous valve transplantation interposes a segment of axillary or brachial vein, containing a competent valve, into an incompetent deep vein, usually the popliteal. Procedures using synthetic, mixed, and animal valves are still experimental. An incompetent superficial femoral vein can be transected and anastomosed end to end or end

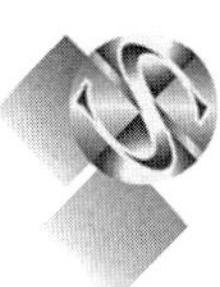

to side to a profunda femoris or long saphenous vein that has a competent valve (vein transposition). An obstructed femoral segment may be bypassed by anastomosing a transected, competent LSV to the side of the popliteal vein. Again, satisfactory long-term patency rates have been reported in small series.

Conclusions

Although the most difficult cases of leg ulceration are multifactorial in origin, CVI is the single most common underlying pathology. As such, there is hope that the prevalence of CVU may decline in the future as a result of improved thromboembolic prophylaxis and treatment. For the moment, however, CVU is a common and disabling condition that is often resistant to conservative therapy, prone to recurrence, and very expensive to manage. There needs to be a low threshold for referral to a vascular surgeon, preferably through a one-stop assessment clinic where a thorough venous and arterial duplex-based assessment can be performed. This will enable patients who might benefit from surgical intervention to be identified and treated early. It will also enable ongoing outpatient treatment to be based on an in-depth understanding of the pathophysiological mechanisms responsible in each patient. Great progress in the management of CVU has been made over the last decade because of an increased understanding of the pathophysiology and the availability of data from clinical trials that have provided a scientifically robust platform on which to base treatment algorithms. Despite all this, further research is required into the epidemiology and natural history of CVU, models of care, primary prevention, and pathogenesis.

Lymphedema

The Lymphatic System

The lymphatic system performs the following functions:

1. It removes water, electrolytes, low-molecular-weight moieties (polypeptides, cytokines, growth factors), and macromolecules (fibrinogen, albumen, globulins, coagulation and fibrinolytic factors) from the interstitial fluid (ISF) and returns them to the circulation.
2. It permits the circulation of lymphocytes and other immune cells.
3. It returns intestinal lymph (chyle), which transports cholesterol, long chain fatty acids, triglycerides, and the fat-soluble vitamins (A, D, E, and K), directly to the circulation, bypassing the liver.

Lymph from the lower limbs and abdomen drains via the cisterna chyli and thoracic duct into the left internal jugular vein at its confluence with the left subclavian vein. Lymph from the head and right arm drains via the right lymphatic duct into the right internal jugular vein. Lymphatics accompany veins everywhere except in the cortical bony skeleton and central nervous system, although the brain and retina possess cerebrospinal fluid and aqueous humor, respectively. The lymphatic system comprises lymphatic channels, lymphoid organs (lymph nodes, spleen, Peyer's patches, thymus, tonsils), and circulating elements (lymphocytes and other mononuclear immune cells).

Lymphatics originate within the ISF space from specialized endothelialized capillaries (initial lymphatics) or nonendothelialized channels such as the spaces of Disse in the liver. Initial lymphatics are unlike arteriovenous capillaries in that they are blind-ended, are much larger (50 μm) and allow the entry of molecules up to 1000 kd in size. This is because the basement membrane of these lymphatics is fenestrated, tenuous, or lacking intra- and intercellular endothelial pores. Lymphatic capillaries are anchored to interstitial matrix by filaments. In the resting state they are collapsed, but when ISF volume and pressure increases, they are held open by these filaments to facilitate increased drainage. Initial lymphatics drain into terminal (collecting) lymphatics that possess bicuspid valves and endothelial cells rich in the contractile protein actin. Larger collecting lymphatics are surrounded by smooth muscle. Valves partition the lymphatics into segments (lymphangions) that contract sequentially in order to propel lymph into the lymph trunks. Terminal lymphatics lead to lymph trunks comprising endothelium, basement membrane, and a media of smooth muscle cells that are innervated with sympathetic, parasympathetic, and sensory nerve endings. About 10% of lymph arising from a limb is transported in deep lymphatic trunks that accompany the main neurovascular bundles. The majority of lymphatic flow, however, is conducted against the venous flow from deep to superficial in epifascial lymph trunks. Superficial trunks form lymph bundles of various sizes, are located within strips of adipose tissue, and tend to follow the course of the major superficial veins.

The distribution of fluid and protein between the vascular and ISF spaces depends on hydrostatic and oncotic pressures (Starling's forces), together with the relative impermeability of the blood capillary membrane to molecules over 70 kd. In healthy subjects there is net capillary filtration, which is removed by the lymphatic system. Small particles enter the initial lymphatics directly; larger particles are phagocytosed by macrophages and transported through the lymphatic system intracellularly. Lymph flows against a small pressure gradient due to transient increases in interstitial pressure secondary to muscular contraction and external compression, the sequential contraction and relaxation of lymphangions, and the prevention of reflux due to valves. Lymphangions respond to increased lymph flow in much the same way as the heart responds to increased venous return in that they increase their contractility and stroke volume. Transport in the main lymph ducts also depends on intrathoracic (respiration) and central venous (cardiac cycle) pressures. In the healthy limb, lymph flow is largely due to intrinsic lymphatic contractility augmented by exercise, limb movement, and external compression. However, in lymphedema, where the lymphatics are constantly distended with lymph, these external forces assume a much more important functional role.

Definition and Pathophysiology

Lymphedema may be defined as abnormal limb swelling due to the accumulation of increased amounts of high-protein ISF secondary to defective lymphatic drainage in the presence of (near) normal net capillary filtration (Szuba and Rockson, 1997). In order for edema to be clinically detectable, the ISF volume has to double. About 8 L of lymph is produced and, following resorption in lymph nodes, about 4 L enters the venous circulation. In one sense, all edema is lymphedema in that it results from an inability of the lymphatic system to clear the ISF compartment. However, in most types of edema this is because the capillary filtration rate is pathologically high and overwhelms a normal lymphatic system, resulting in the accumulation of low-protein edema fluid. By contrast, in true lymphedema, capillary filtration is normal and the edema fluid is relatively high in protein. Both mechanisms frequently coexist, as in patients with CVI.

Lymphedema can result from lymphatic aplasia, hypoplasia, dysmotility (reduced contractility with or without valvular insufficiency), obliteration by inflammatory, infective or neoplastic processes, or surgical extirpation (Table 10.4). Whatever the primary abnormality, the resultant physical or functional obstruction leads to lymphatic hypertension and distention with further secondary impairment of contractility and valvular competence. Lymphostasis and lymphotension lead to the accumulation in the ISF of fluid, proteins, growth factors and other active peptide moieties, glycosaminoglycans, and particulate matter, including bacteria. As a consequence, there is increased collagen production by fibroblasts, an accumulation of inflammatory cells (predominantly macrophages and lymphocytes), and activation of keratinocytes. The end result is protein-rich edema fluid, increased deposition of ground substance, subdermal fibrosis, and dermal thickening and proliferation. Lymphedema, unlike all other types of edema, is confined to the epifascial space. Although muscle compartments may be hypertrophied due to the increased work involved in limb movement, they are characteristically free of edema.

Two main types of lymphedema are recognized:

- Primary, in which the cause is unknown (or at least uncertain and unproved) but often presumed to be due to congenital lymphatic dysplasia
- Secondary, in which there is a clear underlying cause such as inflammation, malignancy, or surgery

Primary lymphedema is usually further subdivided on the basis of the presence of a family history, age of onset, and lymphangiographic findings (see below).

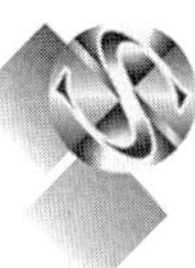

Table 10.4. Differential diagnosis of the swollen limb

Nonvascular or lymphatic	General disease states	Cardiac failure from any cause; liver failure; hypoproteinemia due to nephrotic syndrome, malabsorption, protein losing enteropathy; hyperthyroidism (myxedema); allergic disorders including angioedema and idiopathic cyclic edema; prolonged immobility and lower lib dependency
	Local disease processes	Ruptured Baker's cyst; myositis ossificans; bony or soft tissue tumors; arthritis; hemarthrosis; calf muscle hematoma; Achilles tendon rupture
	Retroperitoneal fibrosis	May lead to arterial, venous and lymphatic abnormalities
	Gigantism	Rare; all tissues are uniformly enlarged
	Drugs	Corticosteroids; estrogens; progestogens; monoamine oxidase inhibitors; phenylbutazone; methyldopa; hydralazine; nifedipine
	Trauma	Painful swelling due to reflex sympathetic dystrophy
	Obesity	Lipodystrophy, lipoidosis
Venous	Deep venous thrombosis	There may be an obvious predisposing factor such as recent surgery; the classical signs of pain and redness may be absent
	Postthrombotic syndrome	Swelling, usually of the whole leg, due to iliofemoral venous obstruction; venous skin changes, secondary varicose veins on the leg and collateral veins on the lower abdominal wall; venous claudication may be present
	Varicose veins	Simple primary varicose veins are rarely the cause of significant leg swelling
	Klippel-Trenaunay syndrome and other malformations	Rare; present at birth or develops in early childhood; comprises an abnormal lateral venous complex, capillary nevus, bony abnormalities, hypo(a)plasia of deep veins, and limb lengthening; lymphatic abnormalities often coexist
	External venous compression	Pelvic or abdominal tumor including the gravid uterus; retroperitoneal fibrosis
	Ischemia- reperfusion	Following lower limb revascularization for chronic and particularly chronic ischemia
Arterial	Arteriovenous malformation	May be associated with local or generalized swelling
	Aneurysm	Popliteal; femoral; false aneurysm following (iatrogenic) trauma

Epidemiology

Lymphedema is estimated to affect around 2% of the population and causes significant physical symptoms and complications, as well as emotional and psychological distress, which can lead to difficulties with relationships, school, and work. Many sufferers choose not to seek medical advice because of embarrassment and a belief that nothing can be done. Patients who do come forward, especially those with non–cancer-related lymphedema, often find they have limited access to appropriate expertise and treatment. Lymphedema is often misdiagnosed and mistreated by doctors, who frequently have a poor understanding of the condition, believing it to be primarily a cosmetic problem. However, early diagnosis and treatment are important because relatively simple measures can prevent the development of disabling late disease, which is often very difficult to treat.

Clinical Assessment

In most cases the diagnosis of primary or secondary lymphedema can be made, and the condition differentiated from other causes of a swollen limb, on the basis of history and examination without recourse to complex investigation. Unlike other types of edema, lymphedema characteristically involves the foot. The contour of the ankle is lost through infilling of the submalleolar depressions; a "buffalo hump" forms

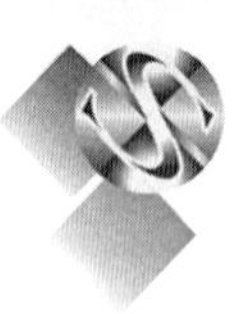

on the dorsum of the foot, the toes appear square due to confinement of footwear, and the skin on the dorsum of the toes cannot be pinched due to subcutaneous fibrosis (Stemmer's sign). Lymphedema usually spreads proximally to knee level and less commonly affects the whole leg. In the early stages, lymphedema "pits," and the patient reports that the swelling is down in the morning. This represents a reversible component to the swelling, which can be controlled. Failure to do so allows fibrosis, dermal thickening, and hyperkeratosis to occur. In general, primary lymphedema progresses more slowly than secondary lymphedema. Chronic eczema, fungal infection of the skin (dermatophytosis) and nails (onychomycosis), fissuring, verrucae, and papillae (warts) are frequently seen in advanced disease. Ulceration is unusual except in the presence of chronic venous insufficiency.

Lymphangiomas are dilated dermal lymphatics that blister onto the skin surface. The fluid is usually clear but may be blood stained, and in the long term they thrombose and fibrose, forming hard nodules, raising concerns about malignancy. If they are <5 cm across, they are termed lymphangioma circumscriptum; if more widespread, lymphangioma diffusum. If they form a reticulate pattern of ridges, they are termed lymphedema ab igne. Lymphangiomas frequently weep (lymphorrhea, chylorrhea), causing skin maceration and act as a portal for infection. Protein-losing diarrhea, chylous ascites, chylothorax, chyluria, and discharge from lymphangiomas suggest lymphangiectasia (megalymphatics) and chylous reflux.

Ulceration, nonhealing bruises, and raised purple-red nodules should lead to suspicion of malignancy. Lymphangiosarcoma was originally described in postmastectomy edema (Stewart-Treves syndrome) and affects about 0.5% of patients at a mean onset of 10 years. However, lymphangiosarcoma can develop in any long-standing lymphedema but usually takes longer to manifest (20 years). It presents as single or multiple bluish/red skin and subcutaneous nodules that spread to form satellite lesions that may then become confluent. The diagnosis is usually made late, and confirmed by skin biopsy. Amputation offers the best chance of survival, but even then most patients live less than 3 years. It has been suggested that lymphedema leads to an impairment of immune surveillance and so predisposes to other malignancies, although the causal association is not as definite as it is for lymphangiosarcoma.

Primary Lymphedema

It has been proposed that all cases of primary lymphedema are due to an inherited abnormality of the lymphatic system, sometimes termed congenital lymphatic dysplasia. However, it is possible that many sporadic cases of primary lymphedema occur in the presence of a (near) normal lymphatic system and are actually examples of secondary lymphedema for which the triggering events have gone unrecognized. These might include seemingly trivial (but repeated) bacterial or fungal infections, insect bites, barefoot walking (silica), DVT, or episodes of superficial thrombophlebitis. In animal models, simple excision of lymph nodes or trunks leads to acute lymphedema that resolves within a few weeks, presumably due to collateralization. In animals, the human condition can only be mimicked by inducing extensive lymphatic obliteration and fibrosis. Even then, there may be considerable delay between the injury and the onset of edema. Primary lymphedema is much commoner in the legs than the arms. This may be due to gravity and a bipedal posture, the fact that the lymphatic system of the leg is less well developed, or the increased susceptibility of the leg to trauma or infection. Furthermore, loss of the venoarteriolar reflex (VAR), which protects lower limb capillaries from excessive hydrostatic forces in the erect posture, with age and disease (CVI, diabetes) may be important.

Primary lymphedema is often classified on the basis of apparent genetic susceptibility, age of onset, or lymphangiographic findings (Table 10.5). None of these is ideal, and the various classification systems in existence can appear confusing and conflicting as various terms and eponyms are used loosely and interchangeably. This problem has hampered research and efforts to gain a better understanding of underlying mechanisms, the effectiveness of therapy, and prognosis. Primary lymphedema, where there appears to be a genetic susceptibility or element to the disease, may be further divided into those cases that are familial (hereditary), where typically the only abnormality is lym-

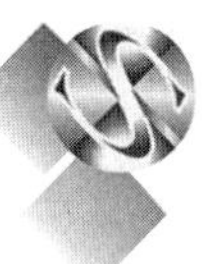

Table 10.5. Lymphangiographic classification of primary lymphedema

	Congenital hyperplasia (10%)	Distal obliteration (80%)	Proximal obliteration (10%)
Age of onset	Congenital	Puberty (praecox)	Any age
Sex distribution	Male > female	Female > male	Male = female
Extent	Whole leg	Ankle, calf	Whole leg, thigh only
Laterality	Uni = bilateral	Often bilateral	Usually unilateral
Family history	Often positive	Often positive	No
Progression	Progressive	Slow	Rapid
Response to compression therapy	Variable	Good	Poor
Comments	Lymphatics are increased in number, although functionally defective; there is usually an increased number of lymph nodes; may have chylous ascites, chylothorax, and protein-losing enteropathy	Absent or reduced distal superficial lymphatics; also termed aplasia or hypoplasia	There is obstruction at the level of the aortoiliac or inguinal nodes; if associated with distal dilatation, the patient may benefit from lymphatic bypass operation; other patients have distal obliteration as well

phedema and there is a family history, and those cases that are syndromic, where the lymphedema is only one of several congenital abnormalities and is either inherited or sporadic. Syndromic lymphedema may be sporadic and chromosomal [Turner's (XO karyotype), Klinefelter's (XXY), Down (trisomy 21) syndrome], or clearly inherited and related to an identified or presumed single gene defect [lymphedema-distichiasis (autosomal dominant)], or of uncertain genetic etiology (yellow-nail and Klippel-Trenaunay-Weber syndromes). Familial (hereditary) lymphedema can be difficult to distinguish from nonfamilial lymphedema because a reliable family history may be unobtainable, the nature of the genetic predisposition is unknown, and the genetic susceptibility may translate into clinical disease only in the presence of certain environmental factors. Although the distinction may not directly affect treatment, the patients are often concerned lest they be passing on the disease to their children. Two main forms of familial (hereditary) lymphedema are recognized: Noone-Milroy (type I) and Letessier-Meige (type II). It is likely that both eponymous diseases overlap and represent more than a single disease entity and genetic abnormality. Milroy's disease is estimated to be present in 1 in 6000 live births and is probably inherited in an autosomal-dominant manner with incomplete (about 50%) penetrance. In some families, the condition may be related to abnormalities in the gene coding for a vascular endothelial growth factor (VEGF) on chromosome 5. The disease is characterized by brawny lymphedema of both legs (and sometimes the genitalia, arms, and face) that develops from birth or before puberty. The disease has been associated with a wide range of lymphatic abnormalities on lymphangiography. Meige's disease is similar to Milroy's disease except the lymphedema generally develops between puberty and middle age (50 years). It usually affects one or both legs but may involve the arms. Some, but not all, cases appear to be inherited in an autosomal-dominant manner. Lymphangiography generally shows aplasia or hypoplasia.

Lymphedema congenita (onset at or within 2 years of birth) is commoner in males, more likely to be bilateral and to involve the whole leg. Lymphedema praecox (onset from 2 to 35 years) is three times commoner in females, has a peak incidence shortly after menarche, is three times more likely to be unilateral than bilateral, and usually only extends to the knee. Lymphedema tarda develops, by definition, after the age of 35 years and is often associated with obesity, with lymph nodes being replaced by fibrofatty tissue. The cause is unknown. Lymphedema develop-

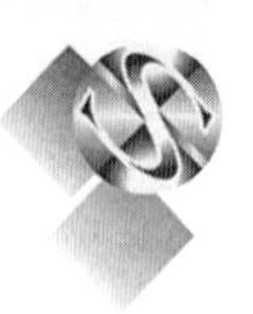

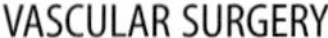

ing for the first time after 50 years should prompt a thorough search for underlying (pelvic, genitalia) malignancy. It is worth noting that, in such patients, lymphedema often commences proximally in the thigh rather than distally.

Secondary Lymphedema

This is the most common form of lymphedema. There are several well-recognized causes, including infection, inflammation, neoplasia, and trauma.

Filariasis is the commonest cause of lymphedema worldwide, affecting up to 100 million individuals. It is particularly prevalent in Africa, India, and South America, where 5% to 10% of the population may be affected. The viviparous nematode *Wucheria bancrofti*, whose only host is humans, is responsible for 90% of cases and is spread by the mosquito. The disease is associated with poor sanitation. The parasite enters lymphatics from the blood and lodges in lymph nodes, where it causes fibrosis and obstruction, due partly to direct physical damage and partly to the immune response of the host. Proximal lymphatics become grossly dilated with adult parasites. The degree of edema is often massive, in which case it is termed elephantiasis. Immature parasites (microfilariae) enter the blood at night and can be identified on a blood smear, a centrifuged specimen of urine, or in lymph itself. A complement fixation test is also available and is positive in present or past infection. Eosinophilia is usually present. Diethylcarbamazine destroys the parasites but does not reverse the lymphatic changes, although there may be some regression over time. Once the infection has been cleared, treatment is as for primary lymphedema. Public health measures to reduce mosquito breeding, protective clothing, and mosquito netting may be usefully employed to combat the condition.

Endemic elephantiasis (podoconiosis) is common in the tropics and affects more than 500,000 people in Africa. The barefoot cultivation of soil composed of alkaline volcanic rocks leads to destruction of the peripheral lymphatics by particles of silica, which can be seen in macrophages in draining lymph nodes. Plantar edema develops in childhood and rapidly spreads proximally. The condition is prevented, and its progression slowed, by the wearing of shoes.

Lymphangitis and lymphadenitis can cause lymphatic destruction that predisposes to lymphedema complicated by further acute inflammatory episodes (AIEs). Interestingly, in such patients lymphangiography has revealed abnormalities in the contralateral, unaffected limb, suggesting an underlying, possibly inherited, susceptibility. Lymphatic and lymph node destruction by tuberculosis is also a well-recognized cause of lymphedema, especially in developing countries.

Treatment (surgery, radiotherapy) for breast carcinoma is probably the commonest cause of lymphedema in developed countries but is decreasing in incidence as surgery becomes more conservative. Lymphoma may present with lymphedema, as may malignancy of the pelvic organs and external genitalia. Kaposi's sarcoma developing in the course of human immunodeficiency virus (HIV)-related illness may cause lymphatic obstruction and is a growing cause of lymphedema in certain parts of the world.

It is not unusual for patients to develop chromic localized or generalized swelling following trauma. The etiology is often multifactorial and includes disuse, venous thrombosis, and lymphatic injury or destruction. Degloving injuries and burns are particularly likely to disrupt dermal lymphatics. Tenosynovitis can also be associated with localized subcutaneous lymphedema, which can be a cause of troublesome persistent swelling following ankle and wrist sprains and repetitive strain injury.

It is important to appreciate the relationship between lymphedema and CVI. As both conditions are relatively common and often coexist in the same patient, it can be difficult to unravel which components of the patient's symptom complex are due to each pathology. There is no doubt that superficial venous thrombophlebitis (SVT) and DVT can both lead to lymphatic destruction and secondary lymphedema, especially if recurrent. Lymphedema is an important contributor to the swelling of the postphlebitic syndrome. It has also been suggested that lymphedema can predispose to DVT and possibly SVT through immobility and AIEs. Certainly, tests of venous function (duplex ultrasonography, plethysmography) are frequently abnormal in patients with lymphedema.

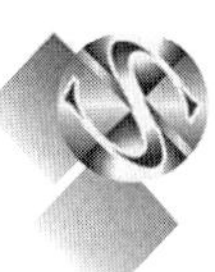

It is not uncommon to see patients (usually women) with lymphedema in whom a duplex ultrasound scan has revealed superficial reflux (such reflux is present subclinically in up to a third of the adult population). Although isolated superficial venous reflux rarely, if ever, leads to limb swelling, such patients are frequently misdiagnosed as having venous rather than lymphedema, and mistakenly subjected to VV surgery. Not only does such surgery invariably fail to relieve the swelling, it usually makes it worse as saphenofemoral and saphenopopliteal ligation, together with saphenous stripping, compromise still further the drainage through the subcutaneous lymph bundles (which follow the major superficial veins) and draining inguinal and popliteal lymph nodes.

Rheumatoid and psoriatic arthritis (chronic inflammation and lymph node fibrosis), contact dermatitis, snake and insect bites, and retroperitoneal fibrosis are all rare but well-documented causes of lymphedema. Pretibial myxedema is due to the obliteration of initial lymphatics by mucin. Factitious lymphedema is caused by application of a tourniquet (a "rut" and sharp cut-off is seen on examination) or "hysterical" disuse in patients with psychological problems. Generalized or localized immobility due to any cause leads to chronic limb swelling that can be misdiagnosed as lymphedema. Examples include the elderly person who spends all day (and sometimes all night) sitting in a chair (armchair legs), the hemiplegic stroke patient, and the young patient with multiple sclerosis.

Lipedema presents almost exclusively in women and comprises bilateral, usually symmetrical, enlargement of the legs and, sometimes, the lower half of the body due to the abnormal deposition of fat. It may or may not be associated with generalized obesity. There are a number of features that help to differentiate the condition from lymphedema, but lipedema may coexist with other causes of limb swelling. It has been proposed that lipedema results from, or at least is associated with, fatty obliteration of lymphatics and lymph nodes.

Investigation

It is usually possible to diagnose and manage lymphedema purely on the basis of the history and examination, especially when the swelling is mild and there are no apparent complicating features. In patients with severe, atypical, and multifactorial swelling, investigations may help confirm the diagnosis, inform management, and provide prognostic information. A full blood count, urea and electrolytes, creatinine, liver function tests, chest radiograph, and blood smear for microfilariae may be indicated. Direct lymphangiography involves the injection of contrast medium into a peripheral lymphatic vessel and subsequent radiographic visualization of the vessels and nodes. It remains the gold standard for showing structural abnormalities of larger lymphatics and nodes. However, it can be technically difficult, is unpleasant for the patient, may cause further lymphatic injury, and has largely become obsolete as a routine method of investigation. Indirect lymphangiography involves the intradermal injection of water-soluble nonionic contrast into a web space, from where it is taken up by lymphatics and then followed radiographically. It shows distal lymphatic but not normally proximal lymphatics and nodes. Isotope lymphoscintigraphy has largely replaced lymphangiography as the primary diagnostic technique in cases of clinical uncertainty. Radioactive technetium–labeled protein or colloid particles are injected into an interdigital web space and specifically taken up by lymphatics, and serial radiographs are taken with a gamma camera. The technique provides a qualitative measure of lymphatic function rather than quantitative function or anatomical detail. A single axial computed tomography (CT) slice through the mid-calf has been proposed as a useful diagnostic test for lymphedema (coarse, nonenhancing, reticular honeycomb pattern in an enlarged subcutaneous compartment), venous edema (increase volume of the muscular compartment), and lipedema (increased subcutaneous fat). Computed tomography can also be used to exclude pelvic or abdominal mass lesions. Magnetic resonance imaging (MRI) can provide clear images of lymphatic channels and lymph nodes, and can be useful in the assessment of patients with lymphatic hyperplasia. It can also distinguish venous and lymphatic causes of a swollen limb. In cases where malignancy is suspected, samples of lymph nodes may be obtained by fine-needle aspiration, needle core biopsy, or surgical excision. Skin biopsy will confirm the diagnosis of lymphangiosarcoma.

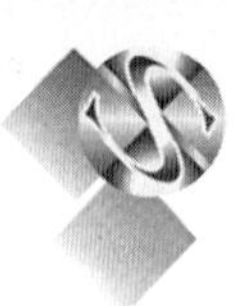

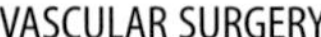

Management

Ideally, a multiprofessional team comprising physical therapists, nurses, orthotists, physicians (dermatologists, oncologists, palliative care specialists), surgeons, and social services should deliver the care. Although surgery itself has a very small role, surgeons (especially breast and vascular) are frequently asked to oversee the management of these patients. Early diagnosis and institution of management are essential because at that stage relatively simple measures can be highly effective and will prevent the development of disabling late-stage disease, which is extremely difficult to treat. There is often a latent period of several years between the precipitating event and the onset of lymphedema. The identification, education, and treatment of such at-risk patients can slow down, even prevent, the onset of disease. In patients with established lymphedema, the three goals of treatment are to relieve of pain, reduce swelling, and prevent the development of complications.

On initial presentation 50% of patients with lymphedema complain of significant pain. The pain is usually multifactorial, and its severity and underlying cause(s) vary depending on the etiology of the lymphedema. For example, following treatment for breast cancer, pain may arise from the swelling itself, radiation and surgery induced, nerve (brachial plexus and intercostobrachial nerve), bone (secondary deposits, radiation necrosis) and joint disease (arthritis, bursitis, capsulitis), and recurrent disease. The detailed treatment of such patients is beyond the scope of this chapter but involves the considered use of nonopioid and opioid analgesics, corticosteroids, tricyclic antidepressants, muscle relaxants, antiepileptics, nerve blocks, physiotherapy, adjuvant anticancer therapies (chemo-, radio-, hormonal therapy), as well as measures to reduce swelling if possible. In patients with non–cancer-related lymphedema, the best way to reduce pain is to control swelling and prevent the development of complications.

Physical therapy for lymphedema comprising bed rest, elevation, bandaging, compression garments, massage, and exercises was first described at the end of the 19th century, and through the 20th century various eponymous schools developed. Although there is little doubt that physical therapy can be highly effective in reducing swelling, its general acceptance and practice has been hampered by a lack of proper research and confusing terminology. The current preferred term is *decongestive lymphedema therapy* (DLT) and comprises two phases. The first is a short intensive period of therapist-led care, and the second is a maintenance phase where the patient uses a self-care regimen with occasional professional intervention. The intensive phase comprises skin care, manual lymphatic drainage (MLD), multilayer lymphedema bandaging (MLLB), and exercises. The length of intensive treatment depends on the disease severity, the degree of patient compliance, and the willingness and ability of the patient to take more responsibility for the maintenance phase. However, weeks rather than months should be the goal.

The patient must be carefully educated in the principles and practice of skin care. The patient should inspect the affected skin daily, with special attention paid to skin folds where maceration may occur. The limb should be washed daily, the use of bath oil (e.g., balneum) is recommended as a moisturizer, and the limb must be carefully dried afterward. A hair drier, on low heat, is more effective and hygienic, and less traumatic, than a towel. If the skin is in good condition, daily application of a bland emollient is recommended to keep the skin hydrated. If the skin is dry and flaky, then a bland ointment [e.g., 50/50 white soft paraffin/liquid paraffin (WSP/LP)] should be used twice daily, and if there is marked hyperkeratosis, then a keratolytic agent such as 5% salicylic acid can be added. Many commercially available soaps, creams, and lotions contain sensitizers, and, as patients with lymphedema are highly susceptible to contact dermatitis (eczema), are best avoided. Apart from causing intense discomfort, eczema acts as an entry point for infection. Management comprises avoidance of the allergen (patch testing may be required) and topical corticosteroids. Fungal infections are common, difficult to eradicate, and predispose to AIEs. Chronic application of antifungal creams leads to maceration, and it is better to use powders in shoes and socks. Ointment containing 3% benzoic acid helps prevent athlete's foot and can be used safely over long periods. Painting at-risk areas with an antiseptic agent such as eosin may be helpful. Lymphorrhea is uncommon but

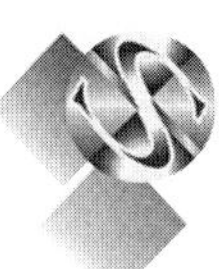

extremely troublesome. Management comprises emollients, elevation, compression, and sometimes cautery under anesthesia.

Apart from lymphangiosarcoma, AIEs are probably the most serious complications of lymphedema and frequently lead to emergency hospital admission. About 25% of primary and 5% of secondary lymphedema patients are affected. The AIEs start rapidly, often without warning or precipitating event, with tingling, pain, and redness of the limb. Patients feel viral, and severe attacks can lead to the rapid onset of fever, rigors, headache, vomiting, and delirium. Patients who have suffered previous attacks can usually predict the onset, and many learn to carry antibiotics with them and self-medicate at the first hint of trouble. This may stave off a full-blown attack and prevent the further lymphatic injury that each AIE causes. It is rarely possible to isolate a responsible bacterium, but the majority are presumed to be streptococcal or staphylococcal in origin. The diagnosis is usually obvious but dermatitis, thrombophlebitis, and DVT are in the differential. Benzyl (intravenous) or phenoxymethyl (oral) penicillin, and flucloxacillin (or clindamycin in severe attacks), are the antibiotics of choice and should be given for 2 weeks. Rest reduces lymphatic drainage and the spread of infection, elevation reduces the edema, and heparin prophylaxis reduces the risk of DVT. Co-amoxiclav can be taken by patients who self-medicate. The use of long-term prophylactic antibiotics is not evidence-based but is probably reasonable in patients who suffer frequent attacks. However, the benefits of scrupulous compliance with physical therapy and skin care cannot be underestimated.

Several different techniques of MLD have been described and the details are beyond the scope of this chapter. However, they all aim to evacuate fluid and protein from the ISF space and stimulate lymphangion contraction. Therapists should perform MLD daily; they should also train the patient or caregiver to perform a simpler, modified form of massage termed simple lymphatic drainage (SLD). In the intensive phase, SLD supplements MLD, and once the maintenance phase is entered, SLD will carry on as daily massage.

Elastic bandages provide compression, produce a sustained high resting pressure, and compress more as limb swelling reduces. However, the sub-bandage pressure does not alter greatly in response to changes in limb circumference consequent upon muscular activity and posture. By contrast short-stretch bandages exert support through the production of a semirigid casing, where the resting pressure is low but changes quite markedly in response to movement and posture.

It is generally believed that nonelastic MLLB is preferable (and arguably safer) in patients with severe swelling during the intensive phase of DLT, whereas compression (hosiery, sleeves) is preferable in milder cases and during the maintenance phase. Whether the aim is to provide support or compression, the pressure exerted must be graduated (100% ankle/foot, 70% knee, 50% mid-thigh, 40% groin), and the adequacy of the arterial circulation must be assessed. As it is rarely possible to feel pulses in the lymphodematous limb, noninvasive assessment of ABI using a handheld Doppler ultrasound device is usually necessary. The details of MLLB are beyond the scope of this chapter; however, it is highly skilled and in order to be effective and safe, it needs to be applied by a specially trained therapist. It is also extremely labor intensive, needing to be changed daily. Compression garments form the mainstay of management in most clinics. The control of lymphedema requires higher pressures (30 to 40 mm Hg in the arm, 40 to 60 mm Hg in the leg) than are typically used to treat CVI. The patient should put the stocking on first thing in the morning before rising. It can be difficult to persuade patients to comply. Donning lymphedema-grade stockings is difficult, and many patients find them intolerably uncomfortable, especially in warm climates. Furthermore, although intellectually they understand the benefits, emotionally they may find wearing them presents a greater body image problem than the swelling itself.

Enthusiasm for pneumatic compression devices has waxed and waned. Unless the device being used allows the sequential inflation of multiple chambers up to 50 mm Hg, it will probably be ineffective for lymphedema. Patient benefit is maximized and complications minimized if these devices are used under the direction of a physical therapist as part of an overall package of care.

Lymph formation is directly proportional to arterial inflow, and 40% of lymph is formed

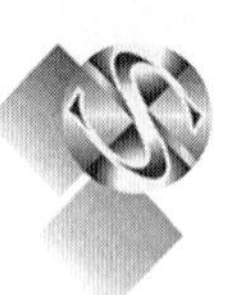

within skeletal muscle. Vigorous exercise, especially if it is anaerobic and isometric, tends to exacerbate lymphedema, and patients should be advised to avoid prolonged static activities, for example, carrying heavy shopping bags or prolonged standing. By contrast, slow rhythmic isotonic movements (e.g., swimming) and massage increase venous and lymphatic return through the production of movement between skin and underlying tissues (essential to the filling of initial lymphatics) and augmentation of the muscle pumps. Exercise also helps to maintain joint mobility. Patients who are unable to move their limbs benefit from passive exercises. When at rest, the lymphedematous limb should be positioned with the foot/hand above the level of the heart. A pillow under the mattress or blocks under the bottom of the bed encourage the swelling to go down overnight.

There are considerable, and scientifically inexplicable, differences in the use of specific drugs for venous disease and lymphedema between different countries. The benzpyrenes are a group of several thousand naturally occurring substances, of which the flavonoids have received the most attention. Enthusiasts argue that a number of clinical trials have shown benefit from these compounds, which are purported to reduce capillary permeability, improve microcirculatory perfusion, stimulate interstitial macrophage proteolysis, reduce erythrocyte and platelet aggregation, scavenge free radicals, and a exert an antiinflammatory effect. Detractors argue that the trials are small and poorly controlled, with short follow-up and soft end points, and that any benefits observed can be explained by a placebo effect. Diuretics are of no value in pure lymphedema. Their chronic use is associated with side effects including electrolyte disturbance and should be avoided.

Surgery

Surgery benefits only a small minority of patients with lymphedema. Operations fall into two categories: bypass procedures and reduction procedures. The rare patient with proximal ilioinguinal lymphatic obstruction and normal distal lymphatic channels might benefit, at least in theory, from lymphatic bypass. A number of methods have been described including the omental pedicle, the skin bridge (Gillies), anastomosing lymph nodes to veins (Neibulowitz),

the ileal mucosal patch (Kinmonth), and, more recently, direct lymphovenous anastomosis. The procedures are technically demanding, not without morbidity, and there is no controlled evidence to suggest that these procedures produce an outcome superior to the best medical management alone. Limb reduction procedures are indicated when a limb is so swollen that it interferes with mobility and livelihood. These operations are not cosmetic in the sense that they do not create a normally shaped leg and are usually associated with significant scarring. Four operations have been described:

1. *Sistrunk:* A wedge of skin and subcutaneous tissue is excised and the wound closed primarily. This is most commonly employed to reduce the girth of the thigh.

2. *Homan:* Skin flaps are elevated; subcutaneous tissue is excised from beneath the flaps, which are then trimmed to size to accommodate the reduced girth of the limb and closed primarily. This is the most satisfactory operation for the calf. The main complication is skin flap necrosis. There must be at least 6 months between operations on the medial and lateral sides of the limb, and the flaps must not pass the midline. This procedure has also been used on the upper limb but is contraindicated in the presence of venous obstruction or active malignancy.

3. *Thompson:* One denuded skin flap is sutured to the deep fascia and buried beneath the second skin flap (the so-called buried dermal flap). This procedure has become less popular as pilonidal sinus formation is common, the cosmetic result is no better than that obtained with the Homan's procedure, and there is no evidence that the buried flap establishes any new lymphatic connections within the deep tissues.

4. *Charles:* This operation was initially designed for filariasis and involved excision of all the skin and subcutaneous tissues down to the deep fascia with coverage using split skin grafts. This leaves a very unsatisfactory cosmetic result, and graft failure is not uncommon. However, it does enable the surgeon to reduce greatly the girth of a massively swollen limb.

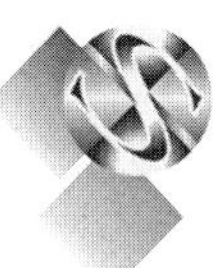

Arteriovenous Fistulas

Classification

Arteriovenous fistulas (AVFS) are broadly classified into congenital and acquired. Acquired fistulas may be traumatic, iatrogenic, or associated with malignancy, aneurysmal disease, and infection. These are not considered further. Congenital AVFs are further classified as hemangiomas or malformations. The former are characterized by endothelial hyperplasia, are not present at birth, and grow in early childhood, but in 90% of cases involute by the age of 5 to 10 years. The latter exhibit normal endothelial cell kinetics, are always preset at birth, grow and continue to grow with the child, and may enlarge dramatically at puberty or in pregnancy. Whenever vascular lesions appear and grow rapidly, it is important to exclude malignancy. Malformations may be high flow (predominantly cardiac and great vessel anomalies) or low flow (arterial, venous, lymphatic, or mixed). The processes leading to the development of the mature vascular tree are largely unknown, but presumably congenital fistulas represent a localized disorder of vessel formation. Occasionally they may be familial, and some abnormalities have been mapped to certain chromosomal loci.

Symptoms and Signs

The clinical presentations are protean and depend on the nature of the lesion, anatomical site, size, and flow.

Malformations

Although malformations are present at birth, they do not usually become symptomatic, and even go unnoticed, until later at life. They typically present at puberty or during pregnancy or following trauma to the part. There is usually an obvious swelling and discoloration, and there may be limb enlargement. Adults typically present with a lump, VVs, (ischemic) ulceration, bleeding, or an inequality in limb length. That which is visible is often the "tip of the iceberg," and the deep component may cause pain, pressure on local strictures, organ dysfunction, and internal bleeding. On examination there is dis-coloration and a lump. If arterial, it is typically firm, pulsates, and is associated with a thrill and a murmur and sometimes pulsatile draining veins. If primarily venous, it is soft and compressible, and reduces in size and enlarges upon elevation and dependency, respectively.

Hemangiomas

Hemangiomas present at or within a few weeks of birth. They are said to be present in 10% of Caucasian children on their first birthday, to be three times commoner in girls, to be multiple in 20%, and to affect the head and neck (60%), trunk (25%), and extremities (10%). If superficial, they are bright (strawberry nevus), and if deep dark (cavernous hemangioma), red. They are firm and rubbery and cannot be emptied of blood on compression or elevation. After an initial phase of rapid growth, they begin to involute at about 6 to 12 months of age when the red color turns to purple, gray/while flecks appear, the lesion becomes softer, and the overlying skin wrinkles. Resolution is typically completed in 50% at 5 years, 70% at 7 years, and 90% or more by 10 years. Apart from cosmetic concerns there may be ulceration and bleeding. On the face they may block vision, and depending on where they are sited may cause mass effects. Large hemangiomas involving internal organs may cause heart failure and anemia.

Diagnosis and Investigation

The diagnosis can usually be made on clinical examination. Handheld Doppler helps to confirm if there is an arterial component, and DU provides more detailed anatomical and functional information. In particular, DU permits detailed assessment of the venous system in patients with Klippel-Trenaunay syndrome where the deep venous system may be hypoplastic or even absent, having been replaced by an abnormal laterally placed venous malformation. Duplex ultrasound has largely replaced venography. Phleboliths may be seen on plain x-rays and are only usually seen in venous lesions. Magnetic resonance imaging, rather than CT, is now regarded as the definitive investigation for assessing the extent of AVF. Angiography is performed only where there is an intention to treat radiologically.

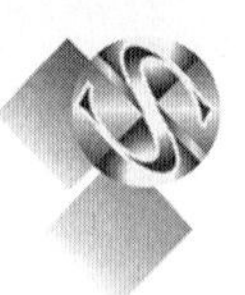

Management

Management is complex, multidisciplinary (vascular, plastic, maxillofacial, and orthopedic surgeons, interventional radiologist, cardiologist), difficult, and highly tailored to the individual patient. Many patients (and parents) simply require reassurance, and in general it pays to be as conservative as possible. Only 10% of hemangiomas fail to resolve spontaneously and many malformations remain asymptomatic. Palliation, not cure, is the principal aim, and it is important to ensure that the treatment is not worse than the disease. Venous lesions may be treated with compression bandaging and hosiery. A small minority of patients are suitable for excisional surgery. Complete excision is rarely possible, and usually the aim is to remove the most symptomatic part. Such surgery can be difficult and bloody, and recurrence is common. For these reasons, most patients are treated radiologically either by transcatheter emboliza-tion (arterial lesions) or by direct injection (venous lesions), usually under general anesthesia. This is a highly skilled and specialized branch of interventional radiology, and great care must be taken to avoid collateral damage. Extremities are particularly vulnerable. Surgical skeletonization of the arterial inflow to the lesion is now avoided, as recurrence is inevitable and such intervention prevents radiological intervention. Strong indications for intervention are hemorrhage, distal ischemia due to steal, and ulceration due to ischemia or venous hypertension.

References

Cornu-Thenard A, Boivin P, Baud JM, De Vincenzi I, Carpentier PH. (1994) J Dermatol Surg Oncol 20:318–26.
Dwerryhouse S, Davies B, Harradine K, Earnshaw JJ. (1999) J Vasc Surg 29:589–92.
Szuba A, Rockson SG. (1997) Vasc Med 2:321–6.

11

Vascular Trauma

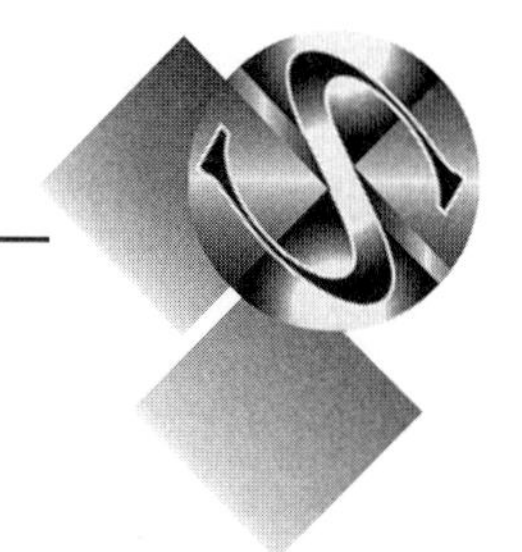

Kathleen J. Ozsvath, R. Clement Darling III,
Laila Tabatabai, Sacha Hamdani, Alun H. Davies,
and Meryl Davis

Trauma is the leading cause of death in patients under the age of 44 in the United States. North American trauma centers have an incidence of penetrating trauma of 35% as compared with 5% to 8% in Europe, the difference being explained by the higher rate of weapon-related crimes in North America. The treatment of traumatic vascular injuries today is based on principles gained during the military conflicts of the 20th century; previously treatment of vascular injuries was limited to the staunching of bleeding by cautery, compression, and ligature. The concept of repair was documented in anecdotal reports only. William Hunter in 1759 recounts the first successful vascular repair on a brachial artery using a farrier's stitch.

Reports of vein grafting were available in the early 20th century; however, these techniques were not suitable for the injuries encountered during World War I, in which the amputation rate was noted to be 72.5%. In 1946 DeBakey and Simeone published a review of World War II experiences with vascular surgery. They concluded that ligation was "of stern necessity," required to control hemorrhage; attempts at vascular repair were superior to ligation and led to an amputation rate of 49%.

The application of vessel reconstruction in the Korean War, despite the mean lag time of over 6 hours between injury and repair, reduced the lower limb amputation rate to 13% (Hughes, 1959); a comparable figure was achieved during the Vietnam War. The Vietnam Vascular Regis-

try was established during the Vietnam War; surgeons were able to document and analyze the long-term management and outcome of vascular trauma (Rich and Hughes, 1969). The significantly improved long-term results of vascular repair were attributed to faster evacuation of casualties within 3 hours of injury, thereby allowing surgeons to treat injuries that had previously been otherwise fatal. Operations were performed by experienced surgeons using autologous vein grafts.

The rise of civilian trauma in the United States has resulted in surgeons becoming more adept and experienced at dealing with vascular injuries (Mattox et al., 1989). Penetrating injuries have been the number one cause of vascular trauma in both urban and rural communities, whereas blunt trauma has accounted for approximately 50% of vascular injuries, most commonly secondary to road traffic accidents.

Regardless of the etiology of the vessel injury, the essential principles of treatment are emergency resuscitation at the scene, triage and rapid transport to an appropriate hospital, vigorous resuscitation, diagnosis, and definitive surgery. Ideally, vascular injuries should be treated by surgeons with expertise in vascular reconstruction and trauma, in an environment with the necessary ancillary support services to allow the best results.

This chapter reviews the workup and treatment of traumatic vascular injuries involving the head and neck, chest, abdomen, and extrem-

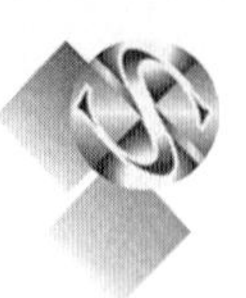

ities, and discusses the approach to iatrogenic injuries and the endovascular treatment of vascular injuries.

Mechanisms of Injury

Vascular injuries can be divided into penetrating and blunt. Penetrating injuries include stabbing and gunshot wounds. Stab wounds are usually clean with minimal soft tissue injury; however, in the neck and upper limb concurrent nerve damage must also be suspected.

Gunshot wounds are classified according to the bullet velocity. Low velocity bullets have a velocity of less than 250 m/s, whereas 750 to 900 m/s represents the speed of high-velocity bullets. Low-velocity bullets injure the tissue through which they pass, whereas high-velocity bullets create a cavitational effect, thereby causing a suctional effect contaminating the entire wound. If a high-velocity bullet strikes bone, there is extensive comminution with a large exit wound. Shotgun injuries particularly to a limb can cause vascular damage at several levels. Bombs, mines, and rocket-propelled grenades produce complex injuries that frequently result in amputation.

Blunt vascular trauma is often caused by deceleration in road traffic accidents and is frequently associated with other injuries. Femoral shaft fractures and fracture dislocations of the knee carry a 10% to 40% incidence of vascular injury. It is important to realize that although the artery can remain intact, intimal damage with concomitant thrombosis risk can occur. Blunt trauma to the upper limb is often associated with avulsion injuries to the brachial plexus. Extensive crush injuries to the limbs are associated with a poor prognosis due to soft tissue damage and reperfusion injury.

Iatrogenic injuries are increasing in incidence as a consequence of invasive procedures. Cardiological and radiological catheterization cause between 60% and 76% of all iatrogenic injuries. Orthopedic procedures including joint replacements may cause vascular injury, commonly to the external iliac, common femoral, or popliteal arteries. In such cases where iatrogenic arterial injury is suspected, expeditious referral to a vascular surgeon must be made.

Diagnosis

The clinical manifestations of vascular injury are divided into hard and soft signs (Table 11.1). The management of penetrating limb trauma in the presence of one hard sign is exploration in the operating room. In blunt trauma, closed head injuries, spinal damage, and cervical and brachial plexus injuries may complicate the clinical findings; a careful neurological examination is mandatory.

Clinical examination in blunt and complex penetrating trauma may be unreliable, and trauma centers advise early angiography. The role of duplex ultrasound in vascular trauma is less clear; currently it has a major role in the diagnosis of occult vascular injuries and in postoperative assessment. Doppler arterial pressure index (API) is a useful tool. It is the systolic arterial pressure in the injured extremity divided by the arterial pressure in a noninjured arm. A result of <0.90 has been found to have a sensitivity of 95% and specificity of 97% for major arterial injury (Johansen et al., 1991).

Once the diagnosis of major vascular injury has been made, the majority of patients require exploration and repair. The principles of emergency vascular repair are to control bleeding and prevent limb ischemia. Hemorrhage is usually apparent, but ischemia may be insidious and must be sought. Time is paramount; it is generally accepted that more than 6 to 8 hours of warm ischemia time makes limb survival unlikely. If there is significant concurrent nerve damage, then limb reconstruction may not be appropriate and amputation should be performed. The input of multidisciplinary teams is vital to ensure optimal treatment.

Table 11.1. The clinical manifestations of vascular injury are divided into hard and soft signs

Hard signs	Soft signs
No pulse	Hematoma (small)
Thrill or bruit	History of bleeding at scene
Active bleeding	Hypotension
Hematoma (large/ expanding)	Nerve damage
Distal ischemia	

Vascular Injuries in the Neck

Wounds of major vessels are often lethal, and frequently these patients have multiple injuries. This is particularly true in penetrating injuries of the brachiocephalic vessels, where airway compromise, hemorrhage, and neurological damage secondary to impaired brain blood flow may occur, along with associated injuries to the pharynx, esophagus, and brachial plexus.

In the neck penetrating trauma is more common than blunt trauma, although vascular injuries caused by blunt trauma can be more difficult to diagnose and treat. Blunt injuries include steering wheel injuries, deceleration forces, and crushing blows.

Injuries to the carotid artery occur in 6% of penetrating injuries to the neck and make up 22% of all vascular neck injuries, whereas 3% to 5% of carotid injuries are secondary to blunt trauma (Demetriades et al., 1996). The mortality rate of patients with penetrating neck vascular trauma is 5% to 20%. Patients presenting with obvious signs of penetrating vascular injury (expanding hematoma, pulsatile bleeding) should be rapidly explored operatively.

Treatment of vascular injuries in the neck is based on dividing the neck into three zones: zone I is 1 cm above the manubrium including the thoracic outlet, zone II extends from the upper limit of zone I to the angle of the mandible, and zone III lies between the angle of the mandible and the base of the skull (Fig. 11.1).

Zone I injuries are best explored through a median sternotomy, which can then be extended superiorly along the anterior border of the sternocleidomastoid muscle as needed. Penetrating trauma to vessels in zone II can be approached directly for definitive repair. Zone III injuries can be difficult to access and sometimes require subluxation of the mandible or mandibular osteotomy. Patients with zone III asymptomatic, angiographically documented injuries are now being managed with endovascular stenting or embolization (Feliciano, 2001).

Arterial defects are repaired with primary repair, transposition, patch, or bypass. Patients found to have an acutely occluded carotid artery are anticoagulated in an effort to prevent clot propagation. Neurologically impaired patients with carotid injuries are aggressively treated surgically. Patients with small intimal defects

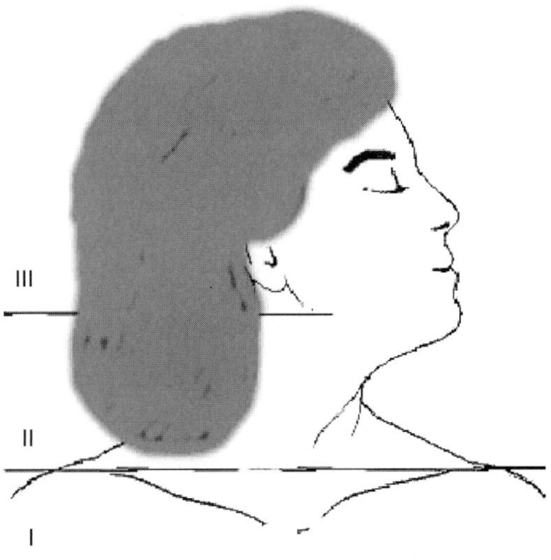

Figure 11.1. Treatment of vascular injuries in the neck is based on dividing the neck into three zones: zone I is 1 cm above the manubrium to include the thoracic outlet, zone II extends from the upper limit of zone I to the angle of the mandible, and zone III lies between the angle of the mandible and the base of the skull.

and dissections of the carotid artery who are otherwise stable may be followed with physical examination and follow-up duplex ultrasound, because these lesions may resolve without intervention. Venous injuries may be dealt with by ligation. In the unusual circumstance of both internal jugular veins having been damaged it is imperative that one vein be reconstructed. Patients with blunt carotid artery injuries can be difficult to diagnose due to either other distracting injuries or altered mental status. Carotid artery blunt injuries are associated with a high mortality and poor neurological outcomes in most patients.

Mechanisms of blunt carotid artery injuries include hyperextension, direct injury, basilar skull fractures, and intraoral injuries. Patients may present with carotid artery dissections, thrombosis, pseudoaneurysms, carotid-cavernous sinus fistulas, or arterial disruption. Carotid artery dissections and thrombosis are treated with anticoagulation. Cogbill et al. (1994) reported that two thirds of patients with carotid dissections eventually have normal studies on follow-up, whereas one third progress. Pseudoaneurysms may be treated surgi-

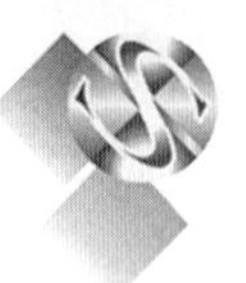

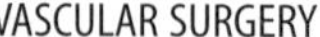

cally or radiologically depending on their size. Carotid–cavernous sinus fistulas are generally treated by endovascular techniques. Complete disruption of the carotid artery is associated with a high mortality.

Injury to the vertebral arteries is rare. The anatomical location of the injury determines the best operative approach when intervention is required. Proximal vertebral artery exposure is performed by a transverse supraclavicular incision or an anterior cervical incision. The cervical vertebral artery is best approached through an incision along the anterior border of the sternocleidomastoid muscle, and can be extended to the posterior auricular area. Once the vertebral artery takes its course from the C2 foramen and enters the skull, the exposure becomes very difficult. Ligation or occlusion of the vertebral artery is usually the treatment of choice. Percutaneous techniques have been successfully employed in managing arteriovenous fistulas, pseudoaneurysms, and occlusions (Halbach et al., 1993).

Thoracic Vascular Injuries

Thoracic vascular trauma constitutes approximately 10% of vascular trauma (Bongard et al., 1990). Although penetrating trauma remains the most common etiology of thoracic vascular injuries, deceleration injuries and crush injuries can result in major thoracic vascular trauma. Injuries to the vessels in the thoracic cavity can lead to rapid blood loss and hemodynamic collapse; many patients die before reaching the hospital. It is often more appropriate to bypass the nearest hospital and transfer the patient to a unit able to manage cardiothoracic problems.

These patients may require immediate treatment for tension pneumothorax or cardiac tamponade. Thoracotomy may be required as an emergency procedure and is usually carried out via a left anterolateral thoracotomy incision (which can be extended across the sternum) or a posterolateral thoracotomy. Access to carotid arteries and innominate artery can be obtained through a median sternotomy. Middle and distal subclavian artery injuries can be controlled with infra- and supraclavicular approaches.

Clinical findings suggesting thoracic injury include external evidence of severe chest bruising, reduced or absent lower limb pulses, raised jugular venous pressure, and unexplained hypotension. The chest radiograph may show a widened mediastinum, fracture of the first or second rib, hemothorax, and thoracic spine injury.

In stable patients the investigations of choice are chest radiographs (suggesting great vessel or aortic injury), spiral computed tomography (CT) with contrast, angiography, and transesophageal echocardiography.

The most common intrathoracic injury caused by deceleration involves disruption of the descending thoracic aorta at the isthmus. Sudden death is common, and it is estimated that 90% die before reaching the hospital; of those who reach the hospital, 25% die within 24 hours.

Commonly the site of aortic disruption is distal to the left subclavian artery. Access is gained via a left posterior thoracotomy with cardiopulmonary bypass. The incidence of paraplegia is approximately 8%. Recent endoluminal treatment has been described and shown to be successful with a lower mortality rate.

The subclavian arteries are relatively well protected from blunt trauma. Patients may present with absent distal pulses, and injury should be suspected in patients with a first rib fracture or traction injury to the brachial plexus. In stable patients, careful clinical assessment of the brachial plexus and magnetic resonance imaging (MRI) should be performed prior to surgical exploration.

Direct repair of the vessel, patch, and prosthetic or autologous interposition grafts are possible choices in repairing aortic and great vessel injuries. Some centers are now opting to use endovascular techniques (Ohki et al., 1997). At present this method of treatment should be pursued only in institutions with adequate surgical and radiological expertise.

Abdominal Vascular Injuries

One third of patients with vascular trauma present with abdominal vascular injuries. These patients are more commonly victims of penetrating injuries, with mortality rates averaging 50%. Deceleration and compression injuries are common blunt injuries and may cause damage to the renal or superior mesenteric arteries and

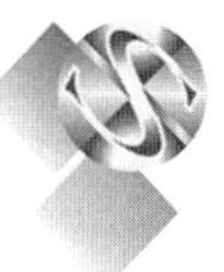

portal vein tributaries. Vessels can be injured by transection or partial transection, or have intimal defects causing thrombosis. Major vascular injury in the abdomen is often associated with injuries to other intraabdominal organs. Of those patients who reach the hospital, the mortality postsurgery remains high (50% to 70% for aortic injury and 30% to 53% for vena caval injury).

Resuscitation is based on Advanced Trauma Life Support (ATLS) guidelines, with unstable patients being transferred promptly to the operating room (Fig. 11.2). Intrathoracic injuries are associated in up to 25% of patients with gunshot wounds of the abdomen.

The assessment of stable patients with intraabdominal pathology has been extensively discussed; ultrasound and CT are the modalities of choice. Angiography in the stable patient with blunt injuries may be useful in documenting unusual injuries.

In unstable patients with significant hemorrhage, laparotomy should be performed and the abdomen packed, and systematic evaluation of the abdomen undertaken. Large defects in the gastrointestinal tract should be temporarily controlled with soft bowel clamps to reduce contamination. If hemorrhage is not controlled, it may be necessary to cross-clamp the proximal supraceliac aorta via the lesser sac; alternatively (via the left thorax) the descending thoracic aorta may be cross-clamped. The goal is to obtain proximal and distal control of the hemorrhaging vessels so that repair or ligation can quickly be undertaken. Hypothermia and coagulopathy is a serious risk; therefore, expeditious control is important. Aortic injuries can be repaired with a transverse primary repair, a

patch with autologous or prosthetic material, or interposition grafting with prosthetic material. The use of antibiotic-soaked grafts may overcome concerns regarding the use of prosthetic material in the presence of penetrating injuries.

The decision to explore a retroperitoneal hematoma depends on the mechanism of injury and stability of the patient. For a retroperitoneal hematoma caused by blunt trauma, a conservative approach is advised especially when it is associated with pelvic fractures. This can be addressed by external fixation of the pelvis, angiography, and coil embolization. In contrast an expanding or pulsatile retroperitoneal hematoma requires immediate exploration.

Retrohepatic caval injuries are difficult to control and carry a high mortality. Mobilization of the liver with division of the right triangular ligament and right thoracotomy with dissection of the diaphragm may be required. Bleeding from the porta hepatis can be controlled by compression of the hepatic artery and portal vein (Pringle's maneuver).

The mortality rate for patients with significant superior mesenteric artery (SMA) injury can be high (58% mortality rate). Injuries to the proximal SMA are technically challenging due to the proximity of the pancreas and the presence of multiple short branches. Control of the supramesocolic vessels can be obtained by medial visceral rotation via the left paracolic gutter. Injuries to the celiac artery and branches may present with an expanding hematoma displacing the stomach and pancreas forward. Celiac axis vessels may be ligated if there is a patent SMA. Retropancreatic SMA control may have to be obtained by transection of the pancreas.

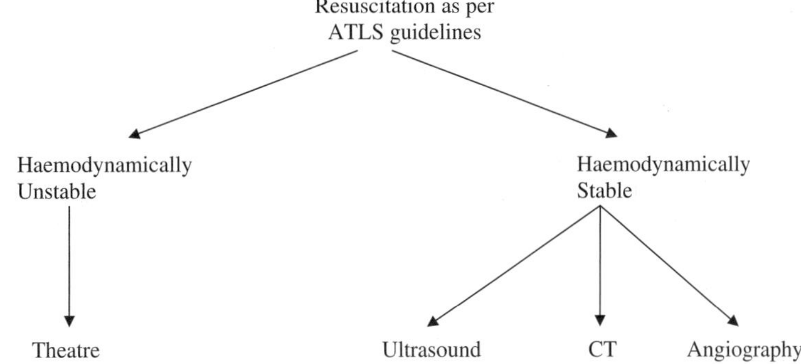

Figure 11.2. Algorithm for the management of a patient with abdominal trauma.

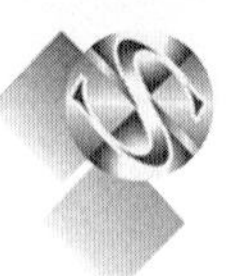

Injury or transection of the SMA may require either autologous or prosthetic bypass. Bowel viability may be difficult to assess intraoperatively; therefore, second-look laparotomy in these patients is advisable.

Inframesocolic vessel injuries can be approached by mobilizing the small intestines and transverse colon superiorly. The inferior mesenteric artery can be ligated in most patients, as collaterals exist that provide adequate blood to the intestine.

Access to the inferior vena cava, right renal vein, suprarenal aorta, and porta may be gained by an extended mobilization of the duodenum, head of pancreas, and right colon (Kocher maneuver). The infrarenal aorta is exposed by retracting the small bowel to the right and incising the retroperitoneum from the root of the mesocolon to the pelvis. Simple stab wounds to the aorta may be closed primarily; more extensive injuries may require a prosthetic patch or bypass graft. In the presence of significant contamination, an axillobifemoral bypass may be preferred after ligation of the aorta. Iliac vessel injuries can be approached via the retroperitoneum; such injuries carry a high mortality (10% to 40%) and morbidity including limb loss.

Renal artery injury may occur after rapid deceleration, resulting in acute renal artery thrombosis or laceration. The diagnosis of thrombosis is often made late, and if explored 12 hours after the injury, renal salvage is often limited. In patients with a functioning kidney on the opposite side, a "watch and wait" policy can be adopted.

The control of venous hemorrhage can be difficult. Simple injuries to the inferior vena cava can be repaired primarily with intermittent digital pressure. In severe hemorrhage, ligation of the infrarenal vena cava may be necessary; in contrast, injury to the suprarenal vena cava requires reconstruction.

Extremity Vascular Injuries

Experience both with trauma patients and with noninvasive techniques are paramount in the management of extremity vascular trauma. A low threshold for angiography should be maintained to diagnose ischemia.

In those patients requiring surgical intervention, vessels are repaired by primary repair, interposition grafting, or bypass with vein (from the uninjured limb) or prosthetic material; 31% of patients with arterial trauma have concomitant venous injuries. Repair of venous injuries has been found to improve the outcome of patients with combined arterial and venous injuries (Martin et al., 1994; Pappas et al., 1997).

Grossly contaminated wounds and massive soft tissue and bone injuries require a multidisciplinary team approach to management. Orthopedic injuries should be reduced with external fixators, and arterial and venous shunts can be used to minimize the ischemia time. Soft tissue coverage either by extraanatomical bypass or muscle flaps may be necessary to protect vascular repairs.

Debridement of devitalized tissue is important for postoperative wound care. Fasciotomies are also of great importance in those patients with extremity injuries who have suffered delayed repair, extensive tissue injury, swelling, elevated compartment pressures, and prolonged hypotension. The development of compartment syndrome can lead to myoglobinuria, renal failure, and skeletal muscle necrosis.

Controversies arise in the presence of extensive tissue damage, vascular injuries, and concomitant nerve injuries. Unfortunate patients may be facing the future with a viable limb that is nonfunctioning and painful after multiple operations. These patients may be best served with a primary amputation. This is a difficult decision to make, and therefore should be made only after extensive discussion with the patient and family, and after the expertise of the combined team has been sought.

Injuries of the subclavian and axillary vessels rarely cause upper extremity ischemia due to the rich collateral network at the shoulder. Penetrating and blunt injuries can both lead to brachial plexus injuries. Brachial artery injuries below the level of the profunda brachii may not present with ischemia due to the collateral supply around the elbow. Isolated injury to the ulnar or radial arteries may be treated with ligation in the presence of a complete palmar arch.

Injuries to the femoral vessels occur in 70% of all arterial injuries, with penetrating trauma being the most common etiology. In 20% to 35% of cases in which the popliteal artery is injured, the popliteal vein and tibial nerve are also involved. Blunt injuries to the knees leading to posterior dislocation can result in popliteal artery injury in 30% to 40% of patients. Single tibial vessel injury can generally be dealt with by ligation; however, if more than one vessel is involved, repair is advocated.

Iatrogenic Vascular Injuries

With an increasing use of percutaneous techniques, there is also a higher risk of iatrogenic vascular injuries. In a survey of 10,500 cases following femoral artery puncture, the incidence of complications was 0.44% (Dorfman and Cronan, 1991). For cardiac catheterization the incidence was 0.55%, whereas peripheral angiography resulted in a complication rate of 0.17%.

The most important risk is bleeding, which may be controlled with direct pressure after a catheter has been removed. Occasionally, surgical repair is undertaken to repair the punctured vessel; direct repair is adequate in most instances. Retroperitoneal bleeding is generally self-limiting; however, when the patient has been taking anticoagulants blood or pharmacological products may be required to correct clotting abnormalities.

Pseudoaneurysms can also complicate punctures in 0.5% to 5.5% of diagnostic femoral punctures. Most of these pseudoaneurysms thrombose spontaneously. Many false aneurysms respond well to ultrasound-guided compression, which has now been superseded by compression with concomitant injection of procoagulant products. Surgical intervention must be undertaken acutely in the presence of a femoral neuropathy, hemodynamic instability, overlying skin necrosis, and extremity ischemia.

Arteriovenous fistulas usually present late and complicate up to 2% of cardiac catheterizations. Although most of these fistulas thrombose, a small percentage can lead to congestive heart failure or limb ischemia requiring either radiological or surgical intervention.

Vascular injury secondary to intraarterial injection of drugs can lead to extensive soft tissue infection, mycotic aneurysm formation, and gangrene.

Endovascular Treatments

With the emergence and development of endovascular techniques, arterial trauma is being treated at some centers with coil embolization, intravascular stent grafts, and covered stent grafts. The use of endovascular techniques has minimized the need for extensive operative dissections and anesthesia; this is especially important in injuries involving vessels difficult to assess. Endovascular techniques are best utilized in institutions equipped and ready to handle trauma in this fashion.

Conclusion

Improvements in patient transport to a level-one trauma center combined with prehospital care have allowed patients to present earlier for treatment. The multidisciplinary team approach to the management of these patients has led to better outcomes.

In vascular reconstructive surgery autologous bypasses should be used wherever possible (vein being harvested from the uninjured limb). In the event of this not being possible, the newer antibiotic-soaked prosthetic grafts is advocated.

Interventional radiology with deployment of endoluminal stents will continue to develop its role in vascular trauma. It is important that vascular surgeons remain involved in all aspects of vascular trauma to facilitate improvements.

References

Bongard F, Dubrow T, Klein S. (1990) Ann Vasc Surg 4:415–8.
Cogbill TH, Moore EE, Meissner M, et al. (1994) J Trauma 37:473–9.
Demetriades D, Asensio JA, Velmahos G, Thal E. (1996) Surg Clin North Am 76:661–83.
Dorfman GS, Cronan JJ. (1991) Radiology 178:629–30.
Feliciano DV. (2001) World J Surg 25:1028–35.
Halbach VV, Higashida RT, Dowd CF, et al. (1993) J Neurosurg 79:183–91.
Hughes CW. (1959) Milit Med 124:30–46.
Johansen K, Lynch K, Paun M, Copass M. (1991) J Trauma 31:515–9; discussion 519–22.

Martin LC, McKenney MG, Sosa JL, et al. (1994) J Trauma 37:591–8; discussion 598–9.

Mattox KL, Feliciano DV, Burch J, et al. (1989) Ann Surg 209:698–705; discussion 706–7.

Ohki T, Veith FJ, Marin ML, Cynamon J, Sanchez LA. (1997) Semin Vasc Surg 10:272–85.

Pappas PJ, Haser PB, Teehan EP, et al. (1997) J Vasc Surg 25:398–404.

Rich NM, Hughes CW. (1969) Surgery 65:218–26.

12

Complications in Vascular Surgery

Jeremy S. Crane, Nicholas J.W. Cheshire, and
Gilbert R. Upchurch, Jr.

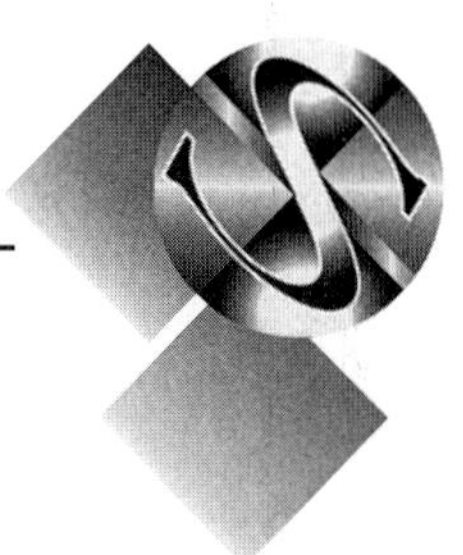

Complications in vascular surgery are often life threatening. However, with treatment options for vascular disease ever widening, patient selection for operative procedures is governed not only by evidence-based treatment options but also by immediate and long-term complications. The major impact complications of vascular surgery, in particular long-term complications, have on patient quality of life, inpatient hospital costs, psychological problems, and health care resources cannot be stressed enough.

A useful working definition of a vascular surgical complication is a procedure-related adverse event that harms a patient (Table 12.1). Many of the same complications that are ubiquitous in general surgery are pertinent to vascular surgery.

Cardiac and Pulmonary Complications

The most important cause of mortality and morbidity after major peripheral vascular surgery is perioperative cardiac complications. Atherosclerosis is a systemic arterial vascular disorder typically involving multiple vascular territories in the same patient. Accordingly, coronary artery disease is the most frequently associated vascular territory affected in patients with peripheral arterial disease. Consequently, cardiac manifestations of atherosclerosis in the

perioperative and postoperative occur, leading to myocardial ischemia. Naturally, the type of surgery is related to cardiac risk; procedures associated with blood pressure and cardiac rhythm changes with significant blood loss are at high risk (e.g., aortic aneurysm repair), whereas carotid endarterectomy carries moderate cardiac risk.

Patients at high risk of a coronary event may be considered for preoperative stress testing or may be directly referred for coronary angiography with possible coronary bypass or angioplasty prior to vascular surgery. Cardiac complications influence the outcome of vascular surgery to such an extent that the existence of cardiac disease may lead the vascular surgeon to pursue an alternative surgical technique, such as extraanatomical bypass to treat aortic disease, or to cancel vascular surgical intervention altogether.

The magnitude of the effect of coronary disease following vascular surgery is such that even 2 years following vascular surgery, 19% of patients experience a late cardiac event (Krupski, 1993).

In addition, many elderly vascular surgery patients have a degree of underlying pulmonary disease. Therefore, postoperative respiratory complications are exceedingly common after major vascular surgery. Predisposing patient risk factors that may give rise to respiratory problems include advancing age, cigarette smoking, and the presence of chronic obstructive pulmonary disease. Predisposing procedure-

Table 12.1. Classification of complications by outcome

Minor complications No therapy, no consequence Nominal therapy, no consequence; includes overnight admission for observation only
Major complications Requires therapy, minor hospitalization (<48 hours) Requires major therapy, unplanned increase in level of care, prolonged hospitalization (>48 hours) Permanent adverse sequelae Death

specific risk factors include emergency procedures, lengthy general anesthesia, thoracic or upper abdominal incisions, massive blood transfusions, and a postoperative period of prolonged immobility. Similar to cardiac disease, screening for pulmonary dysfunction preoperatively can reduce postoperative respiratory morbidity. A thorough history to ascertain whether the patient suffers from dyspnea on exertion or has significant sputum production, coupled with a plain chest radiograph, identifies most respiratory disease. Pulmonary function tests and arterial blood gas samples further aid diagnosis.

Preoperative therapy involving chest physiotherapy, smoking restriction, antibiotics, and bronchodilators can greatly reduce postoperative pulmonary complications. The severity of postoperative pulmonary complications can range from benign minor atelectasis, which is usually self-limiting, to a fulminant acute respiratory failure that carries a very high mortality. Accordingly, recognition and management of postoperative cardiac and pulmonary complications are essential for the vascular surgeon.

Complications of Arterial Reconstruction

Vascular surgical complications arising specifically from peripheral arterial reconstruction are becoming more prevalent. This is due to increasing numbers of operations being undertaken, with up to 50,000 patients being admitted annually to hospitals in the United Kingdom for treatment of lower limb ischemia. Due to the growing aging population coupled with the ever-expanding role of vascular surgery, surgeons will be faced with increasing numbers of complications following lower extremity revascularization. As these complications may be life or limb threatening, treating these complications is one of the most significant challenges facing the contemporary vascular surgeon.

Specific complications associated with peripheral arterial reconstructions usually occur within predictable time frames, and can be classified as immediate, early, intermediate, or late (Table 12.2). For the purpose of this chapter, *immediate* complications refer to those events occurring intraoperatively or within the first 24 hours after surgery, *early* complications occur less than 30 days after surgery, *intermediate* occur within the first year, and *late* occur after the first postoperative year. Complications occurring immediately perioperatively and within the first 30 days after surgery are most often due to technical error or poor patient selection. Technical errors include inadequate anastomotic suturing technique, kinking of the graft, and the injudicious choice of a poor-quality, small-diameter graft. Poor qualities of either inflow or distal run-off are predictors of poor graft longevity. Complications ensuing from these errors are usually anastomotic hemorrhage or a partially or completely

Table 12.2. Time frame for complications of peripheral vascular grafts

Immediate	Early	Intermediate	Late
Anastomotic bleeding	Myointimal hyperplasia	Accelerated atherosclerosis	Graft infection
Graft thrombosis	Graft thrombosis	Myointimal hyperplasia	Atherosclerosis
Embolic sequelae		Vein graft stenosis	Myointimal hyperplasia
		Graft infection	Graft aneurysm formation
			Vein graft stenosis

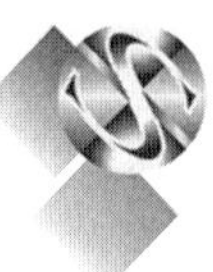

thrombosed graft with possible distal embolic sequelae.

The wide range of vascular grafts now available has revolutionized vascular surgery. However, before a graft is declared competent and durable, long-term follow-up is needed, as graft failure may only become apparent several years after implantation. There are three types of vascular graft: autologous (venous and arterial), prosthetic [e.g., Dacron, polytetrafluoroethylene (PTFE)] and biological prosthetic (e.g., modified human umbilical vein graft). Once functioning in the arterial circuit, each type of graft has its inherent drawbacks, leading to specific complications. These complications can be categorized into two groups. Direct complications involve those where the graft itself fails (e.g., thrombosis), whereas indirect complications are those that relate to a graft that still functions (e.g., graft infection, suture line false aneurysm).

Autologous Grafts

Autologous vein is the conduit of choice for lower limb arterial reconstruction, as this has been repeatedly demonstrated in large retrospective studies (Bergamini, 1991).

Due to its anatomical constancy, the long (or greater) saphenous vein (GSV) is generally considered to be the vein of choice. However, when the GSV has been affected by thrombophlebitis, been removed for previous bypass surgery, or has become dilated and varicosed, the short (or lesser) saphenous vein or upper extremity vein (basilic or cephalic) are often used and have acceptable long-term patency rates. Regardless of the conduit, there remains a significant failure rate in autologous vein graft, which is associated with considerable morbidity and mortality.

The most common cause of autologous vein graft failure in the intermediate and long term is the development of myointimal hyperplastic lesions that lead to vein graft stenosis, subsequent graft occlusion, and ultimately graft failure. Myointimal hyperplasia (MIH) is the morphological lesion that underlies vein graft stenosis. It can be described as an abnormal accumulation of cells and extracellular matrix in the intima of the vessel wall. The mechanical injury caused by a bypass procedure or angioplasty of the peripheral arteries can initiate and maintain the process of MIH. The clinical relevance of MIH is pertinent, as the development of MIH at the outflow anastomosis of a vein bypass placed in the arterial system is responsible for most complications leading to revision surgery. Proliferating smooth muscle cells migrate to the injury-provoked denuded endothelial layer area and forms a hyperplastic lesion, which is associated with vein graft stenosis and obstruction of the vascular lumen. The pathogenesis of MIH remains under investigation. However, it has been established that both mechanical and chemical factors may induce this process. Arterial injury is believed to stimulate the production of growth factors, such as platelet-derived growth factor (PDGF), which have been shown to stimulate the proliferation of arterial smooth muscle cells and the formation of the hyperplastic lesion in the vascular system. A variety of cells, including endothelial cells, macrophages, platelets, and smooth muscle cells, have been shown to secrete growth factors and cytokines. Blocking the effects of growth factors such as PDGF or fibroblast growth factor (FGF), by the administration of antibodies against these growth factors, may limit the development of the hyperplastic lesion (Neville and Sidawy, 1998). The role of hemodynamic changes in the vein graft, including altered vessel wall shear stress and increased particle residence time, has also been shown to play an important part in MIH growth. Investigations aimed at modifying blood flow dynamics within vein grafts to diminish MIH development are currently under way.

It has been theoretically proposed that leaving a vein graft in situ, instead of using the reversed vein graft technique, may lead to fewer subsequent complications. Due to the natural tapering of the vein, an in situ vein graft has a better diameter match between the vein and the native artery at the proximal and distal ends of the vein graft. This makes the construction of both the proximal and distal anastomosis easier to perform and therefore reduces the probability of technical errors. A more suitable diameter match leads to more favorable blood flow features with decreased incidence of graft thrombosis, anastomotic aneurysm, and development of MIH. Also as the blood supply to the vein

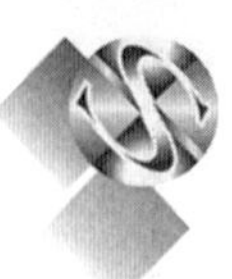
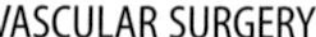

graft through the vasa vasorum is still partially intact, the vein graft remains less hypoxic. Conversely, as the need to use a valvulotome to obliterate the valves is essential, damage to the vessel wall may ensue, possibly leading to increased risk of early graft thrombosis. However, biological studies of the integrity of the vein wall in in situ and reversed vein grafts have failed to show significant differences. It is important to note that several studies have found no significant difference in complication rates resulting from either technique.

Prosthetic Grafts

Once incorporated into the circulation, the luminal surface of a prosthetic graft becomes lined with fibrinogen, followed by fibrin and red and white blood cells. This layer is known as a pseudointima. Whereas prosthetic grafts perform well in a high-flow environment (e.g., in aortic reconstruction), their performance in the infrageniculate position is poor compared with that of autologous vein. The main problem leading to poor long-term graft patency is the increased thrombogenicity of prosthetic distal bypass grafts. Some have advocated the case for primary amputation being first-line treatment when autologous vein is unavailable for a distal bypass.

Originally, Dacron grafts were used as the material of choice for distal bypass. However, due to very poor patency rates, PTFE took over as the prosthetic conduit of choice. As well as the complications resulting from increased thrombogenicity of prosthetic grafts, graft infection has dire consequences, described later in this chapter.

Lower Limb Graft Occlusion

As the majority of vascular grafts in the lower limb are performed for critical limb ischemia, graft occlusion often reverts the limb back to its original critical state or worse. Moreover, ischemia may be compounded due to a reduction in collateral flow caused by division of vessels during surgery, by physiological reduction of collateral flow as a result of a successful graft, or by thrombosis extending distally into the run-off vessels.

Diagnosis

The diagnosis of an occluded infrainguinal graft is made clinically, but can be confirmed by duplex ultrasound. Presentation ranges from a sudden onset of a reduction in pain-free walking distance to acute limb ischemia. From the history, the time of onset of occlusion can be ascertained, and the time frame between original surgery and occlusion can aid in the etiology (Table 12.2).

Management

If a thrombosed graft presents within hours or days of the occlusion, the limb is usually viable and the aim is to restore graft patency. In the absence of contraindications, thrombolysis is indicated. Hemorrhage at the site of catheter thrombolysis insertion occurs in 10% to 30% of cases and is the most common complication. The most catastrophic complication of thrombolysis is intracranial hemorrhage that is often fatal, in particular in elderly patients with a history of stroke. Bleeding into other organs is also commonly recognized. Due to the high complication rate during thrombolysis, if an occluded lesion does not render the patient critically ischemic, it can be argued that thrombolysis is not justified.

If after successful thrombolysis an underlying lesion is identified, the patient should be heparinized and the lesion corrected. Jump grafting or patch angioplasty is an appropriate procedure. When a myointimal hyperplastic lesion postthrombolysis is found, transluminal balloon angioplasty, patch angioplasty, or interposition grafting can be used, as well as jump grafting. Autologous vein is preferable for secondary reconstructions.

An emergency revascularization is the management of a graft occlusion associated with a threatened limb. Loss of neurological function coupled with a tender and tense calf is an indication for urgent surgery. The procedure differs depending on the type of graft. The aim of treatment of a thrombosed vein graft threatening the limb is restoration of graft flow with correction of any underlying abnormality. The distal anastomosis should be opened and the graft and distal vessels cleared of thrombus. On-table angiography should be performed once flow has been restored. Then any abnormality can surgi-

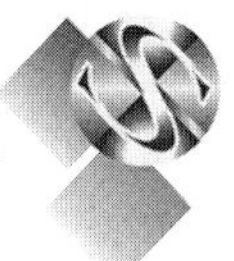

cally be corrected as previously described. With a prosthetic graft, the aim of an emergency procedure is restoration of the original graft function with or without correction of an underlying cause. The long-term patency of salvaged occluded autologous or prosthetic infrainguinal grafts is disappointing, and complete replacement with a new vein graft, reserving graft revision for those patients' with no better bypass options, has been advocated. Following an emergency procedure for lower extremity graft thrombosis, particularly if there has been significant preoperative ischemia, the surgeon should have an extremely low threshold for performing a fasciotomy to prevent muscle necrosis.

Complications of Aortic Reconstruction

Reconstruction of the aorta for atherosclerotic aneurysmal or occlusive disease brings about a different spectrum of complication when compared with lower-extremity revascularization. The aortic graft used is either Dacron or PTFE, as there is no autologous conduit large enough to replace the aorta. Due to the high flow through a large-caliber vessel, prosthetic grafts replacing native aorta perform well and have well-documented excellent long-term results. The two most common local complications after aortic reconstruction are occlusion and graft infection (see Infected Prosthetic Graft, below).

When an aortic graft or the limb of an aortobifemoral graft occludes, the limb is usually viable. Occlusion of a single limb of an aortic graft is most often caused by anastomotic stricture at the femoral anastomosis. If the onset of the occlusion is in the early phase (within 30 days) postsurgery and the graft can be thrombolyzed successfully, subsequent patch angioplasty or distal jump grafting is usually successful. Thrombolysis of retroperitoneal knitted Dacron grafts must be performed with caution because of the risk of extravasation of blood into the retroperitoneum. Thrombectomy using ring strippers or adherent clot catheters is more successful than using ordinary thrombectomy balloon catheters. It is more common that the time of graft failure is not known and is likely to be of several weeks' duration. In these

circumstances, open graft thrombectomy or thrombolysis is not possible, and so common practice involves revascularizing the affected limb with a femoral artery–to–femoral artery crossover graft taken from the contralateral limb. Other extraanatomical reconstructions are also feasible in this situation.

When the body and limbs of an aortic graft are thrombosed, proximal disease advancing into the graft from the proximal aorta is usually the cause. This complication can be avoided by placing the initial graft on the aorta near the level of the renal arteries. However, once a diagnosis of total aortic graft occlusion is made, most surgeons would undertake an axillobifemoral graft as an option; redo aortic grafting is major corrective surgery carrying great risk to the patient. Occasionally, a failed aortic graft will not produce new or acute symptoms because of the development of collateral vessels in a relatively mobile patient or because immobility masks claudication symptoms. If this were the case, it may be that the patient will present many months after the graft has failed, with either nonhealing ulcers or rest pain. In either case, and to thwart the onset of critical ischemia, a complete graft replacement is the only option, as at this stage the graft is usually unsalvageable.

Infected Prosthetic Graft

One of the most challenging complications in vascular surgery is a graft infection. Infection radically changes patient outcomes and is both life and limb threatening. Quantifying incidence of graft infection is not easy, as many reports are anecdotal and this is compounded by the long and variable time period between original surgery and evidence of graft infection. The incidence of graft infection, however, is influenced by anatomical site of graft, indications for original intervention, underlying disease, and the patients' host defense. The literature quotes figures that range between 0.7% and 7% for graft infection after aortic surgery. Prosthetic graft infection is more common after emergency procedures (e.g., ruptured abdominal aortic aneurysm), or when the graft is anastomosed to the femoral artery in the groin or sited superficially (e.g., axillofemoral bypass). When and how a graft becomes infected is often difficult to ascertain, and there are multiple risk

Table 12.3. Risk factors for graft infection

Local factors
Prosthetic graft
Groin invasion
Emergency or lengthy surgery
Leg ulceration or gangrene
Postoperative wound infection

Systemic factors
Diabetes mellitus
Malnutrition or obesity
Chronic renal failure
Malignancy
Steroid therapy

factors for graft infection (Table 12.3). However, there are three modes whereby the graft may become contaminated: (1) the infection may be seeded onto the graft at the time of surgery (perioperative contamination), (2) subsequent bacteremia may seed the graft, and (3) direct spread from a nearby source (e.g., skin or duodenum) may occur.

Presentation

Any symptoms and signs of sepsis in a patient with a vascular graft should alert the clinician to the possibility of a graft infection. With a subcutaneous graft, localized erythema and cellulitis or a discharging sinus may be clinically visible over the length of the graft, or prosthetic material may be visualized eroding through the skin. With a deep infected graft (e.g., an aortic graft), the patient may present with vague symptoms and have pyrexia of unknown origin. An infected aortic prosthesis may form an aortoduodenal fistula and present with upper gastrointestinal bleeding that may be mistaken for peptic ulceration. Less commonly, lower gastrointestinal hemorrhage may be seen from aortoenteric fistulas into distal bowel sites. Alternatively, signs of septic emboli to the extremities may present as a purpuric rash. Other more rare sequelae of a graft infection included metastatic mycotic aneurysm formation, anastomotic pseudoaneurysm formation, or anastomotic hemorrhage. With all these potential sequelae, the clinician must have a high index of suspicion in the presence of a prosthetic graft.

Making a definitive diagnosis of graft infection can be difficult. The presence of a perigraft collection should be determined whenever possible. Determining which organisms are infecting a graft is also imperative to help guide antibiotic choice following graft removal. Once these two factors have been elucidated, the likelihood of infection must be balanced against the general condition of the patient, the extent of the revision surgery required, and the necessity for immediate intervention.

Investigations

Having bacteriological cultures done on swabs taken from a discharging sinus may identify the organism involved. Blood cultures may also be positive, particularly if blood is drawn from the femoral artery, downstream to a possible graft infection. The organisms most commonly isolated from blood or from wounds are gram-positive bacteria, *Staphylococcus* and *Streptococcus* species. A particularly worrying phenomenon is the continued rise in the number of reports of methicillin-resistant *Staphylococcus aureus* (MRSA) isolated from infected grafts. This organism and gram-negative infections are associated with severe systemic sepsis, and experience in our unit and elsewhere has shown these organisms to carry a less favorable outcome in terms of limb salvage and mortality than infection with less virulent organisms. Early graft infection is usually associated with virulent organisms such as *S. aureus*, *Streptococcus faecalis*, *Escherichia coli*, *Klebsiella*, *Pseudomonas aeruginosa*, and *Proteus* or mixed pathogens. Late graft infections are usually caused by less virulent bacteria (e.g., *Staphylococcus epidermidis*, which is a common skin commensal). Interestingly, this organism has been cultured from grafts that have been removed for purposes other than infection, which may signify that only a small proportion of such contaminated drafts develop graft-threatening infection. The type of antibiotic therapy differs between centers, but it is prudent to discuss an appropriate antibiotic regimen with a microbiologist.

There are a few imaging techniques to elucidate the presence and extent of a graft infection. Computed tomography (CT) scanning can help in demonstrating fluid collections around a suspected infected graft. The presence of gas within a perigraft collection is pathognomonic of an infection; however, around an aortic graft, gas

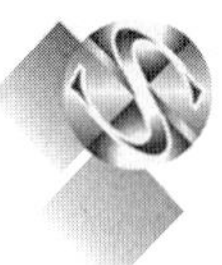

may represent resolving thrombus. Computed tomography scanning may also not be able to differentiate free gas that is around a graft and gas within the bowel that is adhered closely to the graft. Computed tomography–guided aspiration of perigraft fluid may be undertaken to aid in diagnosis; however, this carries the risk of introducing infective seedlings into a potentially sterile field.

A radioisotope-labeled white blood cell scan enables localization of occult sites of infection, as labeled granulocytes concentrate around an infected focus. Magnetic resonance angiography of the aorta is believed to be complementary to a tagged white cell scan and may increase the likelihood of appropriately diagnosing a graft infection. Angiography, even though unable to pinpoint sites of infection, is necessary for preoperative planning for revision surgery. It demonstrates the nature of distal run-off and the state of arteries that may be used in an extraanatomical bypass. Occasionally it may aid diagnosis in an aortoenteric or aortocaval fistula. Gastrointestinal endoscopy to rule out aortoduodenal fistula must be the first-line investigation in a patient presenting with hematemesis or melena.

Management

Graft conservation involves local debridement of infected tissues surrounding a superficial graft, followed by a primary wound closure and local irrigation with gentamicin antibiotic solution via suitably placed drainage catheters or impregnated collagen sponge or beads. Another method of graft preservation involves covering the debrided area and graft with a vascularized omental or muscle flap. This form of management is strongly proposed for localized groin wound infection in the presence of a patent graft and is said to be associated with a low mortality, high limb salvage rate and an acceptable incidence of recurrent infection. The decision to excise an infected graft should be undertaken carefully, and whenever possible the patient's condition needs to be optimized prior to the operation. The best-case scenario is when adequate collateralization has taken place and no further revascularization procedure is required once the graft is removed. More commonly, though, graft removal results in a return to the preoperative state, often rendering one or both legs ischemic, and at the time of removal of the infected graft further revascularization is required.

Complications Related to Disorders of Coagulation

The acute thrombosis of an arterial procedure in the perioperative period is usually seen before the patient exits the operating room and may occur up to 12 hours following surgery. Dealing with unexplained thrombosis intraoperatively or in the immediate postoperative period is one of the greatest uncertainties faced by the vascular surgeon.

Hypercoagulability as grounds for an unexplained vascular thrombosis poses a challenging clinical problem. Graft failure in the perioperative period is presumed to result from technical errors in the construction of the anastomosis, problems with the choice of and quality of vascular conduit, or unsuitable patient selection. Only once these other factors as a cause of failure have been excluded can the diagnosis of abnormal coagulability be formulated. When it becomes apparent there is abnormal coagulation (i.e., heparin is not preventing clotting in the operating field or when there is an immediate thrombosis of a vascular repair), the diagnosis can be confirmed only by the analysis of a blood clotting profile. It therefore stands to reason that detection of clotting disorders prior to surgery is most often associated with a favorable surgical outcome. It is with experience that a surgeon develops an intuition as to which reconstructions are likely to succeed and has some ideas as to the types of complications that may occur. Likewise, with experience a surgeon develops a feel for the characteristic presentations of atherosclerotic occlusive disease. When abnormal or unexplained thrombosis is diagnosed (e.g., a thrombosed suprarenal aorta or upper extremity thrombosis in a patient who is not diabetic and has little evidence of atherosclerotic occlusive disease elsewhere), the surgeon should investigate clotting disorders as a possible cause. Unusual angiographic findings, particularly young patients who present with an occlusion in one limb with pristine vasculature in the contralateral limb, should prompt an investigation into the coagu-

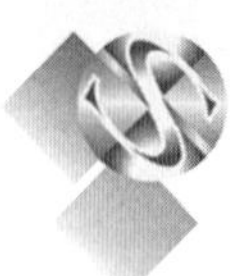

lation system. The role of screening for potential thrombophilic states in vascular surgical patients has been studied. Approximately 10% of all patients scheduled for a variety of vascular surgical procedures had test results indicating a potential hypercoagulable state. The three most common clotting disorders are heparin-induced platelet aggregation, lupus anticoagulants, and protein C deficiency. The incidence of infrainguinal graft occlusion within 30 days was 27% among patients who were in the hypercoagulable group compared with 1.6% in patients who were not in this group. At present, an established screening program does not exist to exclude the wide variety of coagulation disorders present in vascular surgical patients. We depend on taking a careful history and clinical examination to identify those patients who may be at a risk of abnormal clotting due to an inherent thrombophilic status. At this time this is probably the more cost-effective and efficient means to establish a hypercoagulable diagnosis prior to operation.

Complications of Interventional Vascular Radiological Procedures

As more minimally invasive interventional radiological procedures are being used as first-line treatment for occlusive and aneurysmal vascular disease, the incidence of complications is rising accordingly. These complications can be divided into three categories: (1) puncture-site related, (2) catheter related, and (3) systemic complications.

About 0.5% of femoral punctures and 1.7% of axillary punctures have been reported to require treatment for a complication. Hematomas at the puncture site are not usually considered a complication and rarely need surgical treatment. Large hematomas (e.g., retroperitoneal, pelvic, and anterior abdominal wall hematomas) that require surgical intervention occur more often in patients with coagulopathies and in patients who are obese. The risk of puncture-site pseudoaneurysm has been shown to increase with increasing catheter size and when a low puncture site is used. Prevention of puncture-site hematomas and pseudoaneurysms can be achieved by using the smallest-caliber catheter possible to perform the necessary intervention. Accordingly, there are fewer puncture-site complications with angioplasty procedures when compared with stenting, as the catheter needed to place a stent is of a larger caliber.

Catheter-related complications include the formation of arterial dissections, subintimal injections, and embolization from the catheter. Fortunately, as the dissections produced are retrograde and are pushed closed by the direction of blood flow, most of these complications are asymptomatic. However, some acute dissections become extensive chronic dissections or cause acute occlusion. Catheter thromboembolism occurs in less than 0.5% of cases.

There are myriad systemic complications associated with angiographic procedures. Examples include vasovagal syncope, cardiac arrest and arrhythmias, myocardial infarction, and nausea and vomiting. Contrast reactions can be reduced by adequate hydration and by using low osmolar contrast in high-risk patients. Rarely radiation injury in the form of a skin burn occurs when the procedure is lengthy and the patient is exposed to over 2 Gy.

References

Bergamini TM, Towne JB, Bandyk DF, Seabrook GR and Schmitt DD. (1991) J Vasc Surg 13:137–47; discussion 148–9.

Hannon RJ, Wolfe JH, Mansfield AO. (1996) Br J Surg 83: 654–8.

Krupski WC, Layug EL, Reilly LM, Rapp JH, Mangano DT. (1993) J Vasc Surg 18:609–15; discussion 615–7.

Neville RF, Sidawy AN. (1998) Semin Vasc Surg 11:142–8.

13

Vascular Access

David C. Mitchell and C. Keith Ozaki

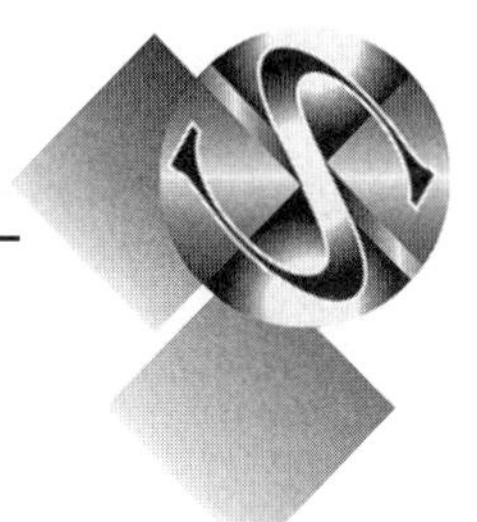

Vascular access is required to assist in the management of patients requiring frequent venous or arterial cannulation. Its principal role is to provide circulatory access for hemodialysis, although such techniques are also used to provide chemotherapy, intravenous nutrition, and access for plasma exchange.

The two techniques used are either implantable synthetic lines, which may have one or more lumina, or a surgically created fistula between the arterial and venous circulation. This latter approach may involve joining artery and vein together, the so-called autogenous arteriovenous (AV) access [arteriovenous fistula (AVF)], or the insertion of a synthetic bridge graft between artery and vein (nonautogenous AV access).

Principles of Vascular Access

The guiding principles of access surgery are to use AVF in preference to synthetic grafts, which are preferred to in-dwelling central venous catheters. Access should be sited as far distally in the chosen limb as possible. The principle is to conserve veins to permit proximal revision if the initial procedure fails. An exception is very old patients, who often have poor distal vessels. Some young patients may have strong wishes to avoid visible forearm scars. The nondominant limb should be used wherever possible.

In patients who may require vascular access, venepuncture, or the insertion of intravenous cannulae in the main named veins of the upper limb, should be avoided. If central venous catheters are required, they should be sited in the jugular and not the subclavian veins to avoid central venous stenosis in the draining veins of the upper limb.

Standards

The United States has led the way in this area with the publication of specific guidelines [National Kidney Foundation-Disease Outcomes Quality Initiative (NKF-DOQI) (www.kidney.org/professionals/doqi/guidelines)]. These guidelines were a response to the rapid growth in patient numbers and costs associated with treatment for renal failure. A multidisciplinary group of nephrologists, nurses, vascular and transplant surgeons, and interventional radiologists reviewed the world literature. The resulting document was approved by all the represented national societies prior to adoption.

The principal recommendations are that the majority of patients starting dialysis should do so using a native vessel AVF at the wrist. Grafts require six times as many interventions as AVF to achieve the same patency, and their use is discouraged. Central catheters have inferior patency and are discouraged for "permanent" access. Their principal role should be for emergency or temporary access. Since the distribution of these standards, placement rates for simple fistulas has increased 35% in the United States.

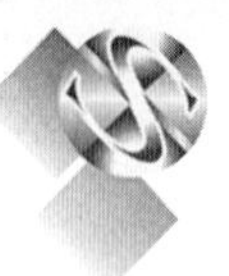

The Europeans have not produced a similar document, although it is hoped that a National Service Framework for renal disease management in the United Kingdom will set standards for vascular access within the National Health Service.

Observational studies have helped to define standards. The Dialysis Outcomes and Practice Patterns Study (DOPPS) was a prospective global study of practice in seven countries involving 309 facilities and over 9500 patients. It showed that there are significant differences between varying health cultures in the developed world. The AVF rates varied from 0% to 87% in the United States, and 39% to 100% in Europe. Graft usage in new hemodialysis patients ranged from 2 to 24%. Central venous lines were particularly common in the United Kingdom and the United States but rare in Japan and Italy.

These differences are not dictated solely by differences between patients, but principally by clinician preference. This study has clarified what is being done at present to provide access. By demonstrating widely differing practice, it informs the debate over ideal practice and can guide future trials to answer questions about treatment where widely differing views are held.

Interpretation of the literature is further complicated by differences in reporting of the results of access surgery. A recent study from the United States should help to standardize reporting in the future (Sidawy et al., 2002).

Types of Access

The principal modes of vascular access are autogenous AVF, synthetic AV bridge grafts (nonautogenous AV access), and in-dwelling synthetic central venous catheters. Consideration of patient demographics, anatomical suitability, and other factors are important in the preoperative planning for access (Table 13.1).

Arteriovenous Fistula

Most clinicians agree that the most durable form of vascular access is the AVF. The preferential site is between the cephalic vein and the radial artery at the anatomical snuffbox, or the wrist, in the nondominant upper limb, the

Table 13.1. Preoperative planning for autogenous or nonautogenous arteriovenous fistula (AVF) placement

Consider patient age, projected life span, time to initiation of dialysis, dominant hand
Elicit history of previous access attempts/subclavian vein cannulations; consider contrast venography to rule out central venous pathologies
Check Allen's test, upper extremity blood pressures, arterial pulse exam → if abnormal then segmental arm pressures, plethysmography → if abnormal then consider ultrasound or angiography
Venous exam with tourniquet → if no clear conduit then duplex; protect that vein from puncture/trauma
Ensure patient is optimized for operation (e.g., address cardiac, metabolic, volume status, nutritional, infectious issues)
Consider risks of steal in elderly and diabetic patients undergoing proximal access construction

Brescia-Cimino fistula (Brescia et al., 1966). The end of the vein is joined to the side of the radial artery, usually under local anesthesia.

The success of this procedure is dependent on the quality of the vein and artery and the technical skill of the surgeon. Where good vessels are not clinically evident, duplex ultrasonography or venography may help to identify the best sites for access formation. The suggested sequence for AVF placement is listed in Table 13.2).

Widely varying success rates are quoted, but about 60% of wrist AVFs mature and become useful for dialysis. The AVFs are robust once established, but may take many (typically 6 to 12) weeks to mature. Many factors may affect

Table 13.2. Suggested sequence for AVF placement

1. Autogenous AVF in hand/forearm (nondominant before dominant)
2. Upper arm autogenous AVF (usually cephalic before basilic)
3. Forearm nonautogenous AVF
4. Upper arm nonautogenous AVF
5. Upper arm or thigh autogenous (using transposed or translocated saphenous/superficial femoral vein) AVF
6. Thigh nonautogenous AVF
7. Central configurations such as axillary artery to contralateral axillary vein, subclavian artery to subclavian vein

maturation, such as the size of artery and vein, change in flow, and the presence or absence of arterial disease (e.g., diabetes). In patients in whom the fistula is failing to become prominent within a few weeks, duplex ultrasound scanning can examine flow rates and identify problems. Surgeons willing to undertake revision may produce higher success rates. The principal reasons for failure are damaged or inadequate veins and (more rarely) inadequate arteries. In such cases, alternative forearm veins may be used. The basilic vein on the ulnar side of the forearm is often large and may not have been traumatized by venesection. This can be mobilized and swung across the forearm to the radial artery, or anastomosed to the adjacent ulnar artery if large enough, although the failure rates for this procedure are higher.

Any vein can be damaged by repeat venesection or placement of in-dwelling catheters. Such veins develop areas of fibrosis that cannot dilate when subjected to arterial flows. For this reason, in those in whom the need for access can be anticipated, every effort should be made to avoid needling the cephalic vein, the antecubital veins, or the subclavian vein.

The radial artery at the wrist is often insufficient in the elderly and particularly those with diabetes. The artery usually shows evidence of arteriosclerosis with calcification. The artery is unable to increase its flow rate in response to fistula formation. The result is failure of the vein to enlarge, or thrombosis. In this situation, it may be better to place the fistula more proximally in the limb, typically at the elbow. Preoperative evaluation can assist in identifying suitable patients for distal AVFs (Malovrh, 2002).

The standard procedure at the elbow is an end of cephalic vein to side of brachial artery fistula. This can usually be fashioned through a transverse antecubital incision or two longitudinal incisions under local anesthesia. The depth of the basilic vein within the arm complicates its use as a direct fistula. This vein, however, may be easily mobilized through a longitudinal incision in the medial arm. The basilic vein is then divided distally, tunneled subcutaneously, and anastomosed to the brachial artery in the distal arm. The procedure can be performed using minimally invasive techniques. Such transposed fistulas may give good service over many years. This technique may also be applied to the lower limb in patients with good arterial circulation, by transposing the long saphenous vein subcutaneously in the thigh and anastomosing it to the distal superficial femoral artery.

Synthetic Access Grafts (Nonautogenous Arteriovenous Access)

Where veins are inadequate, or dialysis is needed urgently (within 2 weeks), AVF may be inappropriate. In such circumstances, access can be rapidly established using synthetic bridge grafts between suitable arteries and veins. The most common material for this is polytetrafluoroethylene (PTFE), which may be cannulated within a week if required. Dacron is not widely used for access as it is difficult to needle, but newer composite grafts that are reported to bleed less after cannulation are available. The role of these grafts has yet to be clearly established.

As veins are often deficient, grafts tend to be placed more proximally in the limb than AVFs. They may be placed in either straight or curved/looped configurations. No data exist demonstrating that one configuration is significantly better than any other. Grafts should be appropriately sized with the arterial anastomosis not bigger than 6 mm to avoid excessive flows and either vascular steal or high output cardiac failure.

Although easier to establish, PTFE grafts are known to have higher thrombotic and septic complication rates, and to need more frequent revision than native AVFs. For this reason, it is advised that AVFs are preferred. This has never been formally tested in a prospective randomized trial. In the elderly patient with limited life expectancy, a rapidly established graft may provide superior access with sufficient durability, compared to several unsuccessful attempts to establish an AVF.

Central Venous Catheters

A well-organized renal failure service should anticipate the need for access in patients approaching end-stage disease, and appropriate access surgery should be planned in advance.

This counsel of perfection is not always realized as patients may present acutely after a long period of stability.

Those requiring emergency access (e.g., immediate need for dialysis) need the insertion of a dual-lumen central venous catheter. These should be left in place for as short a time as possible. Definitive access surgery should follow as a matter of urgency.

Central catheters become infected easily, and often have to be removed or re-sited. In addition, they stimulate fibrosis in the veins and can cause stenosis. For this reason, subclavian lines are to be avoided, as the loss of the subclavian vein prejudices further access in the ipsilateral upper limb. Lines should be placed via the jugular route if at all possible. If access is needed only for a few days, then in the absence of suitable jugular veins the femoral veins may be used.

Patients needing more permanent catheters (longer than 3 weeks) should have tunneled catheters inserted. Placement considerations are the same as for temporary lines. Tunneled catheters should be cuffed, as the cuffs reduce the risk of infection from the site of skin entry.

Complications of Vascular Access

Arteriovenous Fistula

Once the AVF is established, AVF revision rates are low at about 15% or less per annum. Fistulas are robust and withstand multiple cannulations well.

Technical Failure

The most immediate complication of AV access is that the fistula occludes shortly after formation. This may be due to obvious problems such as inadequate vessels or to technical imperfections in the procedure. In the former, re-siting the fistula is the best course of action. In the latter situation, revision, often under local anesthesia, may salvage a functioning AVF. This is rarely an emergency and can be managed during the next available elective operating session.

Failure to Mature

Failure to mature is the most common problem seen in AVFs. Fistulas demonstrate significant increase in flow within 48 hours and enlarge thereafter. Most successful AVFs are capable of being needled in about 6 to 8 weeks after formation, although longer may be required. Detecting those that will fail to mature may be difficult. Ideally, AVFs should be placed well in advance of the time that they are likely to be required. This permits time for assessment and revision if the fistula is not developing satisfactorily. An alternative approach if time is pressing is to scan the fistula with ultrasound soon after formation. Flow rates greater than 500 mL/min signify that the fistula is likely to develop successfully. Scanning can also be used for the early detection of technical deficiencies, stenoses, and other problems. In constructions that are failing to mature, some groups advocate early liberal use of fistulograms to aid in diagnosis and therapeutic planning. Others rely primarily on the diagnostic vascular laboratory, and reserve fistulography for cases in which duplex scanning is equivocal or unavailable.

Vascular Stenosis

Vein stenosis and aneurysmal dilatation are both seen following development of AVFs. The former may compromise both the quality of dialysis and the longevity of the fistula. Some centers advocate routine fistula scanning, but this has not yet been shown to be an effective way of monitoring fistulas for complications. Where obvious stenoses exist, or dialysis is inadequate despite an apparently satisfactory fistula, then ultrasound may reveal a stenosis. Stenoses greater than 50% or AVFs with flows below 500 mL/min are more likely to fail and may need revision. Stenoses within 1 to 2 cm of the anastomosis are most easily dealt with by surgical revision. This can be undertaken under local anesthesia with an occlusive tourniquet. The fistula is ligated and divided and reanastomosed to an adjacent portion of artery. More remote stenoses may often be dealt with by angioplasty. If this fails, then short skip grafts of vein may bypass a stenosis and permit continuous use of the fistula without the need for temporary lines.

Vascular Steal and High-Output Cardiac Failure

Proximal fistulas tend to have higher flow rates and may divert blood from the hand. The risk of vascular steal should be borne in mind in proximal fistula. It is uncommonly seen (about 1% to 8%), but the neurological effects are irreversible if the steal is not quickly corrected (Tordoir et al., 2004). Any suspicion of hand ischemia demands immediate attention, beginning with bedside examination. Temporary finger occlusion of the AVF can assist in determining whether there is an inflow problem, or whether the arterial flow distal to the arterial anastomosis has been interrupted. If hand arterial perfusion returns to baseline with AVF compression, then inflow is inadequate to maintain flow to the hand and through the AVF. If the extremity remains ischemic, then there may be a problem with the arterial anastomosis that occludes outflow, or thromboembolic complications. Segmental arm and finger pressures, followed by repeated exam while the access is occluded, confirm the diagnosis. If inflow is inadequate, then improvement of distal pressures and symptoms should occur while the AVF or graft is compressed.

If steal physiology is demonstrated, then appropriate urgent imaging to screen for occult inflow arterial occlusive disease may be undertaken, and lesions addressed. Fistula revision is often required. If preservation of the fistula is not essential, taking it down and creating a new one is probably the procedure of choice. The alternatives are banding to reduce flow, or bypass from the artery at least 6 cm above the anastomosis to an artery distally and then ligation of the artery immediately beyond the anastomosis. This last procedure is known as the distal revascularization-interval ligation (DRIL) procedure. It is gaining in popularity as it takes flow to the distal arterial tree from above the fistula and prevents steal due to reversed flow in the artery distal to the anastomosis.

Banding is a complex procedure, necessitating intraoperative flow measurement. Flows may fluctuate during the procedure, but ideally the banding should produce a flow between 800 mL and 1.5 L per minute. Success rates for this procedure are low, and it is not recommended if an alternative is available. Postoperative thrombosis is common and may be due to overvigor-ous banding. If this happens, the fistula is usually lost.

High fistula flows can also cause high-output cardiac failure, which is seen more commonly in proximal AVFs. In these cases, fistula revision to reduce flows is required. The choices include sacrificing the fistula and siting new access, or attempting a flow reduction procedure.

Infection

Infection is rare, but if associated with bacteremia, abscess, or aneurysm formation, revision is usually required. The clinical features are of an area of inflammation in relation to the fistula, sometimes with rapid enlargement. Fever and rigors, particularly on dialysis, may be seen, but are not a universal feature. Sudden rapid bleeding can occur at infected needling sites. Immediate pressure and placement of a skin suture will achieve acute control, but should be followed by a definitive revision in most cases.

Thrombosis

Thrombosis is uncommon, but when it occurs it can often be retrieved by acute intervention, with salvage of the fistula and avoidance of temporary central lines. Overdialysis is an uncommon cause of fistula thrombosis, but should be suspected if no stenosis can be found. Imaging of the whole fistula and ipsilateral central veins should always follow surgical or radiological declotting. Dilatation of fistula or central vein stenosis may be required to restore normal function. When the stenosis is in close proximity to the anastomosis, then surgical revision to an adjacent proximal arterial segment is often the best procedure.

The complications associated with transposed fistulas are the same as those seen with other native AVFs. They tend to have high flows, so cardiac failure and steal are more common in these fistulas.

Arteriovenous Access Grafts (Nonautogenous Arteriovenous Access)

Arteriovenous grafts can usually be established easily, with a high technical success rate. However, complications are common, and the frequent need for intervention should prompt the surgeon and dialysis team to undertake regular surveillance.

Thrombosis

Thrombosis is usually the consequence of intimal hyperplasia at the venous end of the graft. This can be recognized by regular intradialysis monitoring of flow or pressure. It has been shown that monitoring of flow or pressure can detect developing graft stenosis. Timely intervention can prolong graft survival. One approach is to use balloon angioplasty where possible, keeping surgical revision to a minimum. Where thrombosis occurs, prompt declotting undertaken by either an endovascular or open approach can retrieve graft function. It is important to identify and correct the cause of the thrombosis or further thrombosis is likely. There is no clear evidence whether open or endovascular approaches are superior in this situation, and each approach has its proponents. As grafts require relatively frequent interventions, many advocate using minimally invasive techniques first and reserving open surgery for those in whom the vascular interventionist fails.

Infection

Like any foreign material, infection is an ever-present hazard, especially as needles are frequently introduced into the graft. Septic episodes in dialysis patients are most likely to originate from the graft. Great care must be taken to use aseptic techniques when cannulating grafts, as once organisms are seeded into a graft the only way to get rid of them is to replace the graft. Eradication of nasal carriage of *Staphylococcus aureus* by use of topical mupirocin has been shown to reduce the rate of graft sepsis.

Grafts are often placed in European practice as a dialysis access of last resort, and there may be limited alternative sites if an infected graft is removed. Clearly if there is inflammation along the length of the graft, then removal is the only option. Where localized sepsis exists, or a small area of the graft is exposed, local

excision with skip grafting through uninvolved tissue may keep the graft functioning. The site of infection should be left open to drain freely, and the patient treated with parenteral antibiotics until the inflammation has completely subsided.

Vascular Steal

This is most commonly seen in arm grafts in older or diabetic patients. Rates vary from between 1% to 19%. The approach is the same as steal in an autogenous AVF, with nonautogenous graft ligation or DRIL being the potential management approaches.

Aneurysm Formation

With repeated cannulation over small areas of a graft, there is a tendency for "aneurysm" formation (actually a pseudoaneurysm). This is a result of longitudinal splitting of the graft. It is not a problem if there is good skin coverage, but if enlarging rapidly or if inflamed, then early revision should be undertaken to prevent rupture and bleeding. The technique is similar to that used for infection, with the exception that excision of the aneurysmal portion of the graft is not always necessary in the absence of infection.

Central Venous Catheters

Infection

Infection is the main problem from central venous (CV) catheters, and rigorous aseptic technique is required to manage dialysis. Newer, totally implantable catheters that are accessed through the skin may reduce the risk of sepsis. The teaching of correct hand and skin preparation prior to needling remains an important part of the management of patients with CV catheters.

Once infected, lines need to be changed. Ideally, the old line should be removed and the patient treated until he or she is well before inserting a new line. This is not always possible. Rotating the line to a new site is to be preferred in such situations, but if the situation is desperate, removing the old line and reinserting in the same location while treating with antibiotics may be successful.

Fibrinous Encasement and Clotting

The tips of catheters become covered with a "biofilm" of fibrin that may contain bacteria. Even if sterile, this film can build up until a large tube of fibrin encases the catheter tip. This can interfere with blood flow and obstruct dialysis. If the line is not infected, removal and replacement may still be necessary to reestablish dialysis. Passing guidewires down the catheter is not usually successful, but snaring the catheter tip radiologically and stripping the fibrin cuff can clear the offending plug. This technique can significantly prolong the life of central lines.

Thrombosis is a common problem, especially if the line is not used frequently. Lines should be flushed with the correct volume of heparin (1000 U/mL) after each use to remove blood from the lumen and prevent thrombosis. Extra care must be paid to this in children, as it is easy to give excessive volumes of heparin and induce systemic anticoagulation and bleeding.

The Avoidance of Complications: Access Surveillance

Concerns about the frequent need for access revision have stimulated inquiry into techniques for the early detection of access complications before symptoms develop. Most techniques concentrate on intradialytic monitoring of flow, pressure, dialysis efficacy, or a combination of these. The advantage of intradialytic monitoring is that it minimizes the need for extra hospital resources for these ill patients. Each technique has its proponents, and the techniques mentioned are not mutually exclusive.

The DOQI guidelines state, "Access flow measured by ultrasound dilution, conductance dilution, thermal dilution, Doppler or other technique should be performed monthly. The assessment of flow should be performed during the first 1.5 hours of the treatment to eliminate error caused by decreases in cardiac output related to ultrafiltration. The mean value of

three separate determinations performed at a single treatment should be considered the access flow. If access flow is less than 600 mL/min, the patient should be referred for fistulogram. Access flow less than 1000 mL/min that has decreased by more than 25% over 4 months should be referred for fistulogram."

This is a counsel of perfection and some centers would advocate duplex ultrasound prior to fistulography. Where there is evidence of a stenosis of >50%, there is a significant subsequent thrombosis rate. Such fistula should undergo endovascular or surgical revision as appropriate. Juxta-anastomotic stenoses are often best dealt with by surgery, with endovascular dilatation being reserved for those in the body of the access.

Desperate Access

Dialysis is becoming more successful in prolonging the lives of patients in renal failure. Unfortunately, this improvement in survival is not being matched by increases in transplantation. As a result, many more people are dependent on long-term dialysis. As successive access procedures fail, the establishment of secure vascular access becomes increasingly difficult.

Surgeons and interventionists have become ingenious at inserting grafts or lines into various veins, sometimes accidentally. Grafts can be placed in necklace fashion between one axilla and the contralateral one. Arteries can be divided and interposition grafts inserted. The superficial femoral vein has been utilized as a hemodialysis access conduit. Lines may be inserted directly into the inferior vena cava (IVC) through the back. Such procedures should be reserved for those in whom no alternative can be found after an extensive search using ultrasound, venography, and magnetic resonance angiography if necessary. It should be made clear to patients undergoing these procedures that the risks involved in establishing such access are high, and the consequence of failure may be fatal.

Although successful arterial access can be obtained for numerous patients with reasonable durability, numerous controversies remain (Table 13.3). These controversies will be resolved with further clinical trials.

Table 13.3. Contemporary controversies

Role of endovascular vs. open management of the failing and failed autogenous AVF and nonautogenous AVF

Construction of upper arm autogenous AVF prior to utilization of forearm nonautogenous AVF

Role of invasive imaging (routine arteriograms and venograms) prior to vascular access constructions

Adjuvant therapies to improve vascular access patency (anticoagulants, antiplatelet therapies, etc.)

Unknown value of new nonautogenous AVF conduits (modified Dacron, homografts, etc.)

Role of duplex surveillance in identifying the failing graft

References

Brescia MJ, Cimino JE, Appell K, Hurwich BJ, Scribner BH. (1966) J Am Soc Nephrol 10:193–9.

Malovrh M. (2002) Am J Kidney Dis 39:1218–25.

Sidawy AN, Gray R, Besarab A, et al. (2002) J Vasc Surg 35:603–10.

Tordoir JH, Dammers R, van der Sande FM. (2004) Eur J Vasc Endovasc Surg 27:1–5.

14

Outcome Measures in Vascular Surgery

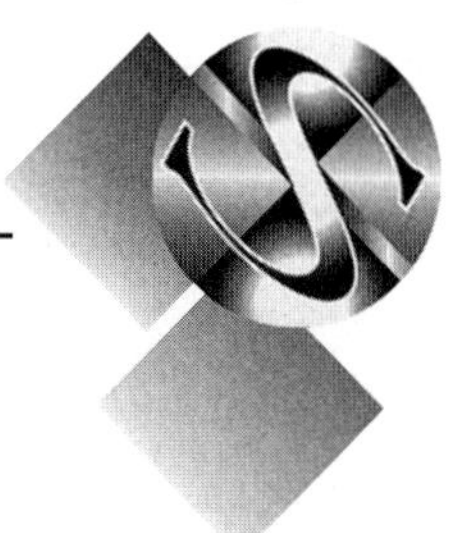

Christopher J. Kwolek and Alun H. Davies

Background

Initial efforts within the health care reform movement in the United States largely focused on reducing cost. This became the preeminent issue as health care expenditures continued to increase on an annual basis, reaching 14% of gross domestic product in 1994. Although some of these expenses can be attributed to improvements in diagnostic and therapeutic regimens, particularly in those areas highly influenced by new technologies, concern has also been expressed about the quality of the product being provided to patients.

The publication of the Institute of Medicine's (IOM) Committee on Quality of Care report, "To Err Is Human: Building a Safer Health System," shifted the focus of attention from cost alone to medical errors within the U.S. health care system and the costs associated with these errors. This has led to an erosion of patient trust in the medical care system. It has been estimated that medical errors are responsible for between 44,000 and 98,000 deaths annually, becoming the eighth leading cause of death in the U.S., ahead of other causes such as breast cancer and motor vehicle accidents. Over 7000 of these deaths were attributed to medication errors alone, with the total cost to society of these errors estimated to be $11637.6 billion a year. Much of the initial research describing the problem of medical errors was performed in the 1990s and supported by the Agency for Healthcare Research and Quality (AHRQ).

The IOM report also led to the establishment of the Quality Interagency Coordination Task Force (QuIC), which was charged with coordinating the quality improvement activities in U.S. federal health care programs. These groups have been responsible for the establishment of standardized guidelines and protocols based on clinical trials, which may decrease variability in the patient care processes while improving care and reducing costs. The vast majority of the errors identified in these studies were systems related and not attributable to negligence or misconduct. In fact, up to 75% of the medical errors and 54% of the surgical errors were found to be preventable.

The U.S. Veterans Administration (VA) hospital system had already begun to look at these quality and outcomes issues through the establishment of the National VA Surgical Quality Improvement Program (NSQIP), which has been responsible for assessing specific surgical outcomes throughout the U.S. VA hospital system, while using risk adjusted data to assess surgical morbidity and mortality and providing specific institutional feedback (Khuri et al., 1998). In fact, this program was so successful that in the late 1990s it was expanded to include three large academic medical centers at the University of Kentucky, the University of Michigan, and Emory University in Atlanta. Currently this program is being expanded to include multiple academic medical institutions across the U.S.

In addition, large companies, which are purchasers of health care for their employees, have

Table 14.1. Current recommendations of the Leap Frog Group

Computerized physician order entry: mandated use to minimize medication errors

Intensive care unit (ICU) physician staffing: use of critical care certified physicians to provide exclusive care of ICU patients

Evidence-based hospital referral: preferential referral of patients undergoing five high-risk surgical procedures to "high volume centers"

Procedure	Annual volume requirement
Coronary artery bypass grafting	500/year
Percutaneous coronary angioplasty	400/year
Carotid endarterectomy	100/year
Abdominal aortic aneurysm repair	30/year
Esophagectomy	6/year

begun to take an interest in improving the quality and potentially decreasing the cost of health care as demonstrated by the activities of the Leap Frog Group (www.leapfroggroup.org). The stated purpose of this group of Fortune 500 companies is to mobilize employer purchasing power to trigger breakthroughs in the safety and overall value of health care to American consumers. Using the results of these and other studies aimed at evaluating medical outcomes, the Leap Frog Group has already identified three areas to decrease errors and improve the quality in U.S.-based health care systems. Health care providers who adopt these recommendations will be rewarded with preferential use and other incentives by this group of health care purchasers. The current recommendations are listed in Table 14.1. It is estimated that implementation of this program would save 60,000 lives with a monetary savings of $3.8 billion a year.

Although these recommendations are supported by reviews of outcome studies in the current medical literature, certain limitations do exist. For example, volume-based outcome studies demonstrate that on average, high-volume centers have better patient outcomes for certain high-risk procedures such as repair of abdominal aortic aneurysm (AAA) or carotid endarterectomy (CEA). However, some high-volume centers may have average or poor outcomes, whereas some smaller centers with low volumes may have excellent outcomes. It may be more important to measure the clinical process for a health care system to identify the reasons and processes that allow one facility to have excellent outcomes so that these can be utilized by other facilities to achieve the same excellent results. This concept was used by the Northern New England Cardiovascular Disease Study Group to improve the outcomes of patients undergoing coronary artery bypass grafting in northern New England (O'Connor et al., 1996).

Outcomes Measures

It has become important that we evaluate the relative value of different treatment regimens to include individual and societal costs and potential risks and benefits. Individual patient perspectives on quality have also become an important part of the evaluation process.

There are several reasons for physicians to participate in this process. Ideally, our participation should lead to an overall improvement in the quality of care that we deliver. In addition, participation in these programs will soon be necessary to qualify for reimbursement from many insurers and purchasers of health care such as the U.S. government and the Leap Frog Group. Finally, as physicians we have a societal responsibility to maximize the good and minimize adverse outcomes in health care, while best utilizing the limited resources that exist. If physicians choose not to participate in this process, then others will make these difficult decisions for us.

These changes have led to the development of "extended outcome assessment" rather than just the traditional physician-oriented outcomes measures that we are used to. The concept of a value compass has been proposed to describe the interplay between traditional medical outcomes, patient satisfaction, functional assessment, and cost/utility outcomes (McDaniel et al., 2000).

Clinical Status

The most traditional group of medical outcomes measures utilized by vascular surgeons usually describes clinical status. These measures are physician oriented and include measurements of morbidity and mortality, graft patency, limb salvage, complications, and laboratory testing such as the ankle–brachial index (ABI)

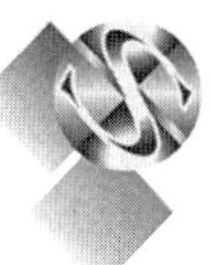

and duplex ultrasound results. Many of these outcomes are important measures of technical success and are easily evaluable by statistical methods such as life table analysis. However, even the long-term results within this category such as patient survival after aneurysm repair, stroke-free survival after carotid endarterectomy, or amputation-free survival after lower extremity bypass grafting do not necessarily correlate with patients' overall well-being, day-to-day functioning, or their perceived quality of life. Physicians are also comfortable with these outcomes since the Society for Vascular Surgery (SVS) and the International Society for Cardiovascular Surgery (ISCVS) have published guidelines for measuring these types of outcomes for commonly performed arterial and venous vascular procedures.

Patient Satisfaction

Patient-oriented outcomes tend to be less frequently measured and not as well defined. None of these outcomes are included in the SVS-ISCVS reporting standards. Patient satisfaction with the health care process is one area being more closely evaluated. Although customer satisfaction surveys have long been used in the world of business, they are now being applied to the area of health care. Two areas being frequently evaluated include patient satisfaction with the physician–patient relationship and satisfaction with the health care delivery process. This may include such issues as timeliness and access to care, provider and staff communication, the physical environment where care is delivered, and courtesy and respect shown to the patient. Managed care plans in the U.S. are now required to assess themselves using standardized patient satisfaction surveys such as the Health Plan Employer Data and Information Set (HEDIS), which was developed by the National Committee for Quality Assurance (NCQA). Many employers and purchasers of health care are now utilizing this information when deciding on which health care providers to include in their panel of providers.

Functional Status

Functional status is another of the patient-oriented outcomes that is being more commonly described in the vascular literature. These health assessment instruments are designed to quantify how illnesses and treatments affect different aspects of patient functioning in everyday life. This will allow physicians to evaluate not only the presence or absence of a leg or the patency of a graft, but how patients are functioning after a specific intervention. These measures are also helpful when evaluating patients' expectations before and after specific interventions. A list of commonly used measures of functional status is included in Table 14.2. There are two types of assessment tools. The specific instrument focuses on a specific disease or client group, and changes in this are more likely to detect subtle changes in quality of life, whereas generic tools give a broader summary of health-related quality of life, hence enabling comparisons with patients suffering from other disease processes (Table 14.3).

The most widely used generic functional health assessment instrument in the United States is the Medical Outcomes Short Form 36 (SF-36). This survey evaluates patient function in physical and social roles, limitations due to health or emotional problems, patient perceptions of general health, mental health, bodily pain, and vitality. In addition, a question concerning change in health status compared to 1 year previously is included in the survey. This survey combines aspects of a Quality of Well-Being Scale and a Functional Status Questionnaire. The reason that this survey has become so useful is that large numbers of patients have been evaluated using this instrument, thus allowing researchers to compare results to the general population or a patient subgroup with specific characteristics. These results may be

Table 14.2. Examples of measures of functional status

General status: quality of life
   SF-36
   Euro-QOL
   Nottingham Health Profile
   Functional Status Questionnaire
   Quality of Well-Being Scale
   Sickness Impact Profile
Disease/symptom specific: quality of life
   Walking Impairment Questionnaire: for patients
      with lower extremity arterial occlusive disease
   Charing Cross Claudication Questionnaire
   Charing Cross Venous Ulcer Questionnaire
   VascQuol

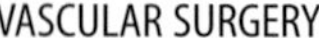

Table 14.3. Advantages and disadvantages of quality of life instruments

Instrument	Advantages	Disadvantages
Generic	Single instrument Detects different aspects of health Enables comparison between different conditions Can be used in cost analysis	May not focus adequately on main problem May lack responsiveness Does not take account of values attributed to levels of quality of life
Specific	Focus on primary are of interest More relevant to clinicians and clinical condition May be more responsive	Not comprehensive May miss side effects Cannot compare across conditions

helpful in predicting long-term functional outcomes in patients. Thus patients scoring above a certain level in the area of bodily pain may have a decreased chance of successfully returning to work, and patients with decreased overall scores in the areas of physical and social function and health may have an increased 5-year mortality. However, the abbreviated form of the SF-36, the SF-12, is growing in popularity.

In addition to general evaluations of functional status, disease-specific instruments have also been developed. One of the most widely used surveys for the evaluation of patients with lower extremity arterial occlusive disease is the Walking Impairment Questionnaire (WIQ); however, there are newer and more specific questionnaires becoming available (Chong et al., 2002). Because peripheral vascular disease has a detrimental effect on quality of life even in patients without the most severe forms of limb-threatening ischemia, these instruments may be very useful in evaluating the benefit to patients undergoing treatment for claudication. These surveys may be even more important for evaluating patients undergoing prophylactic interventions for the management of asymptomatic disease.

Some authors have recommended that a combination of two different surveys such as the SF-36 and the EuroQol be used to evaluate the quality of life outcomes in patients with and without ischemic complications who are undergoing infrainguinal bypass grafting (Tangelder et al., 1999). Tangelder et al. found that the combination of the SF-36 and the EuroQol provided useful information concerning the patients' quality of life after lower extremity bypass grafting. Interestingly, patients' functional outcomes were similar for those with asymptomatic graft occlusions and patent grafts, although the lowest outcomes were found in patients who underwent amputation after failed attempts at secondary revascularization. These results confirm clinical findings that are often well known in clinical practice but that are not shown by primary or secondary patency rates or limb salvage.

Additional concerns have been expressed about the potential for patient bias with self-reporting of health status. However, patient reports of functional health status appear to have good face value validity. Thus patients who suffer from severe strokes report worse functioning in the areas of physical and general health than patients with mild strokes. Similarly, patients with venous ulcers report impaired social interaction, domestic activity, and emotional status with improved functioning after healing of their venous ulcers (Smith et al., 2000). Also, the benefits of varicose vein surgery can be justified in terms of improvements in quality of life scores.

Cost/Utility

Cost outcomes are another important area of recent interest. Increasing pressures are being exerted by the government and insurers to optimize the quality of the health care while minimizing expenditures. True costs to the individual and society must be calculated both for the acute illness and over the long term.

Practice guidelines can often be established based on the results from existing controlled clinical trials. These guidelines can then be used on a regional or national basis to evaluate physicians and health care organizations. Using the same processes of continuous quality improvement (CQI) found in major industrial manufac-

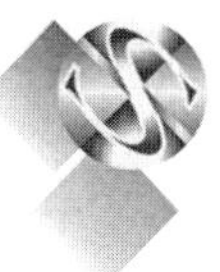

turing plants, these guidelines should reduce variation in the processes of care, thus improving quality while decreasing cost. These guidelines are designed to evaluate processes, with the ultimate philosophy of continuously improving the process to ensure the best possible outcome.

This process is in contradistinction to the more traditional concept of quality analysis (QA), where minimum standards or thresholds are set to ensure a good outcome and only outliers are evaluated rigorously. The pitfall of this approach is that it encourages organizations to be just "good enough" and meet the minimum standards set rather than aim for being the best possible. In addition, it singles out only those groups or individuals doing a poor job rather than rewarding groups that are doing a good job and trying to reproduce those results in other areas.

The value that patients and society place on certain outcomes and levels of functioning can also play a role in evaluating the cost-effectiveness of certain procedures. The cost-effectiveness of a certain intervention can be expressed as the net benefit to a population by using statistical probabilities of certain outcomes occurring along with specific costs associated with various outcomes as documented from the medical literature. One example of this is the use of the Markov decision model to evaluate the cost-effectiveness of performing carotid endarterectomy in asymptomatic patients with >60% stenosis (Cronenwett et al., 1997). The measurement units in this study are in quality-adjusted life years (QALYs) defined as the fraction of a year in perfect health that the patient believes to be equivalent in value to a year in the health state in question.

In this study, Cronenwett et al. demonstrated that from a societal standpoint, carotid endarterectomy appeared to be cost-effective for the young asymptomatic patient with standard risk factors in the hands of a surgeon with a 2.3% 30-day perioperative stroke and death rate. However, the procedure was not found to be cost-effective for patients older than 79 years of age, those with a high perioperative stroke risk, or those with a particularly low stroke risk with medical management. In this study it is important to note that cost-effectiveness is compared to cost/QALY for other medical interventions, and that a cost of over $100,000/additional QALY was defined as not cost-effective. Interestingly, one could extend the evaluation even further to include the individual's risk aversion and risk taking behavior when defining the cost-effectiveness for that person. This is essentially what occurs every time we obtain informed consent from a person who is about to undergo a high-risk procedure.

Conclusion

The reasons for physicians to utilize extended outcomes assessment include the following: (1) to achieve a better understanding of the effectiveness of our interventions; (2) to provide health care consumers, both patients and insurers, with information that will allow them to make better informed decisions; and (3) to develop public health standards that will allow us provide the most cost-effective care (McDaniel et al., 2000).

In addition, the Accreditation Council for Graduate Medical Education (ACGME) in the United States has mandated that all residency training programs evaluate as part of their core competency requirements six areas, all of which involve some component involving outcomes measures: (1) practice-based learning, (2) systems-based practice, (3) medical knowledge, (4) patient care, (5) interpersonal and communication skills, and (6) professionalism (www.acgme.org/outcomes).

Finally, the incorporation of outcomes measures are now being studied by the task force on competence of the American Board of Medical Specialties to be used in the process of recertification. In fact, recommendations have already been published stating that outcomes measures should be included as part of the requirement for recertification in vascular surgery by the American Board of Surgery (Hertzer, 2001).

References

Chong PF, Garratt AM, Golledge J, Greenhalgh RM, Davies AH. (2002) J Vasc Surg 36:764–71; discussion 863–4.
Cronenwett JL, Birkmeyer JD, Nackman GB, et al. (1997) J Vasc Surg 25:298–309; discussion 310–1.
Hertzer NR. (2001) J Vasc Surg 34:371–3.
Khuri SF, Daley J, Henderson W, et al. (1998) Ann Surg 228:491–507.

McDaniel MD, Nehler MR, Santilli SM, et al. (2000) J Vasc Surg 32:1239–50.

O'Connor GT, Plume SK, Olmstead EM, et al. (1996) JAMA 275:841–6.

Smith JJ, Guest MG, Greenhalgh RM, Davies AH. (2000) J Vasc Surg 31:642–9.

Tangelder MJ, McDonnel J, Van Busschbach JJ, et al. (1999) J Vasc Surg 29:913–9.

15

Carotid Artery Disease

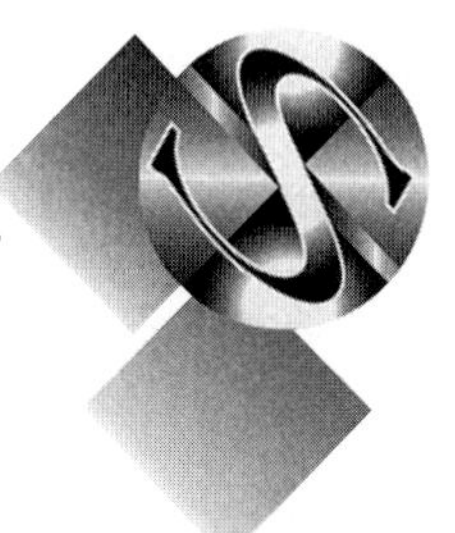

A. Ross Naylor, Peter H. Lin, and Elliot L. Chaikof

Epidemiology

Stroke

A stroke is defined as a focal (occasionally global) loss of cerebral function lasting for more than 24 hours, and which after investigation is found to have a vascular cause. Stroke is responsible for 4.5 million deaths worldwide, with the majority occurring in nonindustrialized countries. In the United States, stroke is the third most common cause of death, with approximately 160,000 Americans dying from the disease each year. Stroke management consumes $45 billion annually, including indirect costs and is responsible for more than one million hospital discharges per annum.

The demographics are remarkably similar in the United Kingdom, where stroke is also the third leading cause of death (12% of deaths overall) and 58,000 Britons die each year. Five percent of the National Health Service budget is used in stroke care (excluding indirect costs), and stroke patients occupy 20% of acute hospital beds and 25% of rehabilitation beds.

The incidence of stroke is 2 in 1000 per annum, but significantly increases with concurrent risk factors of age, sex, and ethnic background. Overall, the 20-year risk for a 45-year-old man is 3%, but this increases to 25% for a 40-year risk (Bonita, 1992). The annual incidence of stroke doubles for each decade over the age of 55 years. For those aged 0 to 44 years, the annual incidence of stroke is 0.09 in 1000, increasing to 2.9 in 1000 for those aged 55 to 64 and 14.3 in 1000 in those aged 75 to 84. The largest incidence is observed in populations aged >85 years, where the incidence is almost 20 in 1000. In both the United States and the United Kingdom, the incidence of stroke is twice as high in blacks as in white. This ethnic difference is thought to be due to the increased incidence in blacks of risk factors such as hypertension, diabetes, smoking, obesity, and sickle cell disease.

Transient Ischemic Attack

A transient ischemic attack (TIA) has the same definition as stroke but it lasts for less than 24 hours. The 24-hour threshold is somewhat arbitrary, as up to 28% of TIA patients have an infarct on computed tomography (CT) scan, of which 36% are bilateral. In the U.S., the prevalence of TIA in men aged 65 to 69 years is 2.7%, increasing to 3.6% for men aged 75 to 79 years. The respective prevalence figures for women are 1.6% and 4.1%. In the U.K., the overall incidence of TIA is 0.4 in 1000, but this varies with age. The incidence is 0.25 in 1000 for those aged 45 to 54 years, increasing to 1.61 in 1000 in the 65- to 74-year age group and 2.57 in 1000 in those aged 75 to 84 years.

Etiology of Ischemic Stroke

Approximately 80% of strokes are ischemic and 20% hemorrhagic. This section deals primarily with the etiology of ischemic carotid territory stroke.

Thromboembolism

Approximately 50% of all ischemic carotid territory strokes follow a carotid thrombosis or embolism from a carotid stenosis (Fig. 15.1) into territories supplied by either the middle cerebral artery (MCA) or the anterior cerebral artery (ACA). The sequelae of carotid thrombosis depend on a number of factors, including the status of the circle of Willis (potential for collateralization), the chronicity of the thrombosis, and the extent of the thrombosis. Once the internal carotid artery (ICA) has thrombosed, the column of thrombus usually propagates distally to the ophthalmic artery. However, the thrombus may occasionally extend beyond the ophthalmic artery and propagate into the circle of Willis.

A very small proportion of strokes (<4%) are secondary to isolated cerebral hypoperfusion. Patients susceptible to this type of stroke include those with critical ICA stenoses, poor collateralization via the circle of Willis, and a secondary trigger such as hypotension following an acute cardiac event.

Rarely, carotid thromboembolism may cause posterior (vertebrobasilar) territory strokes. This arises because, embryologically, the ICA provides the blood supply to the developing posterior cerebral hemispheres and brainstem via the posterior communicating and posterior cerebral arteries. In a very small proportion of the population, this anatomical arrangement persists into adult life.

Intracranial Small-Vessel Disease

Occlusion of the penetrating end arteries (lenticulostriate, thalamoperforate) in the deep structures of the brain causes discrete wedge-shaped infarctions of brain tissue. These ischemic lesions, termed lacunar infarcts, are responsible for up to 25% of ischemic carotid territory strokes. Conditions predisposing toward lacunar infarction include hypertension and diabetes. There is still considerable debate as to whether embolization from a carotid stenosis can cause lacunar infarction.

Cardiac Embolism

Cardiac embolism accounts for 15% of ischemic carotid territory strokes. The emboli consist of fibrin, cholesterol, calcified debris, and atheroma depending on the underlying pathology. Sources include valvular heart disease, prosthetic valves, atrial myxoma, ventricular aneurysm thrombus, cardiomyopathy, and infective endocarditis. However, the commonest causes are atrial fibrillation and embolization of mural thrombus overlying a dyskinetic segment of myocardium following a myocardial infarction (MI).

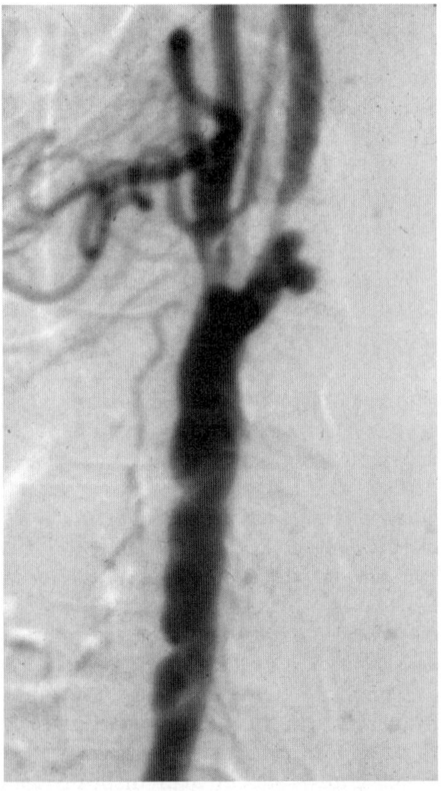

Figure 15.1. Selective intraarterial digital subtraction angiogram of left carotid bifurcation showing diffuse disease of the upper third of the common carotid artery, a stenosis at the origin of the external carotid artery, and a complex severe stenosis at the origin of the internal carotid artery with deep ulceration.

Hematological Causes

A variety of pathologies predisposing toward a hypercoagulable state are responsible for about 5% of ischemic strokes. These include polycythemia, sickle cell disease, leukemia, thrombocythemia, malignancies, functional protein S deficiency, lupus anticoagulant (antiphospholipid antibody syndrome), antithrombin III deficiency, and the paraproteinemias.

Miscellaneous Causes

Miscellaneous causes account for the remaining 5% of ischemic carotid territory strokes. These include migraine, oral contraceptive use, trauma, dissection, giant cell arteritis, Takayasu arteritis, systemic lupus erythematosus (SLE), polyarteritis nodosa, amyloid angiopathy, cocaine abuse, fibromuscular dysplasia, and radiation arteritis.

Pathology of Carotid Artery Disease

Atherosclerosis

Atherosclerosis is the commonest pathology affecting the carotid artery. The typical plaque encountered at carotid endarterectomy (Fig. 15.2) is the culmination of a sequence of pathophysiological processes starting with endothelial dysfunction/damage. The tendency for atherosclerotic plaque to form at the carotid bifurcation is related to a number of factors, including geometry, velocity profile, and shear stress.

It was originally proposed that local turbulence predisposed to high wall shear stress and endothelial injury. This hypothesis, however, was refuted by Zarins et al. (1983), who showed that plaque formation was *increased* within areas of low flow velocity and low shear stress and *decreased* in areas of high flow velocity and elevated shear stress. Postmortem specimens showed that atherosclerosis was particularly pronounced along the outer (lateral) aspect of the proximal ICA and carotid bulb. This zone corresponds to areas of low velocity and low shear stress. The medial or inner aspect of the carotid bulb (associated with high blood flow

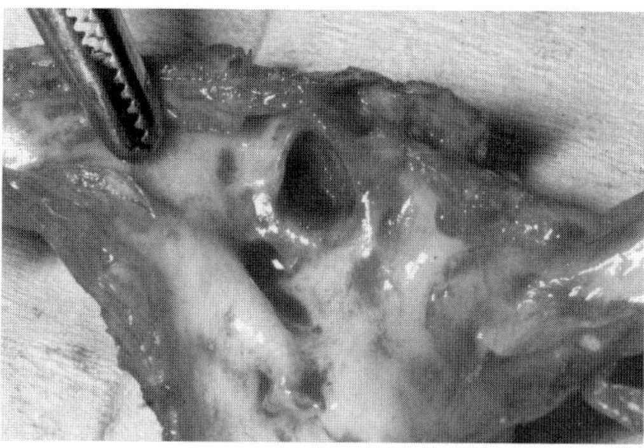

Figure 15.2. Atheromatous plaque excised at carotid endarterectomy. Note the deep area of ulceration in the plaque surface.

velocity and high shear stress in the flow model) were relatively free of plaque formation.

The smooth muscle cell has an important role in the initial stages of plaque development. Smooth muscle cells migrate through the intima, proliferate within the media, and promote accumulation of cholesterol and other lipid molecules within the evolving lesion. Thereafter, the macrophage becomes a source of growth factor production that stimulates further smooth muscle cell proliferation and extracellular matrix production. Smooth muscle cells and macrophages initiate a secondary inflammatory cell reaction and are capable of ingesting lipid and of being transformed into vacuolated foam cells that are characteristic of atherosclerotic lesions.

Besides these cellular components, the majority of carotid plaques have a necrotic core consisting of loose cellular debris and cholesterol crystals. The necrotic core is separated from the carotid lumen by a fibrous cap, which is composed of a rim of variable thickness comprising cellular components and extracellular matrix. The structural integrity of the fibrous cap is crucial to the final stage of plaque disruption and its clinical and pathological sequelae. It is now generally accepted that acute changes within the plaque, notably fissuring/splitting of the fibrous cap (Fig. 15.2), with exposure of the deeper lipid contents predisposes toward thrombosis with or without secondary embolization. It is not known what actually predisposes toward acute plaque disruption, but recent studies suggest that excess matrix metalloproteinase activity or cytokine expression

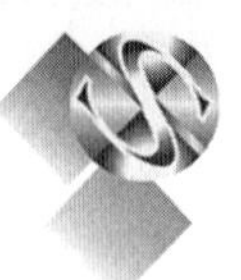

within the plaque may be associated with this process (Loftus et al., 2002).

Another feature characteristic of advanced atherosclerotic plaques is intraplaque hemorrhage that can occur in the absence of a disrupted fibrous cap. Symptomatic carotid disease is associated with increased neovascularization within the atherosclerotic plaque and fibrous cap. These vessels are larger and more irregular and may contribute to plaque instability and the onset of thromboembolic sequelae.

Fibromuscular Dysplasia

Fibromuscular dysplasia (FMD) is the commonest nonatherosclerotic disease to affect the ICA. Approximately one quarter of patients with carotid FMD have associated intracranial aneurysms, and up to two thirds of these patients will have bilateral carotid fibromuscular dysplasia.

Fibromuscular dysplasia can be divided into three pathological subtypes. *Medial fibroplasia* is the most common (>85% of cases) and is usually found in long segment arteries with few side branches. It is characterized by stenoses alternating with intervening fusiform dilatations that resemble a string of beads, particularly in the upper ICA. Pathologically, smooth muscle cells in the outer media are replaced by compact fibrous connective tissue, whereas the inner media contains excess collagen and ground substance in disorganized smooth muscle cells. Because of its prevalence in females, a possible role for estrogen and progesterone has been postulated. Others have suggested that the absence of vasa vasorum in long nonbranching arteries such as the ICA or renal arteries may predispose to mural ischemia that leads to the development of fibromuscular dysplasia.

Intimal fibroplasia accounts for less than 10% of cases of FMD and affects men and women equally. It typically appears as a focal narrowing in older patients and long segmental stenoses in younger patients. The lesion is confined to the intimal layer while the medial and adventitial structures are always normal. Its pathophysiology is due to irregularly aligned subendothelial mesenchymal cells within a loose matrix of connective tissue. *Perimedial dysplasia* is characterized by accumulation of elastic tissue between the media and the adventitia. This subtype predominantly affects the ICA and renal arteries and may be associated with secondary aneurysm formation.

Coils and Kinks of the Extracranial Carotid Arteries

Redundancy of the extracranial carotid artery is thought to be due to abnormalities in development. Occasionally, the ICA may undergo a complete 360-degree rotation. The ICA is derived embryologically from the third aortic arch and the dorsal aortic root. In its early stages, a normally occurring redundancy is straightened as the heart and great vessels descend into the mediastinum. Incomplete descent of the heart and great vessels may result in the development of complex coils and kinks. These are bilateral in approximately 50% of affected patients.

Elongation of the ICA, which can also result in kinking of the ICA, is usually due to degenerative changes associated with increasing age and atherosclerosis. The loss of elasticity of the arterial wall due to the aging process (coupled with hemodynamic shear stresses) predisposes toward kinks of the elongated carotid artery between the proximal and distal fixed points of the skull base and thoracic inlet.

Carotid Artery Aneurysms

As with aneurysms anywhere else in the body, carotid aneurysms may be either true or false. In the past, most true aneurysms (Fig. 15.3) have traditionally been classified as part of the atherosclerotic process, but emerging evidence suggests that aneurysmal disease may be yet another manifestation of abnormalities of matrix metalloproteinase enzyme expression and production, unless associated with other distinct pathologies, for example, arteritis (giant cell, Takayasu) or FMD. False aneurysms may arise as a consequence of iatrogenic injury, blunt trauma, spontaneous dissection, or infection (e.g., prosthetic patch infection after carotid endarterectomy).

Carotid Dissection

Acute carotid dissection can complicate atherosclerosis, FMD, cystic medial necrosis, or blunt

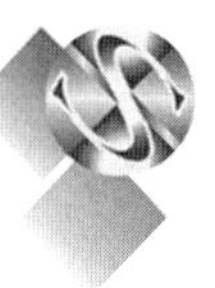

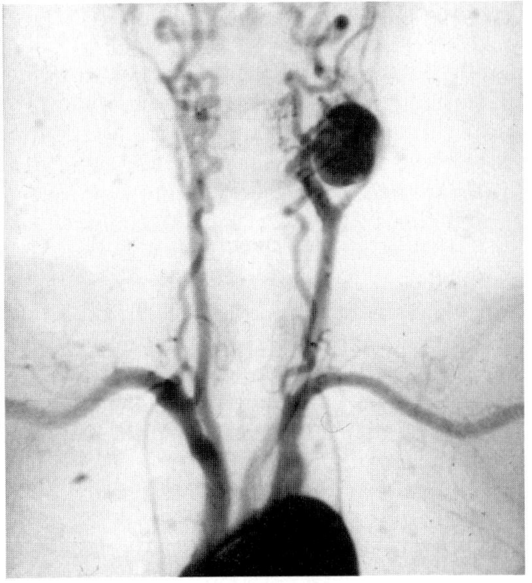

Figure 15.3. Intraarterial digital subtraction angiogram of the aortic arch and great vessels. There is a large aneurysm just beyond the left carotid bifurcation.

more prevalent in Asia and usually affects young females. Its pathogenesis relates to an inflammatory process involving all three layers of the arterial wall with proliferation of connective tissue and degeneration of the elastic fibers. Granulomatous lesions may also develop, and the condition may also be associated with fusiform or saccular aneurysms.

Takayasu's arteritis is classified according to its mode of involvement. Type I involves branches of the aortic arch; type IIa involves the ascending aorta, aortic arch, and branches; type IIb involves the vessels involved in IIa plus the descending aorta; type III involves the descending thoracic aorta and abdominal aorta (with or without renal arteries); type IV involves the abdominal aorta (with or without renal arteries) and type V involves a combination of type IIb and IV.

trauma, or be associated with a collagen vascular disorder such as Ehlers-Danlos syndrome type IV or Marfan syndrome. Angiographic studies suggest that the most likely mechanism is an intimal tear followed by an acute intimal dissection, which produces luminal occlusion due to secondary thrombosis within the false lumen. This appears as a flame-shaped occlusion 2 to 3 cm beyond the bifurcation (Fig. 15.4). Autopsy studies typically reveal a sharply demarcated transition between the normal carotid artery and the dissected carotid segment. The ICA is commonly affected, with the dissection plane typically occurring in the outer medial layer. The classical triad of clinical signs/symptoms following carotid dissection include (1) pain in the face and neck (20%), (2) a partial Horner syndrome (50%), and (3) retinal or cerebral ischemia (50% to 90%). About one in ten will suffer cranial nerve palsy.

Takayasu's Arteritis

Takayasu's arteritis (TA) is a nonspecific arteritis affecting the thoracic and abdominal aorta and their major branches. Although this disease is uncommon in Western countries, it is

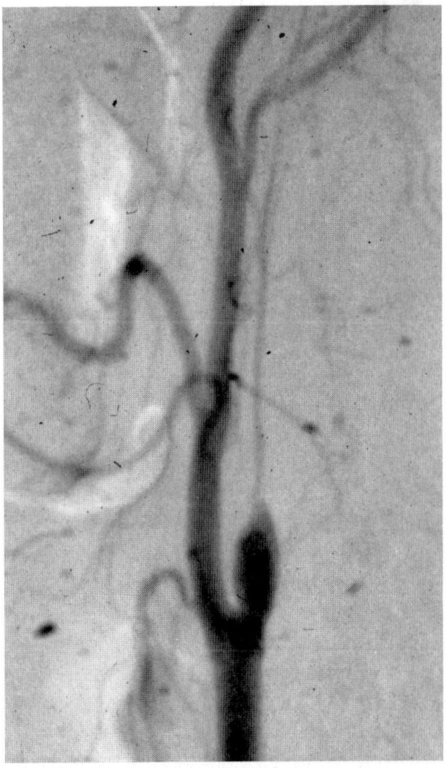

Figure 15.4. Selective intraarterial digital subtraction angiogram in a patient with acute carotid dissection. The internal carotid artery is almost completely occluded 2 to 3 cm beyond the origin of the internal carotid artery. There is virtually no flow visible up the true lumen.

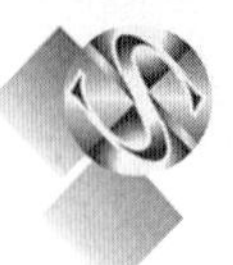

Giant Cell Arteritis

Giant cell arteritis predominantly affects elderly women. Although it commonly involves the temporal arteries, it can involve other major vessels including the carotid artery and upper extremity vasculature. There is usually tenderness over the inflamed artery. Laboratory evaluation generally reveals elevation of C-reactive protein and the erythrocyte sedimentation rate. Biopsy of an affected artery shows characteristic giant cell granulomata with abundant T lymphocytes. However, a negative biopsy does not exclude the diagnosis. Management of giant cell arteritis usually includes the use of high-dose corticosteroids as well as other forms of immunosuppression including cyclophosphamide or azathioprine. Steroids can usually be tailed off after 1 year of treatment.

Radiation Arteritis

The principal effects of radiation on arteries include immediate arterial spasm and endothelial denudation, intimal disruption, subintimal edema, and degeneration of collagen and smooth muscle. These acute changes predispose toward an increase in vessel wall permeability to circulating lipids, which produce a plaque characterized by fibrosis, fatty infiltration, and elastic tissue destruction. Hyperlipidemia and hypercholesterolemia appear to predispose patients who have received radiation therapy to develop accelerated atherosclerotic lesions. The sensitivity of elastic tissue to radiation may account for the mechanism of structural weakening and eventual rupture in elastic arteries.

As a result of the increased use of external radiation to treat neck malignancies, a rise in radiation-induced atherosclerotic disease in association with symptomatic carotid stenosis has been noted. Radiation-induced carotid lesions can present either in a segmental or diffuse manner. The affected carotid segments typically lie within the field of radiation treatment. One or both common carotid arteries may be involved, whereas the carotid bifurcation is often spared. The severity of carotid injury is related to radiation dose. Smaller doses cause less cellular damage, whereas larger doses may even lead to arterial wall necrosis.

Carotid Body Tumor

Carotid body tumors (CBTs) originate from the chemoreceptor cells located at the carotid bifurcation. Because cells of the carotid body typically detect change in the PO_2, PCO_2, and pH, CBTs have been reported to be more prevalent in individuals who live at high altitudes, which suggests that chronic hypoxia may be an etiological factor. A CBT typically presents as a palpable, painless mass over the carotid bifurcation region in the neck. Cranial nerve palsy may occur in up to 25% of patients, particularly involving the vagus and hypoglossal nerves. The differential diagnosis includes cervical lymphadenopathy, carotid artery aneurysm, branchial cleft cyst, laryngeal carcinoma, and metastatic tumor.

The treatment of choice of CBT is surgical excision. Because these tumors are highly vascularized, preoperative tumor embolization has been advocated by some surgeons to minimize operative blood loss when dealing with tumors >3 cm in diameter, but there is no consensus on this strategy. An important surgical principle in CBT resection is to maintain the plane of dissection within the subadventitial space, which enables complete tumor excision without interrupting carotid artery integrity.

Carotid Trauma

Blunt trauma to the neck can cause carotid artery injury either by forceful compression or extension of the artery. Common scenarios include motor vehicle or motorcycle accidents, pedestrian injuries, hanging, or strangulation.

Patients with carotid trauma may present with focal physical findings such as neck hematoma, pulsatile cervical mass, carotid bruit, or localized bleeding. More generalized physical findings include loss of consciousness and lateralizing neurological deficits. Arteriography remains the diagnostic test of choice for carotid trauma, since it has the highest sensitivity and specificity compared to all other imaging modalities. Treatment of all blunt carotid artery injuries usually involves anticoagulation. Antiplatelet therapy should be considered if systemic anticoagulation is contraindicated.

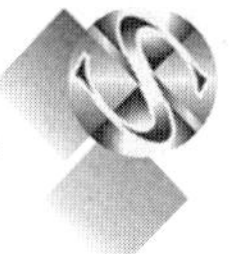

Clinical Presentation of Carotid Disease

Syndromes

Transient Ischemic Attack

A transient ischemic attack is a focal loss of neurological function (lasting <24 hours) that has a vascular cause upon investigation. It is conventional to describe a TIA as being carotid or vertebrobasilar (see below).

Completed Stroke

A completed stroke is a focal (occasionally global) loss of neurological function, lasting for more than 24 hours, that is found to have a vascular cause upon investigation. The term *completed* refers to the fact that the severity of the neurological deficit has now reached its maximum.

Stroke in Evolution

A stroke in evolution is a progressive worsening of the neurological deficit, either linearly over a 24-hour period or interspersed with transient periods of stabilization and/or partial clinical improvement.

Crescendo Transient Ischemic Attacks

This condition has never been properly defined. Traditionally, it refers to a syndrome comprising repeated TIAs within a short period of time with complete neurological recovery in between. At a minimum, the term should probably be reserved for those with daily events.

Hemodynamic Transient Ischemic Attacks

These attacks are focal cerebral events (hemisensory or retinal) that are aggravated by exercise or hemodynamic stress and typically occur after short bursts of physical activity, postprandially or after getting out of a hot bath. It is implied that they are due to severe extracranial disease and poor intracranial collateral recruitment.

Nonhemispheric Symptoms

These are a group of nonfocal symptoms that, on their own, are not indicative of true carotid or vertebrobasilar events. Classical nonhemispheric symptoms include isolated dizziness, isolated vertigo, isolated syncope (drop attacks, blackouts), isolated double vision (diplopia), and presyncope (faintness). In the absence of any corroborative carotid or vertebrobasilar symptoms, they cannot be ascribed to extracranial carotid or vertebral disease alone.

Clinical Features

Ocular Symptoms

Ocular symptoms associated with extracranial carotid and vertebrobasilar disease include amaurosis fugax (transient monocular blindness), Hollenhorst plaques, retinal/optic nerve ischemia, the ocular ischemia syndrome, and visual field deficits secondary to cortical infarction and ischemia of the optic tracts.

The blood supply to the retina originates from two sources. The short posterior ciliary arteries supply the outer two layers, together with the optic disk and optic nerve. The central retinal artery supplies the inner layers of the retina. Amaurosis fugax is a temporary loss of vision in one eye (likened to a shutter coming down), but which can also refer to graying of the vision. The blindness usually lasts for a few minutes and then resolves. Most (>90%) are due to embolic occlusion of the main artery or its upper/lower divisions. It remains unclear, however, why some patients always have repeated episodes of amaurosis and never hemispheric signs.

Monocular blindness progressing over a 20-minute period suggests a migrainous etiology. Hemodynamic amaurosis is rare but can be precipitated by heavy exercise or arising from a hot bath. In this situation, where there is a severe carotid stenosis and poor collateralization, the visual loss tends to start at the periphery and move toward the center. Occasionally, a patient recalls no visual symptoms, but the optician notes a yellowish plaque within the retinal vessels (the Hollenhorst plaque). This is frequently derived from cholesterol embolization from the carotid bifurcation and it warrants further investigation (Fig. 15.5).

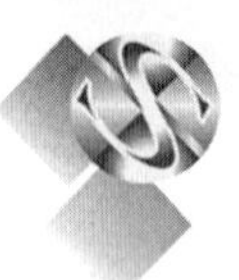

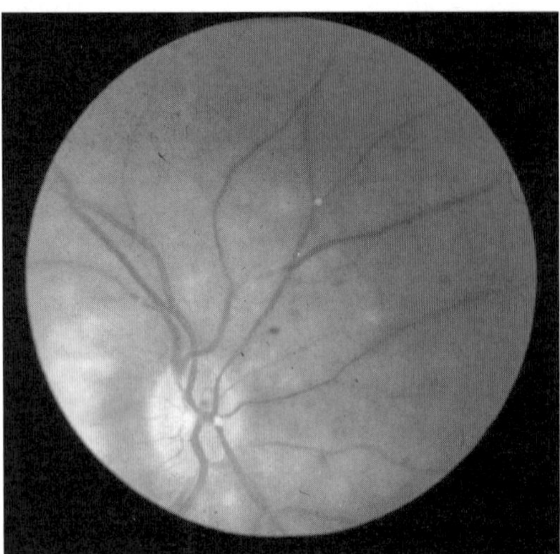

Figure 15.5. Funduscopic examination. Note the two cholesterol emboli within the retinal vessels.

Monocular visual loss due to central retinal artery occlusion, persisting for more than 24 hours is analogous to cerebral infarction, with the occlusive process usually occurring in the intraneural part of the central retinal artery. In addition to an embolic etiology, it is also important to consider microatheroma, and arteritis in occasional patients with other atypical symptoms. Bilateral visual loss (cortical blindness) is due to infarction of the visual cortex in the occipital lobe and therefore is never a carotid territory event.

The optic nerve head can be rendered ischemic by thromboembolic phenomena, although it is rarely due to extracranial carotid artery disease. Optic nerve ischemia is usually due to intrinsic disease of the short posterior ciliary arteries and can present as an acute loss of either central or peripheral vision in one eye. If the upper or lower visual fields are lost, this suggests occlusion of the upper and lower branch divisions of the ciliary artery.

The ocular-ischemia syndrome is a relatively rare condition where there is global under-perfusion of the eye, deteriorating monocular vision, and excessive proliferation of the conjunctival vessels. It is indicative of extremely poor eye collateralization.

Homonymous hemianopia can occur as a consequence of ischemia at varying points in the optic tracts. Occipital lesions cause a congruous homonymous hemianopia (visual field defects exactly overlap in each eye). Homonymous hemianopia involving the lower visual fields is usually due to a parietal infarction and follows ischemia of the upper fibers of the visual pathway that traverse the parietal lobe. Conversely, temporal lobe infarcts can extend to involve the lower fibers of the visual pathways and so cause a hemianopia involving the upper fields. Of practical importance is the observation that homonymous hemianopia secondary to occipital lesions tends to cause a very perceptible visual void to the patient. In contrast, the patient with homonymous hemianopia due to parietal or temporal lobe lesions is often unaware of the deficit and may bump into objects.

Motor/Sensory Symptoms

A number of cerebral pathologies can cause motor or sensory symptoms that may mimic the focal symptoms observed in TIA or stroke. These primarily include intracranial hemorrhage, tumor, migrainous phenomena, and arteritis. Overall, the pattern of onset in conjunction with the distribution and nature of the symptoms enables the clinician to be more discriminating in developing a differential diagnosis.

Ischemic events tend to have an abrupt onset, with the severity of the insult being apparent from the outset. By contrast, motor/sensory signs associated with migraine often progress from one part of the body to the next over a 15- to 20-minute period of time. Ischemic TIAs rarely include positive phenomena. For example, the hemisensory/motor signs with ischemic TIAs are not usually associated with seizure or paresthesia but represent loss or diminution of neurological function. Migrainous or postictal events frequently include seizures, clonic contractions, and enhanced sensory phenomena.

Motor/sensory deficits can be unilateral or bilateral, with the upper and lower limbs being variably affected depending on the site of the cerebral lesion. For example, occlusion of the anterior cerebral artery causes a hemiparesis, with the leg being more severely affected than the arm. The combination of a motor and sensory deficit in the same body territory is suggestive of a cortical thromboembolic event as opposed to lacunar lesions secondary to small-vessel disease of the penetrating arterioles. However, a small proportion of the latter may present with a sensorimotor stroke secondary to small-vessel occlusion within the posterior limb of the internal capsule. Pure sensory and pure motor strokes and those strokes where the weakness affects one limb only or does not involve the face are more typically seen with lacunar as opposed to cortical infarction.

Higher Cortical Dysfunction

A number of clinical phenomena, including speech and language disturbances, can be caused by thromboembolic phenomena within the anterior and posterior circulations. There are a large number of examples of higher cortical dysfunction (dysphasia, apraxia, visuospatial neglect, alexia) that are beyond the scope of this review. However, the most important clinical example for the dominant hemisphere is expressive dysphasia/aphasia, with visuospatial neglect being an example of nondominant hemisphere injury.

Dysphasia is a language disorder as opposed to dysarthria, which is a locomotor speech problem. Differentiation between the two is important, as dysarthria is a vertebrobasilar symptom whereas dysphasia is of carotid origin. In expressive dysphasia, patients know what they wish to say but either cannot find the word or produce seemingly meaningless verbal output. Dysarthria can be defined as a simple inability to "get your tongue" around the word. Visuospatial neglect is the result of injury to the nondominant parietal lobe. Here patients may exhibit inattention to one side of their body.

Carotid or Vertebrobasilar Territory?

Typical carotid territory symptoms (anterior and middle cerebral arteries) include hemisensory/motor symptoms, amaurosis fugax, and evidence of higher cortical dysfunction. Homonymous hemianopia alone is not a feature of injury to the carotid territory. Classical vertebrobasilar symptoms comprise bilateral motor/sensory symptoms, bilateral visual loss, homonymous hemianopia, dysarthria, nystagmus, ataxia and gait problems, dysphagia and dizziness, and vertigo, provided they accompany other vertebrobasilar features.

Discrimination between carotid and vertebrobasilar symptoms is usually straightforward but can be difficult. For example, 10% of patients with vertebrobasilar stroke have hemisensory/motor signs. This is because of anatomical variations in the vascular boundary zones between the carotid and vertebrobasilar system. Similarly, a small number of patients with thromboembolic carotid artery disease present with vertebrobasilar symptoms because the posterior cerebral artery is embryologically derived from the carotid artery as opposed to the vertebrobasilar system. If there is any question regarding interpretation of the clinical picture, advice from a neurologist or stroke physician should be sought.

Clinical Features of Nonatherosclerotic Disease

One of the characteristic features of the nonatherosclerotic pathologies listed earlier is the potential for thrombosis/stenosis and aneurysm formation. Accordingly, each condition can cause ischemic stroke/TIA, but most are relatively rare. The onset of stroke/TIA in a patient exhibiting other atypical features should raise the possibility of a nonatheromatous pathology. Sudden onset of temporal headache or neck pain associated with a neurological or visual deficit is suggestive of carotid dissection. The initial neurological symptoms are thought to be due to acute expansion of the dissection resulting in compression of cranial nerves IX, X, XI, or XII, followed by cerebral ischemia. Horner syndrome can also occur, which is believed to be due to disruption of periadventitial sympathetic fibers adjacent to the carotid artery. Systemic illness, malaise, weight loss, and myalgia suggest an underlying arteritis (Takayasu, giant cell, SLE, polyarteritis). Jaw claudication is an important presentation in giant cell arteritis. Takayasu arteritis patients also present with symptoms attributable to involved vascular beds (renovascular hypertension, TIA/stroke, MI).

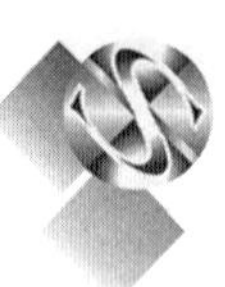

it does not alter management decisions, and it incurs undue cost.

In an ideal world, all patients should undergo functional imaging (preferably MRI) combined with MRA. However, all clinicians would agree that patients presenting with a stroke require imaging within 2 weeks of onset (so as to identify patients with intracranial hemorrhage), as should patients reporting atypical symptoms (seizure, progressive neurological symptoms, headaches, cranial nerve signs). Centers that continue to advocate routine CT/MRI must ensure that implementation of such a policy does not lead to unacceptable delays in planning management strategies.

Management of Occlusive Carotid Artery Disease

Best Medical Therapy

There is more to investigating and treating patients with stroke or TIA than simply identifying those who might benefit from carotid endarterectomy. More importantly, the implementation of the best medical therapy should not be delegated to the most junior member of the team. Although some risk factors (age, sex, gender, family history) are nonmodifiable, there is an increasing body of systematic evidence to guide the clinician with regard to implementing optimal medical therapy in patients with cerebral vascular disease.

Antiplatelet Therapy

Aspirin irreversibly blocks cyclooxygenase-mediated breakdown of arachidonic acid, thereby inhibiting the formation of thromboxane A_2 (platelet aggregator and vasoconstrictor). Meta-analyses have shown no evidence that aspirin has any beneficial role in the primary prevention of stroke. However, in patients with a history of vascular disease, the Antiplatelet Trialists' Collaboration showed that aspirin conferred a 22% relative risk reduction (RRR) in all vascular events (nonfatal stroke, nonfatal MI, vascular death). A more recent meta-analysis has shown that aspirin confers a 15% reduction in stroke alone in patients presenting with symptomatic cerebral vascular disease.

There has been much debate about the optimal aspirin dose. A balance must be struck, as there is a 1.0% annual risk of adverse events associated with aspirin therapy, with the risk increasing as the aspirin dose increases. In Europe, there is a trend toward using low-dose aspirin (50 to 150 mg daily), whereas larger doses have previously been recommended in North America (300 to 1200 mg). Meta-analyses have shown that aspirin doses of <100 mg daily confer a 13% RRR in subsequent vascular events in patients with a presenting history of stroke or TIA, falling to 9% for medium doses (300 mg daily) and 14% for daily doses in excess of 900 mg. The North American Symptomatic Carotid Endarterectomy Trial (NASCET) originally observed that the incidence of perioperative stroke was significantly higher in patients receiving lower-dose aspirin. However, a subsequent randomized trial in more than 2500 patients undergoing carotid endarterectomy indicated that the 30-day risk of stroke, MI, or death was significantly lower in patients taking 81 mg or 325 mg aspirin as compared with 650 to 1300 mg.

Dipyridamole inhibits platelet aggregation by partially blocking the adenosine diphosphate (ADP) receptor on the platelet and by elevating levels of cyclic adenosine monophosphate (cAMP) and cyclic guanosine monophosphate (cGMP). Dipyridamole on its own does not significantly reduce the risk of secondary stroke, but a number of studies have suggested that combination therapy with aspirin is more effective. This has been confirmed in a recent meta-analysis that showed that aspirin and dipyridamole conferred a 23% RRR in stroke. However, the benefit was slightly offset by the fact that about a quarter of patients experienced adverse side effects, necessitating dipyridamole withdrawal.

Ticlopidine and clopidogrel have similar modes of action. Both inhibit platelet activation through inhibition of ADP binding to its platelet receptor, thereby blocking the GpIIb-IIIa receptor complex that is the principal receptor for platelet fibrinogen binding. Although some studies showed a beneficial reduction in the risk of stroke, an overview by the Antiplatelet Trialists' Collaboration suggested that ticlopidine conferred no extra benefit over aspirin alone in terms of reducing the risk of all vascular events. However, ticlopidine was associated with a 20% incidence of adverse complications including neutropenia in 2% and a tendency to increased cholesterol levels. Overall, 6% of patients had to stop the drug.

Clopidogrel is the newest antiplatelet agent and has a greater antiplatelet effect than ticlopidine. Although the CAPRIE study observed a significant reduction in the incidence of vascular events in favor of clopidogrel (75 mg daily), as compared with aspirin (325 mg daily), it should be borne in mind that the relative risk reduction was 8.7%, the absolute risk reduction only 0.5%, and subgroup analyses failed to show a significant reduction in stroke risk relative to all vascular events (CAPRIE Steering Committee, 1996). In the U.K., a course of clopidogrel is 30 times more expensive than aspirin.

In summary, aspirin remains the antiplatelet agent of choice. The dose should be between 75 and 300 mg daily, and therapy should continue throughout the perioperative period in patients undergoing carotid endarterectomy. Medically treated patients who suffer repeated thromboembolic events while on aspirin should either have dipyridamole (200 mg) added to the aspirin regime or convert to clopidogrel (75 mg daily). Clopidogrel is preferable to dipyridamole alone in patients who are aspirin intolerant. Surgeons, however, should be aware that clopidogrel trebles the bleeding time whereas a combination of aspirin and full-dose clopidogrel increases the bleeding time by a factor of five as compared with aspirin alone.

Treatment of Hypertension

A systematic review of randomized trials comprising 48,000 hypertensive patients found that a sustained reduction of 5 mm Hg in diastolic blood pressure over a 3-year period was associated with a 38% reduction in the risk of late stroke (Collins and MacMahon, 1994). However, relatively few of these patients had a prior history of stroke or TIA. More recently, the Antithrombotic Trialists' Collaboration performed a review of the randomized trial data from 150,000 patients with cerebral or coronary events, and found that for every 5 mm Hg reduction in the diastolic blood pressure, there was a 15% relative reduction in the risk of stroke. Interestingly, there was no evidence of a lower diastolic threshold below which the risk of stroke did not fall.

There remains some controversy over the threshold for therapeutic intervention in patients with hypertension. In the U.S., the recommendation is to maintain blood pressure less than 140/90 mm Hg, whereas in the U.K. the advice is for control to also reflect the age of the patient. The exception might be the diabetic patient with hypertension who warrants more careful control of blood pressure (see below). The one other golden rule is that patients undergoing carotid endarterectomy should not undergo surgery with uncontrolled hypertension, as this is associated with a twofold excess risk of perioperative stroke.

Smoking

For obvious reasons, there have never been any randomized trials comparing stroke risk in patients who continue to smoke! A meta-analysis of epidemiological and cohort studies indicates that the relative risk of stroke is doubled in smokers as opposed to nonsmokers. The excess risk of stroke declines with time after smoking cessation and is equivalent to that of nonsmokers after about 5 years.

Diabetes

Diabetes is associated with a twofold excess risk of stroke, and, intuitively, one would have thought that careful glycemic control would be associated with a significant reduction in stroke risk. However, one of the few randomized trials to address this issue showed that the risk of late stroke appeared to be unchanged in patients randomized to aggressive glycemic control. The available evidence suggests that it is the *hypertensive type 2 diabetic* who is most at risk of late stroke. The U.K. Prospective Diabetes Study Group randomized hypertensive, type 2 diabetic patients to strict antihypertensive therapy (mean blood pressure 144/82 mm Hg) or less stringent control (mean blood pressure 154/87 mm Hg). During follow-up, the former strategy was associated with a 44% reduction in late stroke.

Treatment of Atrial Fibrillation

About 20% of all strokes are secondary to nonvalvular atrial fibrillation (NVAF). Approxi-

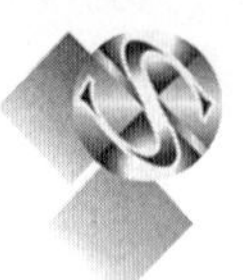

mately 5% of the population aged >65 years have NVAF, incurring a 3% to 5% annual risk of stroke. Treatment with warfarin reduces the risk of stroke by 68% but decisions regarding the role of anticoagulation must take into account the potential hemorrhagic risks. The annual risk of significant bleeding in anticoagulated patients is 1.3%, including a 0.3% incidence of intracranial hemorrhage. Patients at increased risk of significant hemorrhage include those with the following findings: a previous history of bleeding, age >75 years, an international normalized ratio (INR) >3.0, fluctuating INRs, and uncontrolled hypertension.

Although each case must be considered individually, it is generally recommended that patients considered high risk for embolic stroke be warfarinized with a target INR of <3.0. High-risk patients (6% annual stroke risk) include (1) those of any age with a past history of TIA or stroke, rheumatic heart disease, ischemic heart disease, and evidence of impaired left ventricular function on echocardiography; and (2) patients aged >75 years with hypertension and/or diabetes. Low-risk patients (1% annual stroke risk), including patients aged <65 years with no risk factors, should be treated with aspirin. The medium-risk group (2% annual stroke risk) are more difficult to categorize. It comprises (1) those aged <65 years with a history of diabetes, hypertension, peripheral vascular disease, and ischemic heart disease who should be warfarinized; and (2) those aged 65 to 75 with no risk factors in whom it might be reasonable to treat with aspirin. Aspirin therapy should be considered in all patients with NVAF who are unable to take warfarin.

Treatment of Hyperlipidemia

In a meta-analysis of the available epidemiological studies (450,000 patients), no association was observed between cholesterol level and overall stroke rate. However, meaningful interpretation of these data was confounded by the fact that although a higher cholesterol level was associated with an increased risk of ischemic stroke, this was offset by an increased risk of hemorrhagic stroke in patients with lower cholesterol levels. A subsequent systematic review of randomized trials indicated that statin therapy was associated with a 25% reduction in the risk of late stroke, but only in those patients with coexistent symptomatic ischemic heart disease. The principal problem regarding planning lipid lowering therapy based on evidence is that most of the randomized trials have been undertaken in patients with coronary heart disease. Few have specifically examined the role of statin therapy in patients with TIA or stroke, although several should be reporting in the next year or so.

In the U.K., there is conflicting advice regarding statin therapy. The National Service Framework for Coronary Heart Disease recommends statin therapy (cholesterol to be reduced to <5 mmol/L) in all patients with coronary heart disease or *other occlusive disease* (including those with TIA or stroke irrespective of cardiac status). In contrast, the National Clinical Guidelines for Stroke recommends therapeutic intervention only in patients with symptomatic cerebrovascular disease *and* coronary heart disease. This conflicting advice will almost certainly be revised following the recent publication of the British Heart Protection Study. This trial randomized 20,000 patients with vascular disease (including stroke/TIA) to placebo or simvastatin (40 mg daily). Overall, statin therapy conferred a 12% reduction in all mortality, a 17% reduction in vascular mortality, a 24% reduction in all coronary events, and a 27% reduction in stroke. Of most importance was the observation that there did not appear to be any lower cholesterol limit below which benefit was not observed.

In the U.S., statin therapy is advised in all patients with TIA/stroke and coronary heart disease. In patients with no coronary heart disease and fewer than two vascular risk factors (selected from men aged >45 years, women aged >55 years, family history of heart disease, smoking, hypertension, diabetes, high-density lipoprotein (HDL) cholesterol <35 mg/dL), the advice is to try dietary modification for 6 months and to introduce statin therapy only if the low-density lipoprotein (LDL) cholesterol is >190 mg/dL with a target of <160 mg/dL. The TIA/stroke patients with no history of coronary heart disease (but having more than two risk factors) should undergo dietary modification for 6 months followed by statin therapy if the LDL cholesterol is >160 mg/dL with a target of reducing it to <130 mg/dL.

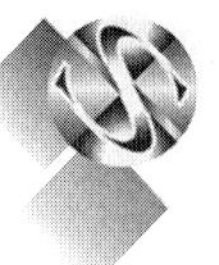

Surgery for Occlusive disease

Carotid endarterectomy (CEA) is one of the few surgical procedures to have been subjected to evidence-based scrutiny with large, multicenter randomized trials. An overview of the principal results from the European Carotid Surgery Trial (ECST), the NASCET, and the Asymptomatic Carotid Atherosclerosis Study (ACAS) is presented below. One other carotid surgical procedure (extracranial–intracranial bypass) has been intermittently advocated for recurrent TIAs/stroke in the presence of a chronically occluded ICA. This procedure was popularized during the 1980s, but a randomized trial thereafter showed no level I evidence of benefit. The methodology of this study has been challenged but few surgeons currently advocate this form of surgery.

Overview of ECST and NASCET

In ECST and NASCET almost 6000 patients in over 200 centers around the world were randomized, comparing "best medical therapy" against "best medical therapy" and CEA. All patients had to have reported ipsilateral carotid territory symptoms within the preceding 6 months; all were seen by a neurologist prior to randomization and all underwent CT scanning and contrast angiography. Follow-up was coordinated by the neurologists and stroke physicians.

The basic results are summarized in Table 15.1. Both trials showed that CEA conferred significant benefit in symptomatic patients with a 70% to 99% stenosis. The ECST found no evidence of benefit in patients with lesser degrees of disease. The NASCET observed a small but significant benefit in patients with 50% to 69% stenoses. The reason for these apparent discrepancies lies in the method for calculating degree of stenosis. The ECST compared the residual luminal diameter against the diameter of the carotid artery at the level of the stenosis (usually the carotid bulb). The NASCET compared the residual luminal diameter against the diameter of the ICA at least 1 cm above the stenosis. As a consequence, the ECST tends to systematically overestimate stenoses (as compared with the NASCET method), particularly in those with mild/moderate disease. In reality, a 50% NASCET stenosis is approximately equivalent to a 65% ECST, whereas a 70% NASCET stenosis equates to an 82% ECST.

The ECST and NASCET have identified predictive factors that are associated with a significantly higher risk of late stroke in medically treated patients. These include male sex, 90% to 94% stenosis, surface irregularity/ulceration, coexistent syphon or intracranial

Table 15.1. Long-term risk of ipsilateral stroke (including perioperative stroke or death)

Trial stenosis (%)	Surgical risk (%)	Medical risk (%)	ARR (%)	RRR (%)	NNT	Strokes prevented per 1000 CEAs
ECST						
<30%	9.8 at 5 y	3.9 at 5 y	−5.9	n/a	n/a	n/a
30–49%	10.2 at 5 y	8.2 at 5 y	−2.0	n/a	n/a	n/a
50–69%	15.0 at 5 y	12.1 at 5 y	−2.9	n/a	n/a	n/a
70–99%	10.5 at 5 y	19.0 at 5 y	+8.5	45	12	83 at 5 y
NASCET						
30–49%	14.9 at 5 y	18.7 at 5 y	+3.8	20	26	38 at 5 y
50–69%	15.7 at 3 y	22.2 at 3 y	+6.5	29	15	67 at 3 y
70–99%	8.9 at 3 y	28.3 at 3 y	+19.4	69	5	200 at 3 y
ACAS						
60–99%	5.1 at 5 y	11.0 at 5 y	+5.9	53	17	59 at 5 y
ACST						
60–99%	6.4 at 5 y	11.8 at 5 y	+5.4	46	19	53 at 5 y

ARR, absolute risk reduction; RRR, relative risk reduction; NNT, number of CEAs to prevent one ipsilateral stroke at specified time interval; n/a = not applicable; y, years.

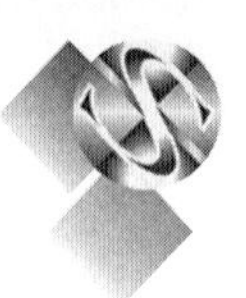

disease, no recruitment of intracranial collaterals, hemispheric symptoms, cerebral events within 2 months, multiple cerebral events, contralateral occlusion, multiple concurrent risk factors, and age >75 years. In contrast, a lower relative risk of stroke is observed in patients with lesser degrees of disease [70% to 79% stenosis (ECST), 50% to 69% (NASCET)], near occlusion with a string sign, smooth stenoses, female sex, retinal symptoms, and those presenting with lacunar stroke.

A pooled analysis of data from the ECST, NASCET, and the Veterans Affairs (VA) trial has recently been performed (Rothwell et al., 2003). All the angiograms were standardized to the NASCET method, and the overall database contained >6000 randomized patients. Table 15.2 summarizes the 30-day death/any stroke rates following endarterectomy for each of the principal trials. Overall, 7.1% of patients [95% confidence interval (CI) 6.3–8.1] in the three trials either died or suffered a stroke within 30 days of surgery. This is an important observation, as the track record for all participating surgeons was vetted before they were allowed to randomize patients.

Figure 15.6 illustrates how the benefit of CEA increases with time and with increasing degrees of stenosis. By contrast, CEA was harmful in patients with <50% stenoses. It conferred a small but significant benefit in symptomatic patients with 50% to 69% stenoses, with the maximal benefit being observed in patients with 70% to 99% stenoses. Note, however, that patients with near-occlusion did not derive any systematic benefit from CEA. Near-occlusion was defined angiographically as severe stenosis with evidence of reduced flow in the distal ICA (delayed arrival of contrast in the distal ICA or recruitment of collateral flow toward the symptomatic hemisphere, or both) and evidence of narrowing of the poststenotic ICA (lumen diameter similar to, or less than, that of the ipsilateral external carotid artery and less than that of the contralateral ICA). Accordingly, there is increasing evidence that patients with subocclusion and distal vessel collapse should be treated conservatively.

Overview of ACAS and ACST

A number of randomized studies have evaluated the role of CEA in patients with severe asymptomatic carotid artery disease (MACE, CASANOVA, VA study), but ACAS and ACST are generally accepted to be the best (ACST, Lancet 2004). The ACAS randomized 1600 patients with asymptomatic 60% to 99% stenoses. Table 15.1 summarizes the principal findings. Although there was a 53% RRR in late stroke, this only equated to a 5.9% actual risk reduction at 5 years. Clinicians in North America and mainland Europe have embraced the findings of ACAS more liberally than their U.K. or Scandinavian colleagues. In the latter countries, concerns remain that the ACAS showed no benefit in women, there was no reduction in disabling stroke, and (unlike ECST and NASCET) no relationship between increasing stenosis and stroke

Table 15.2. Analysis of pooled data from the ECST, NASCET, and the Veterans Affairs trial: 30-day risk of death and/or stroke after carotid endarterectomy

Trial	<50%	50–69%	≥70%	Near occlusion
ECST	73/1044 7.0% (5.4–8.6)	37/371 10.0% (6.9–13.1)	17/249 6.8% (4.0–10.8)	3/78 3.8% (0.8–10.8)
NASCET	43/663 6.5% (4.7–8.6)	30/421 7.1% (4.8–10)	14/261 5.4% (3.0–8.8)	5/70 7.1% (2.4–15)
VA309		2/20 10.0% (1.2–3.2)	5/71 7.0% (2.3–15.7)	
Combined	116/1707 6.8% (5.6–8.0)	69/812 8.5% (6.6–10.5)	36/581 6.2% (4.4–8.5)	8/148 5.4% (2.4–10.4)

Note: The data shown are the observed percents. The 95% confidence interval is shown in parentheses.
Source: Adapted from Rothwell et al. (2003). Here the individual data from each trial were reanalyzed and combined after having standardized all the angiograms to the NASCET method of stenosis measurement.

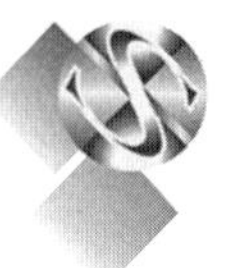

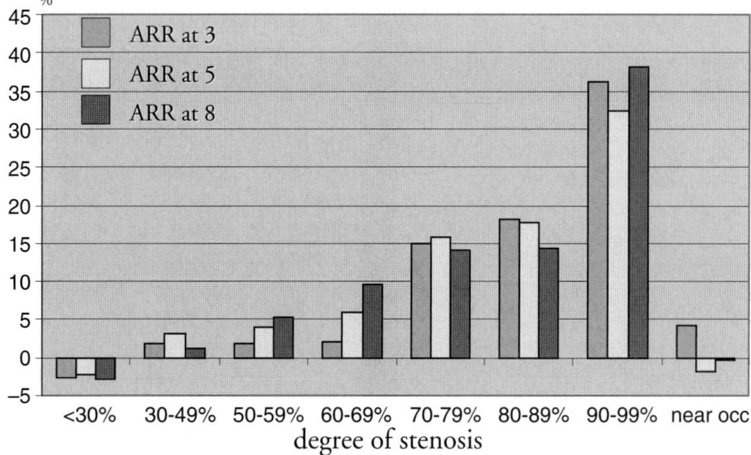

Figure 15.6. Pooled results from European Carotid Surgery Trial (ECST), the North American Symptomatic Carotid Endarterectomy Trial (NASCET), and Veterans Affairs (VA) studies, showing the absolute risk reduction (ARR) in stroke at 3, 5, and 8 years relative to the degree of stenosis at randomization. Note that the maximal benefit was observed in patients with 90% to 99% stenoses, whereas patients with near occlusion and distal vessel collapse or underfilling (string sign) did not benefit from CEA. (From Rothwell et al., 2003.)

risk (in fact there was an inverse relationship). Table 15.1 also summarizes the principal results from the ACST. Note that the results were very similar to those of the ACAS. However, the key finding from ACST was a 50% reduction in fatal or disabling stroke long term.

Carotid Endarterectomy

Operative Principles

The carotid bifurcation is usually approached via a longitudinal incision based on the anterior border of sternomastoid. The upper aspect of the incision angles posteriorly to minimize trauma to the greater auricular nerve. Any superficial veins are ligated and divided. Dissection continues medial to the sternomastoid to reveal the common facial vein. This large tributary of the internal jugular vein often overlies the carotid bifurcation and is a useful landmark. The common facial vein is divided. Round-toothed West retractors open up the space between the perilaryngeal structures and the jugular vein. Dissection continues medial to the jugular vein and the common carotid artery (CCA). Careful dissection is then continued superiorly. The external carotid artery (ECA) can be identified by locating its first branch (the superior thyroid artery). Occasionally the bifurcation is rotated. The surgeon should remember to mobilize the ECA branches toward the first assistant.

There are a number of strategies for mobilizing the bifurcation and distal ICA. Care should be taken to avoid excessive mobilization of the bifurcation, as this leads to functional elongation and distal ICA kinking (predisposing toward postoperative thrombosis) and an increased risk of procedural embolization. Most surgeons prefer to mobilize a discrete segment of ICA well above the bifurcation so as to minimize the risks of dislodging an embolus into the cerebral circulation. The patient is systemically heparinized and the carotid arteries cross-clamped. If the surgeon chooses to shunt the patient, the shunt is inserted now. The plaque is endarterectomized, tacking sutures inserted if required, and the ECA origin cleared of plaque using the eversion technique. The arteriotomy is closed either primarily or by a patch (vein/prosthetic). Flow is restored first up the ECA, then the ICA. Having achieved hemostasis, the wound is closed with absorbable suture to reconstitute platysma (usually over a deep suction drain). Nonabsorbable suture or clips are used to close the skin.

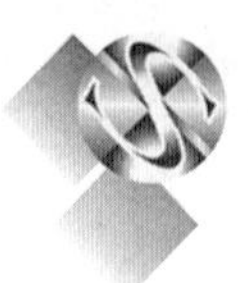

Points for Debate

Despite being a relatively straightforward operation in concept, few operations arouse so much debate regarding content. A summary of the principal debating points follows, which highlights those of most practical concern.

Stop Antiplatelet Therapy or Not?

There is no evidence that aspirin should be withdrawn during the perioperative period. An emerging problem, however, is the effect of the ADP inhibitor clopidogrel on surgical hemostasis, particularly if the patient is receiving combination antiplatelet therapy. Many surgeons have anecdotally observed that suture line bleeding is significantly increased in patients receiving chronic clopidogrel therapy. In the Leicester Royal Infirmary, clopidogrel therapy is stopped 1 week preoperatively and aspirin is restarted.

Locoregional or General Anesthesia?

The rationale for the use of locoregional anesthesia is that the surgeon is immediately aware of any neurological deficit during the procedure. Accordingly, steps can be taken to treat this deficit. Advocates of general anesthesia cite ease of operation, no patient movement, and lower cerebral metabolic requirements to counter this deficit. There is no evidence that either anesthetic technique reduces operative morbidity or mortality. However, meta-analyses of nonrandomized trials suggest that locoregional anesthesia may be associated with lower perioperative cardiovascular morbidity. A further large randomized trial (GALA) is currently underway in the U.K.

Preincision Infiltration with Local Anesthesia and Adrenaline?

No randomized trial data are available. The rationale is to minimize troublesome skin edge bleeding at the beginning of the procedure. Advocates need to be aware that subcutaneous and cutaneous bleeding may occur in the early postoperative period as the adrenaline effect wears off.

Longitudinal or Transverse Incision?

No randomized trial data are available. Transverse wounds probably confer a better cosmetic result, but may be associated with problems relating to access to the distal ICA. Longitudinal incisions inevitably divide more cutaneous nerves, leading to a larger area of anesthesia under the chin. The latter, however, is the approach of choice if there is any question of high carotid disease, especially in male patients with short fat necks!

Anticipating Distal Disease?

Preoperative preparation is mandatory. Nasolaryngeal intubation opens the space between the ramus of the mandible and the mastoid process. Nasolaryngeal intubation should probably not be undertaken in all patients, as there is a not insignificant risk of retronasal bleeding, which can predispose to vomiting (and aspiration) in the early postoperative period. If the surgeon feels that temporomandibular subluxation may be necessary (preferable to dislocation), this must be anticipated in advance and maxillofacial specialists must be involved. This procedure cannot readily be undertaken once the procedure has started. In the Leicester Royal Infirmary, >1200 CEAs have been performed over the last decade without recourse to temporomandibular subluxation. Surgeons unfamiliar with dissecting in the upper reaches of the neck should involve more experienced colleagues. High carotid dissections are associated with an increased risk of operative stroke, bleeding, and cranial nerve injury.

When Should I Clamp the Internal Carotid Artery Early?

Transcranial Doppler (TCD) allows the surgeon to be promptly aware of particulate embolization during the dissection phase of the operation. One or two emboli warn of the likelihood of an unstable plaque. The dissection technique is then made even more meticulous, and early clamping is not usually necessary, provided no attempt is made to injudiciously dissect around the bifurcation. Continued embolization (despite modification in operative technique) is a worrisome phenomenon and merits consideration of early distal ICA clamping. There is usually more than enough time to complete the dissection safely and insert a shunt as necessary.

Blocking the Sinus Nerve?

There is no randomized trial evidence that routine blockade of the sinus nerve with lignocaine significantly influences postoperative cardiovascular morbidity. The rationale is that sinus blockade minimizes intraoperative hypotension. However, this must be offset against the potential for postoperative reinnervation hypertension. In practice, once the ICA has been clamped, intraoperative hypotension is not usually a problem.

Should I Ever Abandon a Procedure at This Stage?

There are few situations warranting abandonment of the operation at this stage. The commonest reason is cardiovascular instability (e.g., electrocardiogram evidence of myocardial ischemia not controlled with simple therapy, unstable arrhythmia). Other reasons reflect an unanticipated change in the risk/benefit ratios for the patient, that is, the benefits quoted to the patient preoperatively are now being exceeded by the potential risks as the procedure becomes ever more complex. Scenarios might include a hypoplastic carotid artery extending to the skull base (this can be evaluated by on-table angiography). Controversy then relates to whether the ICA should be tied off or left alone. Most would probably leave it alone and start the patient on warfarin postoperatively. Other examples include unexpected high disease extension in a patient with a unilateral asymptomatic stenosis. As the annual risk of stroke was only about 2% in the ACAS and ACST trials (where high disease was specifically excluded), it may now be considered best to abandon the procedure, as the operative risks will be in excess of what was quoted preoperatively.

What Dose of Heparin?

Most centers administer 5000 units of intravenous heparin before clamping. There is no evidence that heparin doses tailored to patient weight influences the balance between antithrombotic and hemorrhagic risk.

Should I Shunt?

This is an ever-enduring controversy. There is no evidence that a policy of routine shunting, selective shunting, or never shunting actually alters the operative risk, largely because the trials were small and poorly designed. Most surgeons are either routine or selective shunters, with the choice being most likely to reflect the strategy of their trainer!

What Choice of Shunt?

The most commonly used shunts are the Javid (less flexible, tapered, requiring external retaining clamps) and the Pruitt-Inahara (softer, more flexible, smaller caliber, intraluminal retaining balloons). Alternatives include the Brener in-line shunt. No large randomized trials have compared the effect of shunt type on clinical outcome. Evidence suggests that 90% of patients have flow rates within 10% of preclamp levels using the Pruitt shunt. High carotid dissections probably benefit from using the Pruitt shunt, as the Javid requires a further centimeter or so of distal dissection to position the retaining clamp. This can sometimes be quite difficult to achieve in the upper reaches of the neck.

Proximal or Distal End of the Shunt in First?

No randomized trial has addressed this issue. Most surgeons insert the proximal (CCA) limb first and flush the shunt to clear debris prior to distal insertion. Allowing the distal ICA to backvent before carefully inserting the shunt can also reduce distal embolism. No force should ever be applied during shunt insertion. Resistance should encourage the surgeon to dissect the carotid artery more distally to exclude an impacting coil.

How Do I Know If the Shunt Is Working?

About 3% of shunts malfunction, usually because of impaction of the distal limb against the ICA wall or carotid coil. Unless some form of monitoring is used, this will go unnoticed. Simple techniques include awake testing or TCD. For those without any access to monitoring, the surgeon using the Pruitt shunt can temporarily clamp the CCA inflow and assess backflow from the circle of Willis (i.e., is the

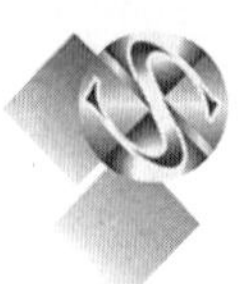

distal channel patent or not) by opening the red tap on the T limb.

The Shunt Is Working But I Am Still Worried About Perfusion

Advocates of TCD recommend trying to maintain mean middle cerebral artery blood flow velocity of >15 cm per second. This threshold broadly corresponds to that equivalent to the level of brain perfusion usually associated with loss of cerebral electrical activity. Note that this threshold does not equate to loss of neuronal function. If flow rates are considered inadequate, check that the shunt limbs are neither impacted nor kinked. If there is no mechanical problem, the anesthetist can then carefully elevate the patient's blood pressure pharmacologically, which usually raises the intracranial blood flow to acceptable levels.

Traditional or Eversion Endarterectomy?

Traditional endarterectomy involves the removal of the plaque through a longitudinal arteriotomy extending from the CCA into the ICA. The plaque is usually transected proximally and removed with cephalad dissection using a Watson-Cheyne dissector. The distal end is feathered or transected. Eversion endarterectomy involves transecting the ICA from the bifurcation. Everting the enclosing media/adventitia then expels a tube of plaque. The CCA is endarterectomized and the ICA reimplanted onto the bifurcation. Potential advantages of eversion endarterectomy include no need for patching and the ability to shorten an elongated ICA. However, neither technique is superior to the other.

Tack the Intimal Step or Not?

No randomized trial data are available, and attitudes usually reflect the policy of the trainer. The NASCET observed that tacking sutures were associated with a higher perioperative risk. This nonrandomized comparison, however, may simply reflect the fact that tacking sutures were more likely to be inserted when the surgeon encountered a more complex case (e.g., difficult to achieve a clean, tapering distal end-point in a thin walled vessel).

Patch or Not?

This is another of the single-issue subjects that have characterized carotid surgery. Options include routine patching, selective patching, and never patching. No randomized trials have compared selective with routine patching. However, a meta-analysis of the six randomized trials comparing routine patching with routine primary closure showed that patching conferred a three- to fourfold reduction in (1) perioperative thrombosis, (2) perioperative stroke, (3) late stroke, and (4) and late restenosis (Counsell et al., 1997). Accordingly, there is little evidence to support continuance with a policy of routine never patching.

Choice of Patch?

A meta-analysis by the Cochrane collaboration has shown that patch type does not influence outcome. There is, however, a perception that prosthetic patches are probably more thrombogenic than vein. A recently published randomized trial addressed this issue and observed no difference in the rates of embolization in the early postoperative period. In reality, patient factors seem more likely to mediate an increased risk of thrombosis than does the patch type. The Achilles heel of prosthetic patching is infection, which complicates approximately 1% of procedures. About half become apparent in the first few months of surgery, the commonest organisms being staphylococci and streptococci. Evidence suggests that removal of the prosthetic material with autologous reconstruction is associated with the lowest risk of stroke and late reinfection. Secondary reconstruction with prosthetic material should be avoided.

Should Vein Be Harvested from Ankle or Groin?

Vein patches are susceptible to rupture. This characteristically occurs on the 5th to 7th postoperative day and is more common in females and in hypertensives where the vein has been harvested from the ankle. Current advice, therefore, is to use groin saphenous vein for patching because of its intrinsically stronger structure. Only about 15% of patients need their saphe-

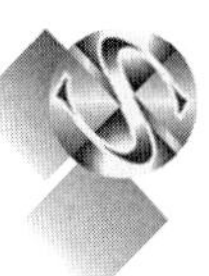

nous vein for alternative cardiovascular reconstructions in the next 5 years.

Carotid Bypass?

Carotid bypasses should not be performed routinely but are indicated if the endarterectomy zone is too thin after plaque removal, if there is extensive atheroma and concomitant kinking, or if there is any question of infection. In common with infrainguinal venous reconstructions, about 20% of carotid bypasses using saphenous vein develop a recurrent stenosis within 24 months. This is significantly higher than that observed with traditional endarterectomy and patching. Accordingly, bypass patients require serial duplex surveillance.

Shorten the Carotid or Not?

Following endarterectomy, particularly if there is a slightly redundant distal ICA, there is a tendency to observe functional elongation of the endarterectomy zone. Uncorrected, this may predispose to perioperative thrombosis. Shortening the endarterectomy zone may reduce this. Options include transection and reanastomosis (may be difficult in thin-walled, narrow-caliber vessels in female patients) or eversion plication. In the latter, stay sutures incorporating the redundancy on either side of the artery are tied, causing the excess arterial wall to be everted. The eversion is then closed with a continuous 6:0 Prolene suture.

Monitor or Not?

There is considerable skepticism as to whether monitoring reduces stroke risk after CEA. Options include electroencephalogram (EEG), somatosensory sensory evoked potentials (SSEPs), TCD, near-infrared spectroscopy, jugular venous oxygen saturation, awake testing under locoregional anesthesia, xenon blood flow measurement, subjective assessment of backflow, and stump pressure. In practice, the most commonly used techniques are awake testing, TCD, and EEG. To date, no randomized trial has been performed to address this issue. However, for any form of monitoring to work, the right questions must be asked. Electroencephalography and SSEP only tell the surgeon that perfusion has dropped below the threshold for maintaining electrical function. Awake

testing identifies any neurological deficit (indicative of perfusion having fallen below the threshold for neuronal viability), but it requires additional strategies (e.g., some sort of quality control) to identify what was actually causing the underlying problem. It has been the experience at the Leicester Royal Infirmary that combining a monitoring method (TCD) with quality control assessment (angioscopy) has been associated with a 60% reduction in the operative risk over the last 10 years.

Quality Control or Not?

Quality control assessment is a slightly different concept from monitoring. Its use is based on the observation that the majority of operative strokes follow inadvertent technical error. Accordingly, detection of technical error should (in theory) reduce the risk. Once again, no randomized trials have evaluated completion angioscopy, angiography, or duplex ultrasound. Advocates of monitoring and quality control assessment have reported significant benefits. However, such a policy is helpful only if the choice of technique addresses the appropriate question. Awake testing does not prevent embolization during carotid dissection. Awake testing remains the only "gold standard" for determining who benefits from selective shunting, but does not prevent a stroke due to embolization of luminal thrombus following restoration of flow unless something like angioscopy is employed.

Drain or Not?

Surprisingly, no randomized trial has addressed this issue. However, most surgeons insert a suction drain into the neck wound for 12 to 24 hours on the basis that it probably does no harm. There is certainly no evidence that drains increase the risk of prosthetic patch infection.

Early Postoperative Management

Establishing the Neurological Status

Following surgery, the patient must be carefully monitored for three clinical variables: neurological status, wound stability, and blood pressure.

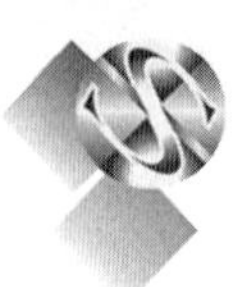

If general anesthesia has been used during the operation, the patient should be closely observed to ensure that cerebral function remains intact upon awakening. The initial assessment should include the patient's response to simple verbal commands and extremity movement. Once the patient becomes fully alert in the recovery room, a more detailed assessment including the vagus and hypoglossal nerve function can be performed.

Neck Hematoma

The neck incision should be regularly monitored for swelling. This is usually a result of hematoma formation, although surprising amounts of tissue edema can accumulate within hours of the procedure. Despite achieving complete hemostasis and placing a closed suction drain in the wound, delayed bleeding resulting in hematoma and airway compromise can occur. Once an expanding hematoma is recognized, the patient should be returned to the operating room promptly to evacuate the hematoma and identify the potential bleeding source. If the patient develops respiratory distress, the neck incision should be opened at the bedside to decompress the hematoma followed by orotracheal intubation to establish an airway if needed. Alternatively, it is useful to have infiltrated the neck incision with local anesthetic agent prior to finishing the procedure. Should a significant neck hematoma occur, it can be released without having to reintubate the patient.

Hypertension and Hypotension

Significant, sustained hypotension is not usually a problem following endarterectomy and tends to respond well to colloid replacement. Early postoperative hypertension is more common and requires careful monitoring and control. As a rule, most anesthetists prefer to maintain blood pressure within 10% of preoperative levels. There is anecdotal evidence from reports documenting outcome for carotid surgery under locoregional anesthesia that postoperative hypertension is less of a problem. Most cases of early postoperative hypertension respond to a single bolus or carefully titrated infusion of beta-blocker (e.g. labetalol). Note

that regular review is required as (quite often) the hypertension is a transient phenomenon and may require therapy only for 4 to 6 hours. Sustained postoperative hypertension at 3 to 5 days requires assessment by a cardiovascular physician. Caution should be exercised in discharging patients before blood pressure is adequately controlled, as these patients are probably at higher risk of suffering seizures in the early postoperative period.

The Patient Suffers a Neurological Deficit

Intraoperative

An intraoperative stroke is defined as having occurred if a neurological deficit becomes apparent as the patient recovers from anesthesia. Usually the first sign is a prolonged delay in awakening. In the absence of any monitoring modality, it should be assumed that the patient has suffered either a carotid thrombosis or embolization into the cerebral arteries, and the patient should be reexplored. The aim of reexploration is to recognize and treat thrombosis before an irreversible neurological deficit occurs. Delay beyond 1 hour is associated with a progressively worsened outcome. The second reason is to identify and correct a source of technical error responsible for platelet accumulation and secondary embolization.

Neurological Deficit Within the First 24 Hours

Focal neurological deficits occurring within the first 24 hours are still usually thromboembolic. In the absence of any monitoring techniques, it is again probably best to return the patient immediately to the operating room. Intracranial hemorrhage is extremely rare within the first 24 hours, and a CT scan is probably unnecessary unless it is done immediately on the way to the operating room.

In the Leicester Royal Infirmary, we have previously observed that the majority of early postoperative neurological deficits were secondary to carotid thrombosis. Subsequent research showed that patients at risk of progressing to thrombosis had a 1- to 2-hour period of increasing embolization on transcranial Doppler before any neurological deficit became appar-

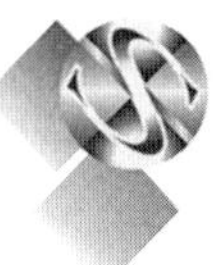

ent. This association has now been corroborated in many centers around the world. This phase of sustained embolization can be arrested by intravenous infusion of Dextran 40 in saline, the dose of which has to be increased in 30% of patients in order to control embolization. No case of stroke due to early postoperative thrombotic occlusion has been encountered following 1000 CEAs in the Leicester Unit since the protocol of 3 hours of TCD monitoring with selective Dextran therapy was instituted in 1995.

The algorithm in Figure 15.7 summarizes the current strategy in the Leicester Royal Infirmary for managing a neurological deficit in the first 24 hours after a successful recovery from anesthesia. Patients with hemiplegia/hemiparesis are more likely to have suffered a major vessel occlusion and are probably more likely to benefit from reexploration. Patients with a monoparesis or isolated dysphasia are highly unlikely to have suffered major vessel occlusion, and there is time for more discriminating investigation and treatment. The aim is to avoid unnecessary reexploration in patients with a normal endarterectomy zones and in those who have suffered embolic occlusion of the middle cerebral artery mainstem. Note that transcranial Doppler is used to detect any evidence of ongoing embolization and can be invaluable in guiding decisions regarding reexploration.

Neurological Deficit After 24 Hours

Strokes occurring after 24 hours have elapsed have a greater number of potential underlying causes. In addition to thromboembolism, the clinician must now consider the likelihood of hyperperfusion and intracranial hemorrhage. Figure 15.8 summarizes the current Leicester protocol in this situation. The key difference from the strategy for managing strokes within the first 24 hours is the importance of performing an emergency CT scan. Intracranial hemorrhage complicates 1% of CEAs and carries a very poor outcome, with up to 80% of patients dying or suffering a major disabling stroke. There is currently very little that can be done to treat these patients, although vascular surgeons may like to ask their neurosurgical

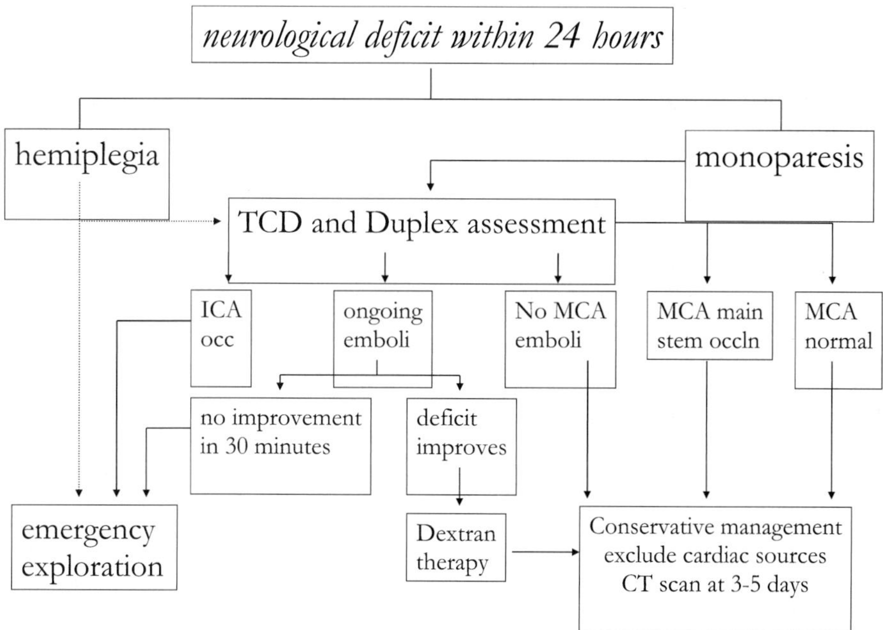

Figure 15.7. Algorithm for the investigation and management of patients at the Leicester Royal Infirmary who have suffered a neurological deficit within the first 24 hours of CEA, having made a normal recovery from anesthesia. CT, computed tomography; ICA, internal carotid artery; MCA, middle cerebral artery; TCD, transcranial Doppler.

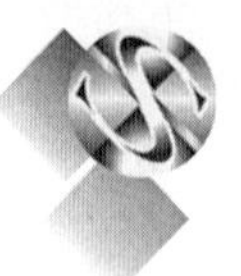

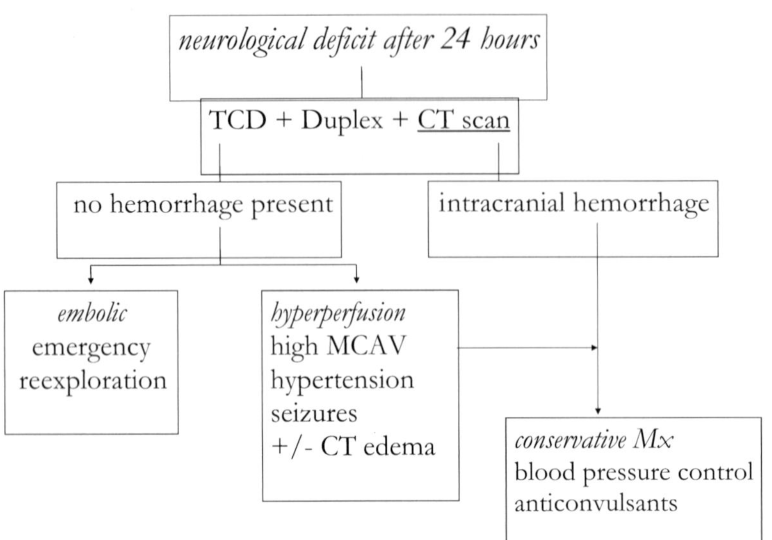

Figure 15.8. Algorithm for the investigation and management of patients at Leicester who have suffered a neurological deficit after 24 hours or more have elapsed after carotid endarterectomy (CEA).

colleagues whether they might ever consider clot evacuation.

Stroke due to hyperperfusion syndrome is another poorly understood entity, and there is considerable controversy as to whether it would be better renamed the "reperfusion" syndrome. More recently, there has been renewed debate as to how much the condition is associated with high flow as opposed to hypertensive encephalopathy or dysautoregulation. Patients at risk of hyperperfusion-related stroke tend to have a history of severe bilateral disease and treated hypertension. Stroke is often preceded by seizure and severe hypertension. The mainstay of management is control of seizures and careful reduction of blood pressure. Early CT scans often show changes consistent with an evolving ischemic infarction, but in fact this is often white matter edema. Paradoxically, a lot of the white matter edema is present in the vertebrobasilar territory.

Late Postoperative Management

There is a surprisingly good transatlantic consensus regarding many of the principal issues relating to carotid surgery. Two, however, serial noninvasive surveillance and reintervention for recurrent stenoses, have aroused considerable debate.

Serial Surveillance and Recurrent Stenoses

In North America and in many centers in mainland Europe, follow-up carotid duplex scanning is considered mandatory. The underlying rationale is to monitor for recurrent lesions, as well as for progressive disease of the contralateral carotid artery. Patients are recommended to return for an initial follow-up visit approximately 1 month following the operation to ensure that adequate wound healing has taken place. A carotid duplex scan is performed at that time to evaluate the carotid reconstruction and to provide a new baseline for future study comparison. This is followed by a subsequent clinic visit at 6 months, at which time a repeat carotid duplex scan is performed. If the duplex scan shows satisfactory results of both carotid arteries, the patient may be seen 1 year following the operation. A bilateral carotid duplex scan should be performed at that visit and at all future annual examinations.

In the U.K., parts of northern mainland Europe, and Scandinavia, the policy is completely different. Here patients are reviewed at 4 to 6 weeks, and unless they are part of an ongoing research program, they are discharged with instructions to return if any new symptoms recur. The rationale underlying this approach is based on the following observations. First, the annual risk of stroke after suc-

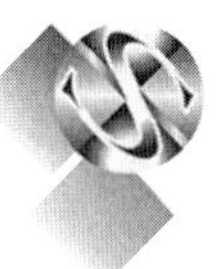

cessful endarterectomy is only about 1% to 2% in the operated hemisphere and 2% in the contralateral hemisphere. Second, it has been difficult to determine the actual risk of ipsilateral stroke in patients with a recurrent stenosis, largely because many of the patients have already been subjected to a prophylactic redo CEA. However, in Frerick's recent overview, 10 published series documented the risk of stroke according to whether the patient had a recurrent stenosis or not. Having corrected for the effects of different lengths of follow-up and study size, a reanalysis of the data suggests that the incidence of ipsilateral stroke in patients with a recurrent stenosis (>50%) is approximately 5.5% at 3 years (i.e., only about 2% per annum). For those with no evidence of a recurrent stenosis, the risk of ipsilateral stroke was 3.3% over 3 years (i.e. only about 1% per annum). These figures correlate closely with the follow-up data reported in the international trials. Third, acute changes in plaque morphology tend to precede onset of symptoms rather than a progressive worsening of stenosis. In short, if one reviews the results of the last surveillance scan before onset of neurological symptoms, it rarely enables reliable prediction of patients at risk of subsequent stroke.

Carotid Angioplasty

Angioplasty is an accepted component of vascular practice apart from the cerebral circulation. The reason for this discrepancy is the potential for procedural embolization and stroke. The first carotid angioplasty was performed in 1980. By 1992, the first overview of balloon angioplasty in the carotid artery was published. In a pooled series of 123 patients from 10 studies, the procedural mortality rate was 0%, the disabling stroke rate 0%, and the 30-day death and any stroke rate was 0.8%. This study was thereafter a catalyst for the increasing interest in the potential for angioplasty to replace endarterectomy as the gold standard treatment for occlusive carotid artery disease.

However, despite the excellent results from these pioneers of angioplasty (particularly as they appeared safer than diagnostic angiography alone), concerns thereafter were voiced that balloon angioplasty alone was probably not safe. This observation was based on concerns that vessel recoil, intimal dissection, plaque dislodgment, and particulate embolization were now major potential problems, despite not having been evident in the original overview. It was proposed that the insertion of a stent would avoid the above problems as well as reduce the rate of re-stenosis. A subsequent overview of outcomes following primary stenting revealed a 4.3% death/stroke rate at 30 days in 2569 patients with either symptomatic or asymptomatic patients and a re-stenosis rate of <5%. Interestingly, there is now a third-generation view that these results can be improved even further with the use of cerebral protection devices. These devices (distal balloon, distal aspiration, distal filters and umbrellas, and retrograde flow during balloon insufflation) are currently under development or clinical evaluation.

To date, the results from voluntary stent registries and single centers around the world have clearly demonstrated that angioplasty is feasible and accepted by patients. It remains to be seen when and where it should replace endarterectomy. The situation regarding carotid angioplasty, therefore, is analogous to that faced by the cardiac surgeons in the 1980s when coronary angioplasty was first introduced. Ultimately, the answer will have to be determined by level I randomized trials, and it is inevitable that angioplasty will have a role in the management of selected patients with cerebral vascular disease. Evidence suggests that the worst procedural outcomes are to be encountered in older patients, symptomatic patients, those with lesions longer than 10 mm, and those with more severe degrees of stenosis.

An overview of the published literature in 2000 indicated that the results of angioplasty were generally poorer than surgery in trials reporting outcomes in symptomatic patients who should, otherwise, form the mainstay of current treatment (Golledge et al., 2000). Angioplasty cannot simply be justified because it is effective in predominantly asymptomatic populations. Using the results of ACAS as a guide, only 58 ipsilateral strokes would be prevented per 1000 angioplasties on asymptomatic patients with 60% to 99% stenoses.

Five randomized trials have now compared CEA and angioplasty in the treatment of symp-

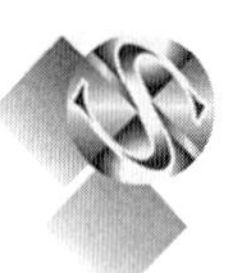

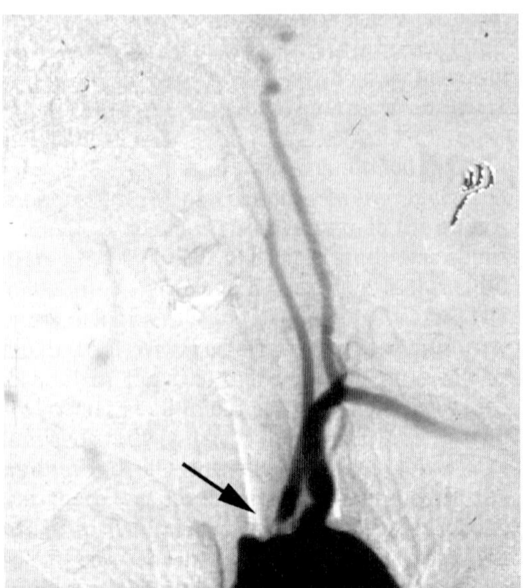

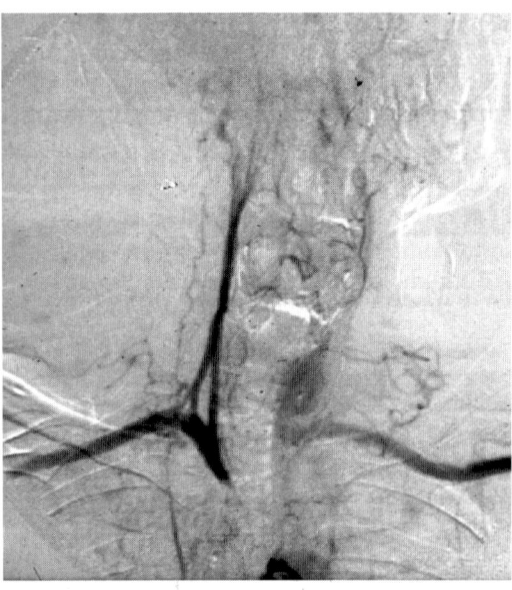

Figure 16.1. A: Arch angiogram showing occlusion of the innominate artery and a severe stenosis at the origin of the left common carotid artery (arrow). B: Delayed films following on from part A. The right subclavian and distal innominate arteries are filled via retrograde flow down the right vertebral artery. The actual innominate occlusion is relatively short.

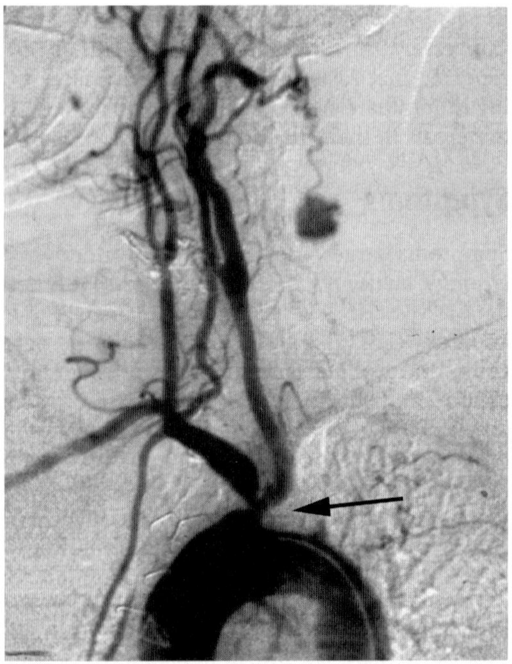

Figure 16.2. Bovine arch anomaly. The innominate and left common carotid arteries have a common origin (arrow). There is a large atherosclerotic lesion causing a severe stenosis of the bovine origin and total occlusion of the left subclavian artery.

Cerebrovascular symptoms [transient ischemic attack (TIA)/stroke] may be due to thromboembolism into the carotid circulation (hemisensory/motor signs, monocular blindness, or higher cortical dysfunction) or the vertebrobasilar system (bilateral sensory/motor signs, dysarthria, ataxia, nystagmus, homonymous hemianopsia, cortical blindness, etc.). Neurovascular symptoms affect 5% to 90% of patients with severe innominate artery disease. Ten percent of patients present with global ischemia involving both the carotid and vertebral territories.

Diagnosis

Many of the clinical features of innominate artery occlusive disease are of equal relevance to subclavian and vertebral artery disease and are reviewed in this section. Atherosclerotic disease of the supra-aortic trunk is suggested by absent pulses in the neck (subclavian, carotid) or arm (axillary, brachial) in one or both sides. Unequal or abnormally low blood pressures in the upper extremity should also be noted. Physical examination should include palpation and ausculta-

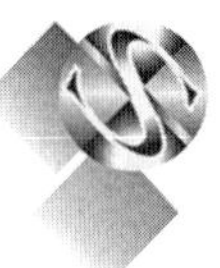

tion of the proximal and midcervical carotid pulses and palpation of the superficial temporal, subclavian, brachial, radial, and ulnar pulses. Carotid or subclavian artery bruits or thrills suggest innominate artery or other supra-aortic trunk stenotic lesions. Absent pulses are suggestive of occlusions.

Blood pressure comparison of both upper extremities is mandatory. If bilateral upper extremity blood pressures are determined to be low, comparison should be made to those in the lower extremity. The hands should be inspected for cyanosis, ulcers, subungual splinter hemorrhages, or livedo reticularis, which may indicate ulcerated proximal lesions predisposing to atheroemboli. In patients with subclavian steal (see later), a pulse delay may be detected in the radial artery.

A computed tomography scan of the brain is an essential part of the workup of any patient with suspected atherosclerotic disease of the supra-aortic vessels. About 80% of the cerebral cortex is clinically silent, and the finding of areas of infarction (in the absence of any previous symptoms) may be helpful in planning management strategies.

Duplex evaluation of the proximal supra-aortic vessels may not be possible because they may be out of the scanning range of most machines. However, an experienced sonographer will warn the surgeon of damped waveforms in the common carotid or subclavian vessels. This should alert the surgeon to the likelihood of inflow disease and the need for employing other imaging modalities.

Arch arteriography remains the gold standard for defining the anatomy of the lesion, extent of disease, and probable etiology (e.g., atherosclerosis versus arteritis). A complete examination should include an arch aortogram, selected carotid views, vertebral imaging, and images of the intracranial circulation.

Concomitant coronary artery disease is present in 40% to 50% of patients with supra-aortic trunk disease. Inevitably, these patients have other cardiovascular risk factors including hypercholesterolemia, history of stroke, TIAs, peripheral vascular disease, hypertension, diabetes, and renal insufficiency. A prior history of smoking is present in 78% to 100% of patients with supra-aortic trunk disease. Accordingly, cardiac evaluation is advisable, especially if any major reconstructions were planned.

Treatment

Historically, supra-aortic trunk disease was treated by direct reconstruction. In 1956 Davis et al. first described transthoracic innominate endarterectomy. Later, in 1958, DeBakey described prosthetic bypass grafting of the great vessels. In appropriately selected patients, both forms of direct reconstruction can give excellent results.

Most patients with supra-aortic trunk atherosclerosis have multiple supra-aortic trunk lesions. Multiple arch vessel involvement occurs in 61% to 84% of patients. The best operative repair of this patient population having multiple arch vessel lesions may therefore be directed reconstruction with bypass grafting.

Bypass grafting has an excellent technical success rate and good early results with relief of symptoms in up to 95% of patients. Long-term relief of symptoms appear equally as good, with primary patency rates of 95% being evident. The two largest series were from Berguer et al. (1998) (100 consecutive patients followed over 16 years) and Kieffer et al. (1995) (148 patients followed over 20 years). Berguer et al. reported 5- and 10-year cumulative primary patency rates of 87% and 81%, respectively. Stroke-free survival rates at 5 and 10 years were 87% and 81%, respectively. Kieffer et al. reported a primary patency rate of 98% and 96% at 5 and 10 years, respectively. The probability of freedom from ipsilateral stroke was 98% and 96% at 5 and 10 years, respectively. Life-table analysis and perioperative events were used to calculate the probability of survival, which was 77% and 51% at 5 and 10 years, respectively. Most patients died from cardiac events.

The excellent outcomes following bypass grafting of supra-aortic trunk disease, however, does not come without a price. Perioperative mortality ranges from 0% to 15%. In the more recent studies, the rate generally is around 5% and is mostly attributable to cardiac causes. The perioperative stroke rate ranges from 0% to 8% giving a combined stroke and death rate of almost 16%. Rhodes et al. (2000) have determined risk factors for early and late complications in these patients. Patients with serum creatinine levels of ≥2 had a significantly higher combined stroke/death rate when compared to patients with normal creatinine (50% versus 7%). Similarly, stroke rates were higher in

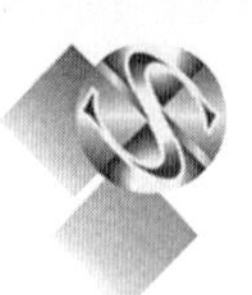

patients with preoperative evidence of a hyper-coagulable state (33% versus 4%).

Although there have been no randomized controlled trials, endarterectomy has been reported to confer the same results as bypass grafting. Bypass grafting of supra-aortic trunk lesions requires the use of prosthetic material, often with multiple limbs, which may be kinked after closure of the sternotomy wound.

Endarterectomy has the advantage of recon-struction without the use of prosthetic material, but is technically intimidating to surgeons who have limited experience of operating in that part of the vascular system. It is essential, therefore, that patients are selected carefully. Anatomical features considered contraindications for endarterectomy include (1) atherosclerosis or calcification of the aortic arch extending into the origin of the innominate artery, and (2) close proximity of the origin of the left common carotid artery, which prevents safe clamping of the innominate artery without increasing the risk of embolization or of compromising cere-bral blood flow. Endarterectomy would not be an appropriate option in patients with bovine arches (Fig. 16.2) as cross-clamping would pre-dispose to inadequate left hemisphere perfu-sion. The San Francisco group has long been proponents of the endarterectomy technique and has partly overcome the problems imposed by multiple vessel disease by performing sepa-rate endarterectomies on each of the affected vessels (Azakie et al., 1998). Certain diseases processes (inflammatory arteritis and radiation arteritis) are best treated with bypass grafting, as the pathological process is a transmural process and development of an endarterectomy plane may be difficult.

The emergence and technical advances in percutaneous angioplasty, however, have ren-dered many of these major reconstructions obsolete. Percutaneous therapy for occlusive lesions of supra-aortic trunk disease has several advantages over a surgical approach. These include its minimally invasive nature, avoidance of general anesthesia, lower cost, and, most importantly, the potential for lower morbidity and mortality. Percutaneous angioplasty for treatment of supra-aortic trunk lesions was introduced in 1980. Since that time more than 30 small series have been published regarding the role of angioplasty or stenting as primary therapy for supra-aortic trunk lesions in more

than 900 patients. None of the reports are ran-domized controlled trials (as is also the case with surgery), and long-term results are still not available.

A comparative trial of stenting and surgical intervention for supra-aortic trunk lesions was reported in 1998 by Whitbread et al. Eighteen patients with symptomatic arch vessel stenosis or occlusion were treated with angioplasty and stenting, and the data compared with the pub-lished results following surgical procedures. The primary success rate was 100%, with no major procedural complications, and at 17-month follow-up all patients were asymptomatic with 100% primary patency. The incidence of stroke and death was 3% and 2%, respectively. The authors therefore concluded that stenting should now be considered the first-line therapy for brachiocephalic obstruction. A review of the available literature suggests that the initial success rate is higher with stenoses (98%), as opposed to occlusions (46%). Both types of lesions were treated with minimal mortality (0.2% for stenoses and 0% for occlusions), the stroke rate was commendably low (0.3% for stenoses, 0% with occlusion), and with no reports of arm embolization. Recurrence of stenoses was similar for both stenotic lesions and occlusions. With a mean follow-up period, 63 months, the incidence of recurrent stenosis was identical: 11% in originally stenotic lesions, 9% for occlusions.

Although the initial results following angio-plasty of supra-aortic trunk lesions are well documented, there is a relative lack of reports describing the long-term results. There are, however, reports of endovascular treatment of patients with supra-aortic trunk lesions with 9- and 15-year follow-up (Henry et al., 1999). These follow-up results are longer than most pub-lished surgical series. Cumulative primary patency was 91% to 95% at 5 years and 81% to 84% at 10 years. Sullivan et al. (1998) prospec-tively studied acute and long-term results of angioplasty and stenting in occlusive lesions of the supra-aortic trunk. The initial technical success rate was 94%, and 80% of the technical failures were due to an inability to cross occlu-sive lesions. With initial failures included, life table analysis revealed 84% patency at 35 months. None of the patients required reinter-vention or surgical conversion for recurrent symptoms. The authors concluded that angio-

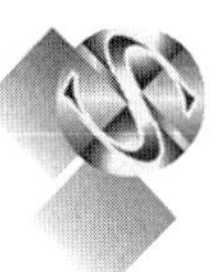

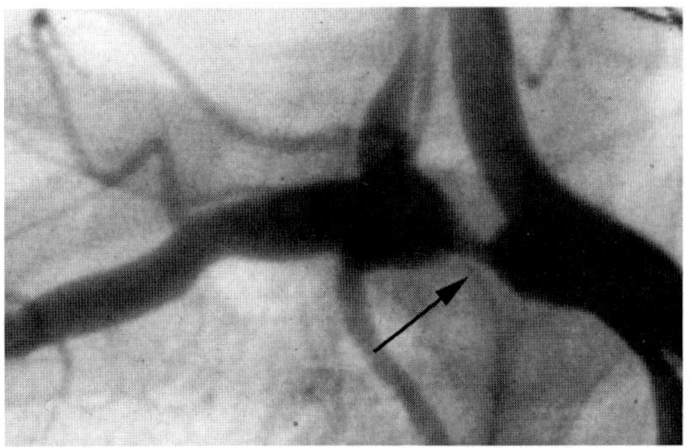
A

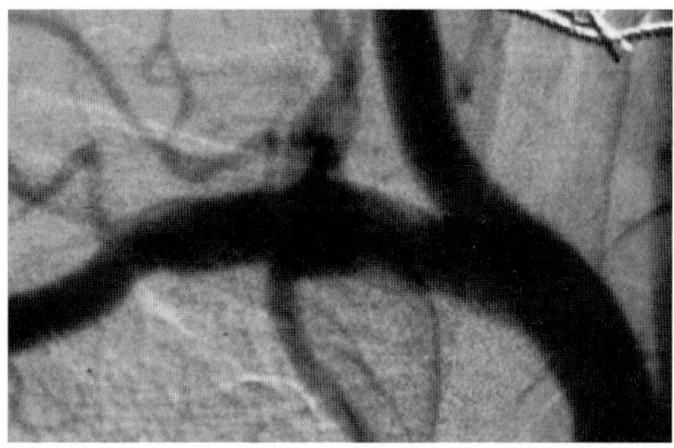
B

Figure 16.3. A: Severe stenosis in the right subclavian artery immediately distal to the vertebral artery (arrow). This produced arm symptoms only and no subclavian steal. This was successfully treated by angioplasty (B).

plasty and stenting of the supra-aortic trunk vessels could be performed with relative safety and satisfactory midterm success.

Endovascular treatment of supra-aortic trunk lesions began prior to the advent of arterial stents. Some groups have advocated the routine use of stents, whereas others use them only when angioplasty produces technically inadequate results. The routine use of stents is supported by nonrandomized evidence documenting improved early and long-term patency rates, especially when treating occlusions.

One further role for endovascular intervention is in the management of the critically ill patient with innominate disruption or false aneurysm formation following trauma. The whole procedure can be undertaken via direct exposure of the right common carotid artery with retrograde cannulation of the carotid and innominate arteries.

The Subclavian Artery
Etiology

Subclavian artery lesions are relatively uncommon, but are encountered more frequently than innominate or proximal common carotid artery lesions. The most common cause is atherosclerosis. In 4748 angiograms performed for signs and symptoms of ischemic cerebrovascular disease, the prevalence of stenosis greater than 30% was 21%, whereas the prevalence of occlusion was 3%. Out of nearly 2000 great vessel reconstructions by Wylie and Effeney (1979),

subclavian artery disease was only found in 4.3%. Isolated subclavian artery stenosis (Fig. 16.3) is most commonly found in patients with systemic vascular disease. The true prevalence of subclavian artery disease, however, is difficult to estimate because most patients are asymptomatic. Only 24% of patients with disease of the subclavian artery arteriography have symptoms. The left subclavian artery, arising directly from the aortic arch, tends to be affected three to four times more frequently than the right.

Other important causes of subclavian artery disease include aneurysm, radiation arteritis, Takayasu's arteritis, and the thoracic outlet syndrome. Thoracic outlet syndrome is due to compression of one or more components of the neurovascular bundle (subclavian artery, subclavian vein, and brachial plexus) by a cervical rib (Fig. 16.4), fibrous band, first rib, and clavicle and anatomical anomalies of the scalene musculature.

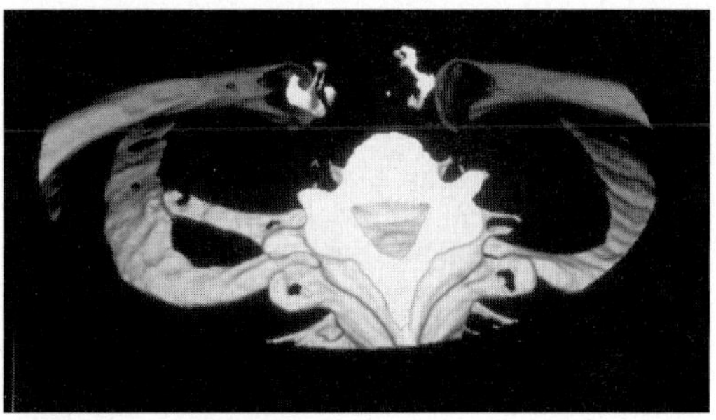

Figure 16.4. Three-dimensional magnetic resonance tomographic image of cervical rib with connection on to first rib.

Symptoms

As with the lower limb, symptoms can be acute or chronic. Thromboembolism from a subclavian artery aneurysm can cause acute upper limb ischemia or more focal digital ischemia. The latter may also originate from poststenotic dilatation distal to (1) an atherosclerotic proximal subclavian stenosis or (2) a damaged artery in patients with thoracic outlet syndrome. The latter is a surgical emergency and must be recognized and treated promptly.

Chronic symptoms depend on the location of the disease. Lesions distal to the origin of the vertebral artery present with forearm claudication with exercise. No neurological signs or symptoms are elicited from the history. Occlusive/stenotic disease proximal to the origin of the vertebral artery produces the subclavian steal syndrome. Here forearm exercise increases the need for increased blood flow, which is produced via reversed flow in the ipsilateral vertebral artery.

Subclavian steal is a vertebrobasilar neurologic symptom that occurs with ipsilateral arm exercise. With the use of the affected arm, the demand for blood flow increases and the arm "steals" blood from the cerebral circulation through the ipsilateral vertebral artery. Interestingly, even if there is reversed blood flow in the ipsilateral vertebral artery on imaging, symptoms of vertebrobasilar insufficiency may rarely be apparent, and the risk of posterior circulation cerebral infarction is extremely low (Hennerici et al., 1988) A rich collateral blood supply is the likely reason why symptoms may not become apparent.

Patients with atherosclerotic subclavian artery disease tend to have a good prognosis, with <20% suffering significant disease progression within 2 years of diagnosis. Moreover, nearly one quarter of patients who presented with steal (i.e., indicating marked hemodynamic impairment) and who were then treated conservatively became asymptomatic over the next 42 months of follow-up (Schillinter, 2002), indicating the potential for developing a collateral circulation in this situation.

A second type of steal, again peculiar to the subclavian artery, is the coronary-subclavian steal syndrome. This phenomenon specifically occurs in patients who have had coronary revascularization using the internal mammary artery. If thereafter they should develop a severe stenosis or occlusion of the proximal subclavian artery, arm exercise can steal blood away from the heart. Most patients present with recurrent angina symptoms or cardiac failure. Treatment (angioplasty or carotid subclavian bypass) produces significant improvements in blood flow to the heart. Clearly, cardiac surgeons should be aware of the potential for this problem and arrange for imaging of the subclavian arteries if there is any evidence of dizziness with arm exercise, forearm claudication, unequal blood pressures in the upper limbs, or weak radial pulses on palpation. Any significant lesion can thereafter be treated (usually with angioplasty) or alternative conduits considered (contralateral internal mammary, radial artery, saphenous vein).

Thoracic outlet syndrome is characterized by symptoms attributable to compression of the subclavian artery, vein, or brachial plexus. Arterial compression can cause claudication with exercise, Raynaud's phenomenon, digital microembolization, and even acute upper limb ischemia. Arterial symptoms are usually associated with bony anomalies (e.g., cervical rib) or compression between the clavicle and first rib. Arterial symptoms secondary to thoracic outlet compression must be treated urgently. Compression of the subclavian vein causes heaviness/blueness of the arm and can predispose to subclavian vein thrombosis (Paget-Schroetter syndrome). Venous compression/thrombosis in this syndrome is often seen in patients participating in demanding fitness regimes. The neurological component of thoracic outlet syndrome depends on whether there is compression of the lower (C8/T1) or upper (C5/C6) trunks of the brachial plexus. Pain or paresthesia predominate, but in severe cases muscle wasting can occur.

Diagnosis

Duplex ultrasound is now the principal imaging modality for examining the subclavian artery. Although the origin of this vessel may be difficult to image directly, an experienced ultrasonographer will be alert to a damped inflow waveform suggestive of significant disease. If required, a corroborative or diagnostic magnetic resonance angiogram (MRA) or digital

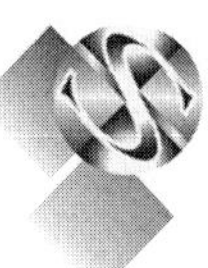

subtraction angiography (DSA) can be undertaken.

Symptoms suggestive of arterial compression (cold arm, fluctuating radial pulse with arm movements, forearm claudication, microembolization) require careful x-rays of the thoracic inlet to look for a cervical rib or a prominent transverse process on C8. The latter suggests that a fibrous band may be present. More modern tomographic imaging can demonstrate the size and location of any cervical rib (Fig. 16.4).

Management

Revascularization of the chronically occluded subclavian artery is possible with either angioplasty or surgery. Surgical options include (1) carotid-subclavian bypass, (2) carotid-axillary bypass, (3) axillary-axillary bypass, and (4) subclavian-carotid transposition. The choice of technique reflects local expertise, clinician preference, and patient presentation.

Primary patency rates following carotid-subclavian bypass have been reported to be 94%, with 87% symptom-free survival at 10 years (Vitti et al., 1994). The principal advantage of subclavian transposition is that no prosthetic material is used. Here the proximal subclavian artery is mobilized, transected, and reanastomosed end-to-side onto the common carotid artery. It is reported to have similar outcomes to carotid-subclavian bypass (primary patency at 5 years, 98%; freedom from recurrent symptoms, 95%). However, these types of revascularization are not without risk: thoracic duct injury (2%), nerve injury (11%), stroke (6%), and wound hematoma (1%). The long-term durability of axillary-axillary bypass is inferior to carotid-subclavian bypass or transposition but may be the treatment of choice in a high-risk patient because it can be performed under local anesthesia. For obvious reasons, this type of reconstruction should be avoided in any patient who might subsequently a median sternotomy.

Angioplasty is the preferred option in the United Kingdom and most European countries. There is, however, no consensus as to whether stents should be routinely used. Angioplasty of the subclavian artery carries a 2% to 3% risk of procedural stroke. This risk can be minimized by passing a protective balloon up the brachial artery and up into the ipsilateral vertebral

artery. This is inflated while the main subclavian lesion is angioplastied, and deflated once it is completed. It is of interest to note that following successful subclavian artery angioplasty, flow reversal in the vertebral artery is not instantaneous. The reason for this delayed reversal of flow is not known.

The Proximal Common Carotid Artery

Etiology

Proximal common carotid disease occurs much less frequently than carotid bifurcation disease, but 1% to 2% of patients with severe bifurcation disease also have significant proximal common carotid disease. Lesions of the right common carotid artery are rare in the absence of innominate artery disease and are rarer compared to left common carotid disease. The principal underlying pathologies include atherosclerotic disease (most common), Takayasu's arteritis, and, rarely, radiation-induced atherosclerosis.

Symptoms

Proximal common carotid lesions present with thromboembolic symptoms that are identical to those of disease at the carotid bifurcation (hemisensory/motor signs, temporary monocular blindness, higher cortical dysfunction).

Diagnosis

The proximal common carotid artery is not within the scanning range of current Duplex technology. However, as with proximal subclavian disease, significant disease at its origin causes significant damping of the waveform and turbulence. If there is any evidence of this (or if the patient is being considered for bifurcation angioplasty), he/she will need to undergo either MRA or DSA. Other emerging alternatives include computed tomography (CT) angiography. Clearly the choice reflects the unit's experience, access, and preference.

Management

In the past, proximal common carotid disease required partial sternotomy and either endarterectomy or bypass off the aortic arch. Other options included carotid-carotid bypass or carotid transposition. However, this is another situation where on-table angioplasty (following exposure of the mid–common carotid artery) affords a balance between minimal risk and prevention of embolization. Venting blood into a sheath or up the external carotid artery can prevent the latter. One advantage of on-table angioplasty is that it can be combined with synchronous bifurcation endarterectomy.

The Vertebral Artery

Etiology

The vertebral arteries arise from the proximal subclavian arteries. The first segment extends from its origin to where it enters the transverse cervical vertebral processes. The second segment is intraspinal. The third segment starts at the upper border of the transverse process of C2 and passes up to the atlanto-occipital membrane. The fourth segment is intradural to its confluence with the contralateral vertebral to thereafter form the basilar artery. The commonest pathology is an atherosclerotic stenosis or occlusion of the proximal vertebral artery (Fig. 16.5). Alternative (less common) pathologies include fibromuscular dysplasia or dissection.

Symptoms

Classical vertebral territory symptoms (vertebrobasilar symptoms) include varying combinations of unsteadiness of gait, diplopia, bilateral motor/sensory impairment, nystagmus, ataxia, bilateral blindness, and dysarthria. These symptoms can be due to either thrombosis or embolism (often very difficult to tell), but the consensus view is that the majority is probably hemodynamic. Tomographic imaging can sometimes help in the difficult task of discriminating between the two etiologies.

There is much controversy about whether nonhemispheric symptoms (isolated diplopia, isolated dizziness, isolated vertigo, syncope, etc.) can be attributed to disease in the vertebrobasilar system. To date, there is no compelling evidence that they are attributable

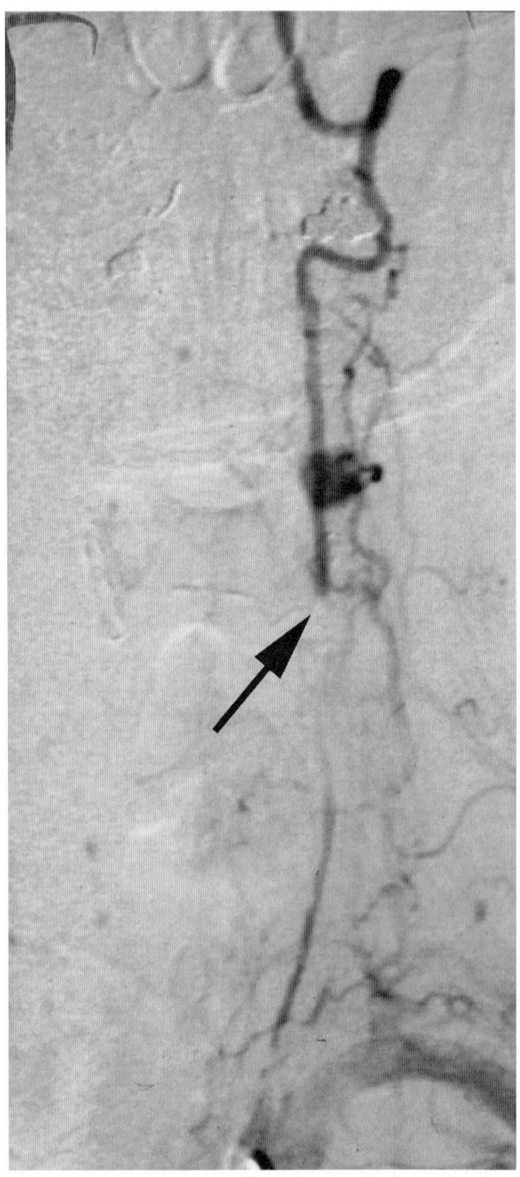

Figure 16.5. Occlusion of the proximal vertebral artery with distal refilling via collaterals. The most likely pathology is thrombosis secondary to atherosclerotic disease.

unless they definitely coexist with other, more typical vertebrobasilar territory symptoms. One other myth is the concept of "nipping of the intraspinal vertebral arteries causing dizziness on head movement." At the Leicester Royal Infirmary, a number of these patients have been examined with transcranial and extracranial

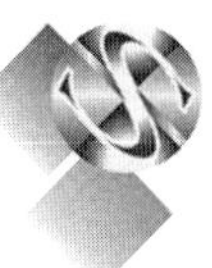

duplex imaging, and none have ever been noted to have any change in flow or direction of flow with head movements. All were subsequently found to have inner ear pathologies. There is also no evidence that coils or kinks in the proximal vertebral artery are responsible for cerebrovascular symptoms unless a coexistent stenosis is present.

Diagnosis

Duplex imaging identifies evidence of damped flow, hypoplastic arteries (not uncommon), and inflow stenoses. It is not, however, particularly good at imaging the entire length of the artery. Accordingly, patients suspected of having vertebrobasilar insufficiency should undergo MRA or intraarterial DSA.

Treatment

The treatment of vertebral artery stenoses/occlusions is to first address the anterior circulation. If there is significant internal carotid artery disease, carotid endarterectomy should be employed first. Some centers have reported huge series of vertebral reconstructions. At Leicester (apart from carotid-subclavian bypass), only three vertebral reconstructions have been performed over the last 8 years, all involving segment 1. Angioplasty is currently the emerging treatment of choice, although some surgeons remain strong advocates of surgical revascularization of segment 2 (endarterectomy and patch, bypass, transposition onto the carotid artery).

Technique

All interventions should be undertaken in a specially equipped operating room with dedicated fluoroscopic/angiographic capabilities. As one of the risks for endovascular treatment of the supra-aortic trunk is distal embolization, local infiltrative anesthesia supplemented with intravenous sedation is optimal. This type of anesthesia allows for continuous monitoring of the patient's neurologic status.

Due to the risk of distal embolization, common carotid lesions are best treated through a limited surgical incision in the neck. This allows for distal control of the common carotid artery and the ability of flushing the artery of atherosclerotic emboli. Flow through the external carotid artery is usually sufficient for cerebral perfusion. If concomitant bifurcation disease is present (around 2% of patients), then the common carotid lesion should be treated first. Once the artery is exposed, intravenous heparin is given prior to obtaining proximal control, placement of the sheath, and crossing the lesion. The artery is accessed with a Potts-Cournand 18-gauge needle in a retrograde fashion and a 0.035-mm wire in advanced with the help of fluoroscopy into the aortic arch. A 35-cm-long sheath may be placed to allow for more distance between the surgeon and radiation field, decreasing exposure to the surgeon's hands. Access of the femoral artery allows for placement of a flush catheter in the aortic arch and more precise localization of the ostium of the vessel. Selection of the innominate artery and selected oblique views to define the right common carotid and right subclavian origin is imperative for precise stent placement. The true location of the ostium is imperative to determine optimal stent placement, with 1 to 2 mm of the stent protruding into the lumen of the aortic arch. Occlusions should be predilated to avoid stent dislodgment during crossing of the lesion or to allow for safe passage of self-expanding stents across the lesion. Whether balloon expandable stents or self-expanding stents are better is unknown, as there are no comparative studies. It would seem logical that if the lesion is tortuous or crosses the clavicle, a self-expanding stent, which is more flexible, would be preferred. Cerebral protection devices may change the need for surgical control of the common carotid artery. These devices could be used for stenoses, but not for occlusive lesions. As in internal carotid artery stenting, the lesion is crossed with the low-profile cerebral protection devise prior to any manipulation of the lesion. This would be impossible with an occlusive lesion. Other limitations of the cerebral protection device use would be common carotid size, not allowing for good apposition of the device to the artery. The device, therefore, would need to be placed in the internal carotid artery.

Subclavian lesion may be treated both from a femoral and brachial approach. Again, a combined brachial-femoral approach allows for placement of a flush catheter in the aorta and therefore more precise placement of the stent. With occlusive lesion, the brachial approach allows for more pushability to cross the lesion. The caveat to this approach is risk of dissection into the aortic arch. In general, stenting allows for tacking of the dissections. Other considerations are posterior circulation embolization. It is therefore imperative to determine flow direction in the vertebral artery by duplex ultrasonography. Antegrade vertebral flow is delayed from 20 to 240 seconds, serving as an effective protective mechanism against embolism in the posterior circulation. Brachial artery cutdown allows for direct repair of the artery after completion of the stenting, thus decreasing the risk of atherosclerotic emboli (allowing for flushing of the artery) and avoiding risk of hematoma.

References

Azakie A, McElhinney DB, Higashima R, Messina LM, Stoney RJ. (1998) Ann Surg 228:402–10.

Berguer R, Morasch MD, Kline RA. (1998) J Vasc Surg 27: 34–41; discussion 42.

Hennerici M, Klemm C, Rautenberg W. (1988) Neurology 38:669–73.

Henry M, Amor M, Henry I, Ethevenot G, Tzvetanov K, Chati Z. (1999) J Endovasc Surg 6:33–41.

Kieffer E, Sabatier J, Koskas F, Bahnini A. (1995) J Vasc Surg 21:326–36; discussion 336–7.

Rhodes JM, Cherry KJ Jr, Clark RC, et al. (2000) J Vasc Surg 31:260–9.

Sullivan TM, Gray BH, Bacharach JM, et al. (1998) J Vasc Surg 28:1059–65.

Vitti MJ, Thompson BW, Read RC, et al. (1994) J Vasc Surg 20:411–7; discussion 417–8.

Whitbread T, Cleveland TJ, Beard JD, Gaines PA. (1998) Eur J Vasc Endovasc Surg 15:29–35.

Wylie EJ, Effeney DJ. (1979) Surg Clin North Am 59:669–80.

17

Aneurysmal Disease

Philip Davey and Michael G. Wyatt

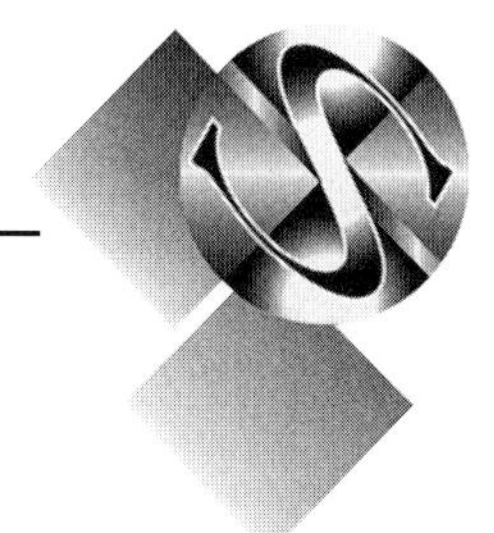

Arterial aneurysmal disease has been recognized now for over 4000 years, with the expression "aneurysm" deriving from the Greek word *aneurysma,* meaning "a widening." Historical review charts a condition in which initially observational experiences of aneurysms have been gradually replaced with the established treatment regimes we see in clinical practice today. Advances made in aneurysm management reflect not only improved surgical acumen and the appliance of innovative technology but also the progress made in our basic scientific knowledge, clinical experience, diagnosis, perioperative care, anesthesia, and follow-up of the disease. Aneurysmal disease constitutes a substantial component of the vascular surgeon's work load, and this chapter reviews the common pathology with reference to contemporary opinion in pathogenesis, diagnosis, and management.

Classification of Arterial Aneurysms

The aneurysm is defined as an abnormal, focal dilatation of a blood vessel. An artery is empirically considered aneurysmal when its diameter becomes 50% larger than its normal vessel segment. This diagnosis is distinct from *ectasia,* which refers to a dilated vessel that has not yet reached this threshold. Similarly, the conditions of arteriomegaly and multiple aneurysms must not be confused. In the former, *generalized* dilated vasculature (>50%) is observed but, unlike the latter condition, normal-caliber vessel segments do not distinguish these conditions.

Aneurysmal disease may be classified as follows:

1. By nature: *true* aneurysms relate to a distinct pathological process involving all three layers of the arterial wall. *False* or *pseudoaneurysms* do not reflect a genuine aneurysmal process at all but rather clinical mimicry true disease. They are, in fact, a vessel-associated contained blood collection and typically result from trauma.

2. By morphology: *saccular* aneurysmal disease is present if only part of the vessel circumference is diseased. Entire circumferential involvement is termed *fusiform.*

3. By etiology: aneurysms are frequently referred to with respect to an antecedent disease process. The list, which is not exhaustive, includes

   a. Degeneration (e.g., atherosclerosis, fibromuscular dysplasia)

   b. Infection (e.g., syphilis, bacterial, fungal)

   c. Trauma (e.g., iatrogenic, penetrating, blunt)

   d. Inflammation (e.g., Takayasu's or Kawasaki disease, polyarteritis nodosa)

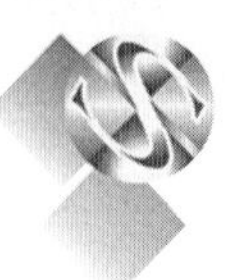

   e. Connective tissue disorders (e.g., Marfan syndrome, Ehlers-Danlos syndrome)

   f. Congenital (e.g., tuberous sclerosis, Turner syndrome)

4. By location: for example, abdominal aortic, popliteal, femoral, subclavian, thoracoabdominal, etc.

Pathogenesis of Aneurysmal Disease

Despite extensive research, the exact mechanisms underlying aneurysm pathogenesis remain unclear. It appears the process is multifactorial, involving variable components of altered biochemistry, immunological, mechanical, and genetic importance (Wassef et al., 2001). Much of our understanding of the disease relates to work performed on the abdominal aorta, and it is assumed that nonaortic aneurysmal disease results from a similar pathological sequence of events.

Aneurysmal disease ultimately results following gradual proteolytic degradation of arterial vessel walls. Structural integrity of arterial wall is dependent on adequate functional connective tissue elements including elastin and collagen. Loss of these elements weakens the vessel wall and thus predisposes to aneurysm formation. Research into abdominal aortic aneurysms (AAAs) has discovered local increased levels of matrix metalloproteinases (MMPs) that result in this observed connective tissue breakdown. Four MMP subtypes are thought to be of importance in this process: gelatinases (MMP-2 and MMP-9), matrilysin (MMP-7), and macrophage elastase (MMP-12). In addition to this increased local expression, altered levels of circulating proteases may play a role, and research continues into the contributions to aneurysmal disease from various plasminogen activators, serine elastases, and cysteine proteases (cathepsins S and K). Abnormally low levels of protease inhibitors are suggested to exert the same pathogenic effects, and this has also been the focus of much recent work. Preliminary research into the most abundant serine protease inhibitor, cystatin c, has confirmed that in patients with aneurysmal disease corresponding levels of this protein are indeed lower than normal.

Chronic inflammation plays an important role in aneurysmal disease. Much of the vessel wall destruction is undoubtedly mediated by the inflammatory infiltrate composed of T cells, macrophages, B lymphocytes, and plasma cells, but the antecedent trigger for this cellular migration remains unclear. It has been suggested that aneurysmal disease is in fact an antigen-driven immune disease from work analyzing AAA disease. Proposed antigenic activators to subsequent inflammation include elastin, interstitial collagen, oxidized low-density lipoprotein, cytomegalovirus, and artery-specific antigenic proteins such as AAAP-40. Following T-cell antigen recognition, the inflammatory cascade begins, ultimately resulting in vessel wall degradation and progression to aneurysmal disease.

Arterial wall biomechanical stress is also accepted as being of considerable importance in both aneurysm progression and rupture. Model analysis of wall stress variation in different anatomical locations implies that altered hemodynamic profiles may explain the varying susceptibility of an arterial wall to become aneurysmal (e.g., increased disease incidence in abdominal as opposed to thoracic aorta). It is suggested that mechanical failure from excessive stress initiates and promotes aneurysmal pathogenesis first by the aggregation of humoral factors, and then by a consequent focal inflammatory response and finally wall breakdown.

The familial clustering of aneurysmal disease has led to interest in determining a possible genetic explanation for the process. Supporting evidence is derived from observations regarding the altered disease characteristics of "familial" and "spontaneous" aortic aneurysmal disease. Cases of familial AAA present significantly younger, carry a greater rupture risk (especially in females) and are 18 times more likely to be present in other family members than is seen with spontaneous pathology. Affected sibling pair DNA linkage studies aims to identify the putative AAA-susceptibility gene, whose expression or mutation promotes progression to aneurysmal disease. This approach to pathogenesis may eventually form the basis of genetic testing of specific increased-risk populations, allowing more focused surveillance and early intervention.

Abdominal Aortic Aneurysms

In the 16th century the anatomist Vesalius first recognized aneurysmal disease affecting the infrarenal aorta. Limited progress was made over the following centuries in the treatment of AAA, and it was not until 1952 that Dubost reported the first successful treatment of the condition by surgical repair. In the past 50 years, increased experience and advancement of surgical techniques have rendered elective AAA repair a routine albeit major operative procedure with expected mortality rates of less than 5% (Hallin et al., 2001). Exciting developments in the endovascular arena over the last decade have offered further options for treatment in elective AAA disease and promises to revolutionize management for many patients.

The natural history of AAA is to gradually expand and eventually rupture. Ultimately, the aim of elective surgery is to prevent this from happening by excluding the aneurysm from the circulation by means of either prosthetic graft insertion or endovascular stent deployment. Unfortunately, even with improved perioperative management and operative technique, the great advances made in elective AAA repair have not been witnessed in the emergency setting for AAA rupture, and consequently mortality rates remain high at approximately 50%.

Definition

Aneurysms are arbitrarily defined as a segment of vessel dilatation that is at least 50% larger than the expected normal vessel diameter. In practical terms this diameter refers to the nonaneurysmal adjacent vessel segment. We accept a "normal" abdominal aorta to be approximately 20 mm in diameter, and therefore an aorta wider than 30 mm would suggest aneurysmal disease.

Epidemiology

In all epidemiological analysis, statistical variation can exist as a result of inconsistent definitions of disease, and AAA is no exception. Population screening surveys and postmortem studies have been used to estimate a current prevalence of AAA of between 1.3% and 12.7% in England (Wilmink and Quick, 1998). Marked increases in the prevalence of the disease are seen if the definition of AAA is relaxed to even 1 mm less than stated earlier (30 mm), but little difference exists between the two methods of prevalence estimation in this condition.

The incidence of asymptomatic AAA has been reported at 3 to 117 per 100,000 person-years. These estimations are derived from the number of hospital admissions for elective asymptomatic AAA repair and have been observed to increase by 7% to 26% over the past 15 years. This basically reflects changes in improved disease awareness, referral patterns, and diagnosis, more specifically the increased availability and use of ultrasound scanning in recent years. The reported incidence of ruptured AAA is much more inaccurate due to high prehospital mortality, but quoted values are between 1 and 21 per 100–000 person-years. Data also suggests that this value is continuing to increase by 2.4% per year. In the United Kingdom, ruptured aortic aneurysms have been reported as the 13th commonest cause of death accounting for 1.2% of male and 0.6% of female mortality.

Abdominal aortic aneurysm is typically a disease of the male population, being five times more common than in women. A sharp increased incidence is seen after the age of 50 years, rising to a peak at 80 years of age. Abdominal aortic aneurysm in females does not tend to occur until about 10 years later than in men, and then increases linearly from the age of 60.

In a more general sense, 5% of the over-60 population will have an AAA, and at the age of 67 a man is ten times more likely to die from a ruptured AAA than is a woman.

Risk Factors for Abdominal Aortic Aneurysm

Factors associated with an increased risk of aneurysmal development in the infrarenal aorta include increasing age, male sex, ethnic origin, family history, smoking, hypercholesterolemia, hypertension, and prior vascular disease. Studies suggest that of these, male sex and smoking are the most important, increasing the chances of AAA development by 4.5 and 5.5 times, respectively. A positive family history (first-degree relative affected) alone doubles the risk of AAA presentation and is more likely if the affected relative is a female. Interestingly,

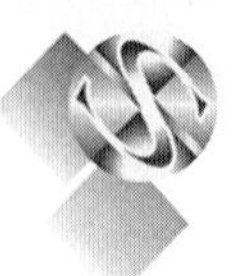

diabetes mellitus, which is a major risk factor for occlusive arterial disease, is associated with less risk (compared to nondiabetics) in the development of aortic aneurysmal disease.

Clinical Features

The vast majority of AAAs are asymptomatic, and the diagnosis is usually made on clinical abdominal examination or following ultrasound investigation for other pathology. If symptoms are present, they usually relate to the complications of infra-aortic aneurysmal disease both locally and systemically.

Abdominal or back pain may be experienced, and this must alert the clinician to the possibility of posterior erosion of the aneurysm into the neighboring vertebral bodies. Classically in this situation, the history of pain follows a nonspecific and indolent course. Appropriate subsequent investigations should distinguish erosion from the diagnosis of inflammatory AAA (see later). Sudden onset of severe abdominal or back pain in a patient with a known AAA who is hemodynamically unstable suggests aneurysm rupture. The pain may radiate into the hips, and the patient will be pale, anxious, clammy, tachycardic, and hypotensive. An aneurysm rupture that is contained within the retroperitoneum is often seen with a similar but less pronounced symptom profile, affording more time for preoperative optimization than uncontained ruptures.

Symptoms of distal ischemia may result directly from the presence of AAAs. Embolization of contents from the aneurysmal sac may present with acute or chronic limb ischemia, whereas a similar picture may be witnessed if the AAA thromboses in situ. In the latter case one would expect symptoms of bilateral leg ischemia.

Less common presentations of infra-renal aortic aneurysmal disease relate to fistulation. Cases of aortoduodenal fistulas present classically with intermittent, unexplained gastrointestinal bleeding and melena or massive uncontrollable hematemesis. The diagnosis is confirmed by upper gastrointestinal endoscopy prompting urgent surgical repair. Isolated aortocaval fistulas are rare but present with symptoms of high output cardiac failure. More commonly, an aortocaval fistula results as a consequence of aneurysm rupture, and the operative finding at laparotomy is that of massive venous hemorrhage requiring rapid control to avert on-table death due to exsanguination.

Detection of an AAA can potentially be made by careful abdominal palpation during clinical examination. The reliability of this technique alone is questionable, its sensitivity governed by a variety of factors such as aneurysm size, examiner's skill, patient's body habitus, and the purpose of the clinical examination itself. Even after acknowledgment of these variables, a correct diagnosis is achieved in only approximately 50% of cases. Smaller aneurysms and obesity increase the likelihood of a missed diagnosis, whereas an false-positive diagnosis of AAA may be made in thin patients, tortuous aortas, or in those with more prominent vessels as a consequence of lumbar lordosis. Similarly, the success of manual examination in the assessment of aneurysm size and proximal extent in relation to the renal arteries is poor. Subcutaneous fat and overlying intestine tend to cause an overestimation of size, and the ability to admit an examining hand between the costal margin and pulsatile mass will not indicate infrarenal disease in all cases.

Investigations for Abdominal Aortic Aneurysm

Plain Film Radiography

Plain abdominal x-rays are cheap and widely available but of little use in the routine diagnosis of the AAA. Occasionally, calcification may be observed in the wall of the aneurysmal vessel or there may be loss of the psoas major shadow. In the preoperative setting their use is limited to exclusion of an alternate diagnosis to AAA. They do, however, play an important role following endovascular stent graft repair of AAA for observation of long-term outcome and graft integrity.

Ultrasonography

Abdominal ultrasound examination is responsible for the detection of the majority of asymptomatic AAAs and it is also used to confirm the suspected clinical diagnosis (Fig. 17.1). In addition, this modality is employed to observe aneurysmal expansion in patients with disease

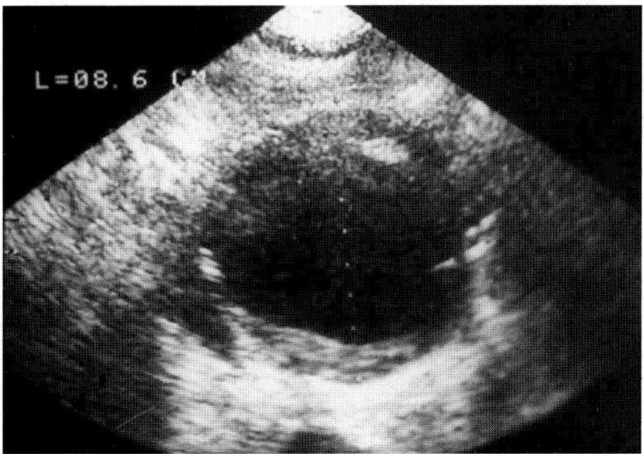

Figure 17.1. An abdominal ultrasound showing an aortic aneurysm.

under surveillance. Ultrasound is cheap, relatively quick, widely available, and noninvasive. Visualization of the aorta is achieved in 97% of patients, and current figures demonstrate minimal interobserver variability. The availability of mobile ultrasound machines allows assessment of the critically ill patient who ideally should not be transferred to the radiology department.

Ultrasound, however, does have its limitations. Unfortunately, cases of suprarenal, visceral artery aneurysmal disease and iliac vessel extension cannot be accurately assessed by ultrasound. In obese, ventilated patients, or those patients with excessive bowel gas, this unreliability is further exaggerated. Furthermore, this modality is poor at confirming the presence of aneurysm rupture and hence plays no role in the emergency setting.

Computed Tomography Scanning

Computed tomography (CT) scanning remains the investigation of choice for the most accurate assessment of AAA disease. The procedure allows visualization of the upper extent of the aneurysm and its nature (i.e., noninflammatory or inflammatory), and provides reliable information regarding iliac artery involvement. Interobserver variation in the measurement of aneurysm size is superior to ultrasound, with over 90% of studies exhibiting a discrepancy of less than 5 mm. Computed tomography scanning with 3-mm cuts can also be used to determine if the patient is a candidate for

endoluminal stent grafting. The imaging, however, is invasive, time-consuming, and expensive, and it entails substantial radiation exposure for the patient. It is therefore restricted for preoperative assessment in those suspected to be imminent candidates for surgical repair, follow-up of endovascular stent graft repairs, and for patients with suspected AAA rupture who are stable enough for deferment of laparotomy.

The advent of spiral CT scanning in some centers has led to increased speed of assessment (a single breath hold) with the ability to reconstruct CT images in a three-dimensional manner, resulting in a more user-friendly and informative imaging. The use of CT scanning must be judicious in patients with a prior history of contrast reaction, high blood pressure, and preexisting renal impairment. As with ultrasound, CT scanning cannot detect visceral artery involvement or the presence of renal artery stenosis, and this must be remembered in assessment of the generated images.

Magnetic Resonance Imaging

Magnetic resonance imaging (MRI) for AAA offers comparable results to CT scanning in terms of assessment of aneurysm size, proximal extent, iliac extension, and etiology (e.g., inflammatory), and has the added advantage of being noninvasive and safe because no contrast administration is required. The procedure, however, is not well tolerated by claustrophobic patients, and its limited availability and expense have relegated its use to a second-line investigation for AAA, reserved for those patients for whom CT scanning is inappropriate (e.g., iodinated contrast allergy, chronic renal failure, or claustrophobia).

Angiography

Contrast arteriography offers little information regarding the possible diagnosis or sizing of an AAA, as it is only the vessel lumen (not the aneurysmal sac) that is delineated in this examination. For these reasons, this investigation plays little role in the management of the routine infrarenal AAA. It does, however, offer detailed information with respect to possible visceral or renal artery disease, and allows adequate vessel anatomy analysis for planning prior

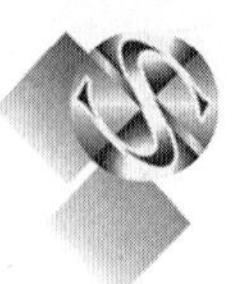

to surgical repair. Indications for arteriography, therefore, include aneurysms with possible suprarenal involvement or suspected visceral artery disease, renal stenosis, and in patients with coexistent peripheral vascular or nonaortic aneurysmal disease (e.g., popliteal). Again, the investigation is invasive, involves the use of substantial amounts of contrast agent, and carries with it the risks of embolic and renal complications.

Screening for Abdominal Aortic Aneurysm

There is currently much debate about the merits about introducing a national screening program for the detection of aneurysmal disease affecting the abdominal aorta (Table 17.1). The nature of AAA is such that the majority of patients have the condition silently, until they present at the hospital under the most extreme circumstances: aneurysm rupture. Because the prevalence of this disease is relatively high (5% of the over-60 population), it has been suggested that a simple ultrasound-screening test at about this age would uncover the asymptomatic pathology at an early stage. Appropriate follow-up and elective repair could then be planned, thus diminishing the frequency of ruptured aneurysm presentation and its inherent cost implications.

Recent studies in the U.K. have shown that a screening program would indeed fulfill these expectations, observing a reduction in the AAA rupture rate by 50%. Other groups suggest a screening program would have a greater diagnostic yield and hence prove more cost-effective if only the specific, high-risk populations were targeted, such as elderly male smokers. Whatever the proposal, it would certainly appear that a timely ultrasound examination may be beneficial in the early management of AAA, but a large multicenter trial is needed to obtain adequate numbers of patients with the power to demonstrate the cost-effectiveness of this approach to AAA disease.

Management of the Elective Abdominal Aortic Aneurysm

The basic goal underpinning the management of the asymptomatic and symptomatic non-ruptured AAA is to avert the presentation of aneurysm rupture. As with all surgery, a surgeon must balance the risks of the required major operation in terms of mortality and morbidity against that of a possible rupture-related death with nonoperative "conservative" management. With appropriate case selection and surgical expertise, mortality following elective AAA repair should be between 2% and 5%. Important issues to be taken into account, which enable the surgeon to make the correct decision whether or not to operate, are discussed in the following subsections.

Aneurysmal Size

The maximum diameter of AAA is without doubt the most important factor in predicting the ruptured risk of an aneurysm. The 5-year rupture risk of an aneurysm less than 4 cm in diameter is approximately 15%, and this rises to nearly 95% if the aneurysm grows to 7 cm in diameter. Unfortunately, vascular surgery is not an exact science, however, and small aneurysms will continue to rupture and many people with large aneurysms will outlive the disease and die of an unrelated cause.

The recently completed U.K. small aneurysm trial aimed to provide guidelines regarding when to offer elective surgery on the basis of aneurysm size (Lancet, 1998). Comparison of surgical repair of small aneurysms (4 to 5.5 cm) with nonoperative ultrasound surveillance suggested that there was no survival benefit to be gained from operative management of the AAA. The trial researchers recommended that aneurysms should be considered for surgical repair when the maximal diameter exceeded 5.5 cm or the aneurysm became symptomatic or tender. It was at this stage the operative risk of repair was less than the risk of rupture associated with nonoperative management.

Table 17.1. Why screen for aneurysms?

Abdominal aortic aneurysms (AAA) are asymptomatic
Major complication of AAA is rupture
Morbidity and mortality of repair of ruptured AAAs:
    50% to 70%; elective AAAs, 1% to 5%
Patients who survive repair have a similar life
    expectancy as the general population
Ultrasound is inexpensive and noninvasive

Treatment protocols for small aneurysms remain less clear-cut, but as a general rule all AAAs greater than 30 mm in diameter should be kept under ultrasound surveillance. Aortas less than 40 mm in diameter should probably be monitored with annual ultrasound scans, whereas if there is growth to between 40 and 55 mm the frequency of observations should increase to every 6 months. Other measures in management include encouragement to stop smoking, aggressive blood pressure control, and possibly the administration of propranolol unless contraindicated (see later). If an aneurysm under surveillance appears greater than 50 mm in diameter, a CT scan should be obtained to formally size and delineate aneurysmal anatomy in preparation for operative repair. At some centers, it is at this stage that the patient may be considered for endovascular treatment as opposed to open repair of their aneurysm.

Expansion Rate

Aneurysmal expansion rate is considered an important factor as it enables the clinician to estimate the timing of elective surgery governed by the size of the AAA. Much evidence suggests that the larger the aneurysm, the quicker the expansion rate, so that aneurysmal growth can be considered as exponential function of aneurysm size. Small aneurysms between 40 and 60 mm are expected to expand "normally" at an annual rate of around 10% (4 to 5 mm). Growth patterns that exceed this reflect unpredictable pathology and may warrant earlier surgical intervention. It is generally accepted that if the aneurysm expansion rate is greater than 10 mm, this is an indication for operative repair, regardless of the aneurysm size.

The exact reasons for the vast differences witnessed in aneurysm expansion remain unclear. Studies have shown that smoking, advancing age, cardiac disease, and hypertension are all independent predictors of an increased expansion rate, and that administration of certain beta-blocker drugs may reduce this phenomenon. Recently, much interest has been directed toward the medical management of small aneurysms with the drug propranolol, which is observed to reduce the rapid expansion of AAA by nearly 40%. The exact mechanism of this finding could simply be explained by improved blood pressure or heart rate control, but some groups suggest that since propranolol blocks circulating tissue plasminogen activator (tPA), there is a direct effect on the aortic wall by diminished plasmin-mediated MMP activation and therefore reduced expansion rate. Whatever the pharmacological explanation, it would certainly appear that unless contraindicated (e.g., asthma, severe cardiac failure), a good argument can be made for the administration of propranolol while the aneurysm is under surveillance.

Proximal Extent of Abdominal Aortic Aneurysm

The relationship of the aneurysm to both the renal and visceral arteries must be elicited prior to surgical repair. Juxtarenal aneurysms commence immediately below the renal arteries and thus do not permit a clamp to be placed infrarenally, as is also the case with suprarenal aneurysms, which may or may not involve the superior mesenteric artery or coeliac axis. If the pathology commences higher than the coeliac trunk, the aneurysm is deemed to be thoracoabdominal. Repair of all these aneurysms carries significantly increased patient mortality or morbidity with requirement for higher levels of surgical expertise. Hence, referral to a tertiary vascular center is mandatory and repair should not be attempted at a district general hospital.

Patient Comorbidity

Full patient assessment prior to proposed AAA surgery should aim to identify medical factors to be addressed in the preoperative workup. Aneurysmal surgery is obviously not appropriate in those patients with widespread advanced malignancy and limited life expectancy or those with neurological degenerative disease. Other conditions that do not preclude surgery should be appropriately treated in order to optimize the patient for the operating room and so minimize the risks of aneurysm repair. Specific preoperative conditions associated with poor outcome following elective AAA surgery include renal dysfunction, cardiac failure, myocardial ischemia, and respiratory impairment. The presence of one or more of these conditions may indicate the need for extensive preoperative investigation and appropriate referral to other medical specialties.

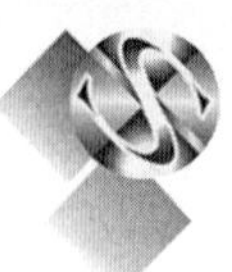

Individual Surgeon's Audited Results

In the current climate of clinical governance and accountability, it is no surprise that the decision to operate in AAA does not entirely depend on the patient but also on the ability of the operating surgeons themselves. Advances in operative technique and vascular anesthesia in major centers have been reflected in a fall of operative mortality following elective AAA repair to around 2% to 5%. Unfortunately, the death rate at some district general hospitals after the same operation by personnel without specialist knowledge has been reported in excess of 10% and poses the question of whether this surgeon-specific discrepancy warrants the shift of all elective AAA repairs to be performed at recognized major vascular centers.

Aneurysmal Symptomatology

Symptomatic and suspected ruptured aortic aneurysms are usually in themselves an indication for surgical intervention. The rationale for this decision is explained by the high mortality rate of a presumed imminent rupture, and predicted morbidity following embolism from the aneurysmal sac.

Preoperative Assessment of the Elective Abdominal Aortic Aneurysm

One of the cornerstones of the successful management of the elective AAA is adequate preoperative preparation. An extensive patient history and full examination should be performed, followed by a set of basic investigations for all patients. These measures should aid the decision of whether or not operative intervention is appropriate and may uncover any subclinical pathologies that can be corrected, or at least optimized prior to surgery. We consider the required analysis as of two distinct types, examining both general health status with quality of life and also aneurysm-specific factors.

General Health Status

After initial assessment of an apparently medically fit patient, it is essential to gain an appreciation of that person's quality of life. This loose term is difficult to define but encapsulates all aspects of the patient's daily living, involving not only physical status but mental and social aspects also. Operation for AAA should both prolong and preserve quality of life. Due to the nature of the disease, it is unlikely that AAA repair will lead to any physical improvement in the preoperative condition with the risk of a drastic deterioration in health. On the other hand, for many, quality of life is still vastly improved by elimination of the cause of much psychological torment that was the "time bomb" ticking in their abdomen. There is little doubt that issues pertaining to a subject's quality of life can raise difficult and emotive questions. The astute clinician should enlist help with management decisions from not only the patient but also the family, nursing staff, and caregivers.

Basic laboratory investigations to be performed on all patients considered for AAA surgery include a full blood count, erythrocyte sedimentation rate (ESR), blood glucose, serum urea, and electrolytes. Hematological disorders and anemia may well be uncovered at this stage, prompting further investigation before surgery. An elevated ESR might be the only indicator of an inflammatory AAA or even reflect ongoing chronic infection or inflammation elsewhere. Hyperglycemia may expose the unknown diabetic and has implications for both peri- and postoperative patient care. Silent renal or endocrine dysfunction is suggested with abnormal urea and electrolyte values, and these would necessitate further investigation and optimization before surgery.

In addition to these tests a 12-lead electrocardiogram (ECG), chest x-ray, arterial blood gas analysis, and pulmonary function tests should be performed. These reflect the importance of adequate cardiorespiratory reserve on the successful outcome of AAA surgery. Depending on the results obtained, it may well be the case that further investigations such as an exercise ECG, echocardiography, and even coronary angiography should be performed before surgery. The presence of significant cardiac disease may indeed require significant intervention such as angioplasty, stenting, or even bypass grafting before the patient is considered fit enough elective AAA repair.

Aneurysm–Specific Factors

It is most likely that by this stage an ultrasound scan will have been performed confirming the

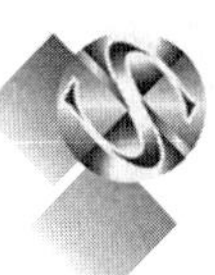

presence of an AAA. Unless contraindicated, the aneurysm should now be imaged by means of CT scanning for accurate sizing, proximal and distal extension, relationships to other abdominal vasculature, and possibly an assessment for endovascular stenting. In those patients where CT scanning is not an option, MRI offers an alternative method of gaining the required preoperative information.

In the majority of cases, this constitutes all that is required radiologically to appropriate plan operative intervention. However, in juxtarenal or suprarenal aneurysms, or patients with peripheral vascular disease or aneurysmal disease elsewhere, angiography should be considered.

Operative Management of the Elective Abdominal Aortic Aneurysm

Assuming the patient workup is completed and the patient is suitably optimized, elective AAA repair can now be attempted. Broadly speaking, there are two techniques used for aneurysm repair, and consideration will be given to each in turn.

Open Repair of Elective Abdominal Aortic Aneurysm

It is now over half a century since the first reported successful open repair of an AAA, and the technique remains well established today. Informed patient consent for the procedure is obtained and adequate (8 to 10 units) type-specific blood is cross-matched before surgery. Invasive monitoring is mandatory in AAA repair, requiring insertion of a urinary catheter and also arterial and central venous cannulation. A nasogastric tube is inserted for stomach decompression, and the anesthetist may decide to float a pulmonary artery catheter (Swan-Ganz) in those patients with significant cardiac disease. It is at this stage that an epidural catheter may be inserted to minimize postoperative pain. A single bolus dose of a wide-spectrum antibiotic (e.g., cefuroxime 1.5 g) is usually given to reduce the risk of prosthetic graft infection and this dose may be repeated in long operative procedures. The general anesthetic is administered and the airway is secured

by endotracheal intubation so that artificial ventilation can commence. Once the vascular anesthetist is satisfied, the stable patient is then transferred into the main operating room.

Elective AAA repair may proceed by either a transabdominal or retroperitoneal approach as long as adequate exposure to gain proximal and distal control is achieved. The patient is thus appropriately positioned, draped, and prepped. A relative indication for retroperitoneal access is the case of a "hostile" abdomen either due to adhesions from a previous laparotomy or the presence of an abdominal wall stoma. In the majority of elective repairs, however, it is a standard transperitoneal approach that is preferred. Laparotomy is performed by standard full-length midline incision offering a generous exposure, although some surgeons advocate a transverse incision in cases with no iliac aneurysmal involvement. Advantages of the latter are a better cosmesis and a decreased incidence of respiratory complications postoperatively as a result of reduced wound pain. Long-term wound disorders, however, are seen more frequently with a transverse incision.

Following skin incision the peritoneum is divided from a point just left to the base of the small bowel mesentery extending distally as far as the iliac artery. A self-retaining retractor is then positioned so that the surgeon has adequate exposure of the aneurysm, with the small bowel usually "stored" in a sterile bag for protection and facilitation of access. The neck of the aneurysm is dissected free followed by each of the iliac arteries prior to application of vascular clamps. Intravenous heparin is given just before aortic cross-clamping in order to reduce the risk of thrombotic complications, and this dose may be repeated in prolonged procedures.

After allowing enough time for systemic anticoagulation, the clamps are applied in a manner so that the possibility of distal complications are minimized. In practice this requires clamping of the least-diseased vessels first, taking care to avoid vessel damage and mural plaque disruption. The proximal clamp should be as close to the renal arteries as possible so that the residual native infrarenal aortic segment is minimal, therefore limiting the risk of subsequent aneurysmal recurrence. Once proximal and distal control has been achieved, the sac of the aneurysm is incised longitudinally along its anterior surface, taking care not to damage the

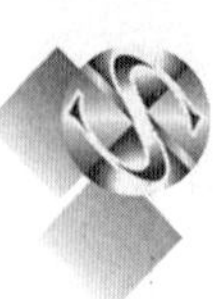

inferior mesenteric artery (IMA) that arises just to the left of midline from the aorta. Problematic bleeding may be encountered at this stage from patent lumbar arteries, and these are oversewn by vascular sutures. Back-bleeding from the IMA should be temporarily controlled with a small vascular clamp (e.g., bulldog clamp) during aneurysm repair, and the need for possible reimplantation should be assessed later in the operation.

An appraisal can now be made regarding the type of graft to be used and appropriate sizing performed. In 60% of cases a straight "tube" synthetic inlay graft may be used, requiring aorto-aortic anastomosis. The remainder of cases require a bifurcated graft due to either iliac extension of aneurysmal disease or concomitant occlusive pathology. In this situation the distal anastomosis should be performed into a normal vessel, distal to the affected artery. This usually requires iliac anastomosis, but if there is extensive iliac artery disease or technical difficulties, a femoral anastomosis must be considered. It should be remembered in the latter scenario that the patient will be at an increased risk of infection and false aneurysm formation as a result of opening the groin. The graft is sutured with 2–0 or 3–0 nonabsorbable stitches, ensuring to take deep-enough bites in the proximal anastomosis for adequate strength. In cases of friable aortic tissue, the surgeon may wish to consider the use of pledgets in the suture line in order to reinforce the anastomosis. Integrity of the proximal anastomosis is confirmed by careful release of the proximal clamp against resistance offered by prior application of a clamp across the graft. Minimal bleeding suggests successful anastomosis, and the proximal clamp is reapplied to its original position so that attention can now be given to the run-off vessel(s).

Distal anastomosis should be to the appropriate vessel as outlined earlier, with the aim to preserve at least internal iliac artery for maintenance for colonic and neural blood supply. After completion of the first iliac (or distal aortic) anastomosis, blood flow into the supplied limb should be restored after confirmation of anastomotic integrity. Close lesion with the anesthetic team is required at this stage, and release of the distal clamp should be very gradual. Sudden clamp release could lead to precipitous falls in blood pressure ("declamping hypoten-

sion") as a result of rapid volume redistribution into the large dilated distal ischemic vascular beds. This phenomenon is further exaggerated by systemic release of accumulated vasoactive metabolites from the clamped limb, and therefore timely intravenous fluid "loading" is necessary following surgical alert before clamp release.

With the graft in situ and hemostasis ensured, attention returns to the IMA. In the majority of cases the IMA may be simply ligated with a vascular suture. This practice, however, requires at least one patent internal iliac artery, a disease-free superior mesenteric artery, pink healthy large bowel, and finally good back-bleeding on release of the bulldog clamp. If these criteria are not met or colonic perfusion appears suboptimal at the end of the procedure, the IMA may have to be reimplanted into the graft by means of a Carrel patch.

Assuming IMA reimplantation is not necessary, the native aneurysm sac is closed over the graft and loosely sutured, providing physical graft protection from other intraabdominal structures. The bowel is released from the temporary storage bag and a final examination is made to ensure adequate organ perfusion and also to allow correction of any iatrogenic injury. The patient's limbs are also assessed to ensure adequate distal perfusion and exclude immediate graft thrombosis or embolism that would require prompt surgical correction. The self-retaining retractor is removed and the abdomen closed in routine fashion.

Following the operation the patient should be transferred to an intensive care or high dependency unit for close monitoring. Return to the ward is usually possible the following day if there have been no complications.

Discharge following elective AAA repair is variable but can be expected at between 7 and 14 days depending on preoperative comorbidity, operative difficulty, patient determination, and postoperative complications.

Complications Following Open Abdominal Aortic Aneurysm Repair

Despite extensive preoperative workup and improvements in anesthesia and surgical technique, complications following elective open repair of AAA still occur. All possible measures must be taken to minimize them, as often morbidity following aneurysm repair can translate to mortality. An acceptable mortality rate of less than 5% justifies prophylactic AAA repair in appropriate aneurysms as compared to the risk of rupture and subsequent near-100% mortality with a conservative approach. The nonfatal complications are considered as early or late.

Early Complications

Cardiorespiratory

Cardiorespiratory complications account for 25% to 30% of all morbidity following elective open AAA repair. The majority of cardiac ischemic events take place in the initial 48 hours postoperatively, myocardial infarcts accounting for a third of these. Measures that can be taken by the surgical team to reduce the incidence of these complications include appropriate fluid management to optimize preload and reduce myocardial stress, administration of oxygen therapy, and adequate postoperative pain relief. Chest infections complicate approximately 5% of AAA repairs and can be minimized by appropriate analgesia without sedation, chest physiotherapy, and early mobilization.

Hemorrhage

Problematic hemorrhage intraoperatively is usually due to bleeding from the proximal suture line or inadvertent iatrogenic vessel injury. The renal and iliac veins are particularly susceptible to damage during initial exposure, and all attempts should be made to address this before proceeding to aneurysm repair. Difficult dissections in freeing the iliac arteries for clamping are probably best managed with intraluminal balloon occlusion rather than potentially hazardous clamp application.

Generalized postoperative hemorrhage is most often due to an acquired coagulopathy rather than a direct consequence of surgery. Massive transfusion and hypothermia lead to clotting factor deficiencies, low platelet counts, an impaired coagulation cascade, and altered platelet function. Appropriate blood product and platelet transfusion with rewarming is necessary to reverse these problems and should be guided by serial laboratory coagulation studies and hematology advice.

Renal

Impaired renal function post open AAA repair accounts for 5% to 12% of all early complications, and of these nearly half require renal replacement therapy with dialysis. These figures reflect a substantial decrease in the incidence of renal morbidity and are attributed to the improvements made in its pre- and perioperative management. Advancing knowledge and understanding of radiological contrast-induced nephrotoxicity has led surgeons to defer surgery following such investigations in order to allow renal recovery. Current perioperative fluid management regimes that are guided by sensitive invasive indicators of circulating volume (e.g., Central Venous Pressure (CVP) lines) have also improved the perioperative maintenance of a normal cardiac output and renal blood flow. The exact cause of renal failure despite these measures after AAA repair remains unknown. It is highly probable that the damage is a consequence of debris embolizing from the diseased aortic wall that is dislodged during proximal aortic cross-clamping. Meticulous preoperative image analysis may highlight this potential complication before surgery and thus allowing modification of the surgical technique.

Patients presenting for elective open AAA repair with known renal impairment are at the greatest risk of postoperative renal failure. Administration of renoprotective agents such as mannitol, frusemide, or dopexamine in these patients may limit this risk, but substantial evidence for this is lacking.

Limb Ischemia

Limb ischemia attributable to AAA surgery is seen in 1% to 4% of cases. This is due to either distal embolization of debris from the aneurysm sac or more rarely graft thrombosis. The microemboli released following AAA repair are usually too small for surgical intervention to be warranted, triggering a variety of limb symptoms such as persistent pain, cold, and blue toes. Rarely, larger emboli may cause postoperative problems, and in this situation operative exploration is mandatory.

Gastrointestinal

A degree of intestinal dysmotility after laparotomy ("ileus") is very common and usually

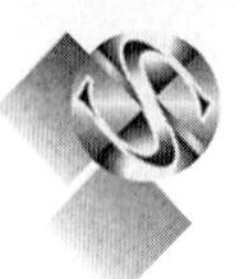

settles with bowel rest and fluid management. Removal of the nasogastric tube should not be too premature, and reintroduction of a normal diet must not occur until there is objective evidence of returning bowel function (e.g., flatus).

The most severe gastrointestinal following open AAA surgery is colonic ischemia. This condition, fortunately, occurs much less often then ileus, in about 1% of open AAA repair. The cause of this potentially fatal complication is explained by inadequate colonic perfusion via the IMA or internal iliac artery. It may occur due to inappropriate IMA ligation (see earlier), inadvertent collateral vessel damage during IMA ligation distant from its origin, or internal iliac artery thrombosis or embolism. Sinister postoperative symptoms include bloody diarrhea, left iliac fossa pain, and an explained high intravenous fluid requirement.

In cases of colonic ischemia, urgent colonoscopy is indicated, and management is dependent on the findings. Patchy areas of partial bowel wall ischemia and sloughing may well settle with conservative bowel rest and intravenous antibiotics. Severe bowel ischemia, which is evident as a full-thickness infarction, requires urgent resection of the affected colon with end-colostomy.

Venous Thromboembolism

The incidence of deep venous thrombosis (DVT) and pulmonary embolism following open AAA surgery is less than is seen with other general surgical operations. This is probably explained by the intraoperative heparin anticoagulation administered during surgery. Nevertheless, DVT still occurs in 8% of patients, and that risk should be addressed with subcutaneous prophylactic low-molecular-weight heparin, compression stockings, and early patient mobilization where appropriate.

Neurological

The most devastating and feared complication after open AAA repair is that of paraplegia. Fortunately, this is a rare event in infrarenal surgery as compared to thoracoabdominal aneurysm repair. It results following ligation of an abnormally low accessory spinal artery (of Adamkiewicz), which is usually found in a descending thoracic or upper abdominal aorta. Interruption of spinal blood flow through collateral vessels by compromising internal iliac artery perfusion may also result in paraplegia, but this is more frequently seen in conjunction with systemic hypotension as experienced during ruptured AAA.

Careless dissection may damage the important autonomic neural pathways found on the left side of the infrarenal aorta. The true incidence of impotence and retrograde ejaculation after elective AAA surgery is unknown, but may approach 20%.

Late Complications

Delayed complications arising from open AAA surgery are infrequent and can be classified as graft or wound related.

Graft-related late complications include false aneurysms (0.2% to 1.2% at 3 years) due to anastomotic disruption, graft infection, and aortoenteric fistulas. Data suggest that the combined likelihood of infection or fistula at 10 years is approximately 5% and is much more likely if a femoral anastomosis is used.

Long-term wound disorders such as poor cosmesis requiring revision or hernia depend on both surgical technique and perioperative factors such as wound infection, nutritional status, diabetic management, etc. Surgical attention is not required in the vast majority of cases, and each presentation should be assessed individually on its merits.

Endovascular Repair of Abdominal Aortic Aneurysm

The first successful treatment of an AAA by transfemoral endoluminal repair was reported over a decade ago. Since that time, advances in endovascular surgery coupled with a greater experience and understanding of this technique has led to possibly a viable alternative to open repair in aneurysm management (Woodburn et al., 1998). The basic principle of endovascular management is the exclusion of the AAA from the systemic circulation by means of a preoperatively sized deployed stent graft, thus preventing further aneurysm expansion and elimination of the rupture risk. For this to be achieved, a self-expanding or balloon-

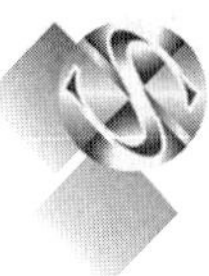

expandable device is advanced into the abdominal aorta to be released at a position so that the seal is generated both proximal and distal to the aneurysmal segment. Depending on the type of repair, the procedure may or may not require a combined surgical bypass for successful treatment.

Suitability for endovascular intervention depends on extensive preoperative investigation of aneurysm morphology, and the limitations of currently available stent graft devices mean that this approach is not an option in all elective or ruptured cases. At present, about 50% to 60% of all elective AAAs could potentially be considered for stenting, but this figure is extremely variable as much debate continues regarding the exclusion criteria for the procedure. With current devices it is generally agreed that the most important morphological features in assessing aneurysms' suitability for stenting are as follows: an adequate length (>15 mm) of infrarenal aneurysm neck with a maximal neck diameter of 30 mm to ensure a good proximal seal; limited vessel tortuosity, defined as vessel angulation (60 degrees at the neck of the aneurysm and 90 degrees at the iliac arteries); and iliac arteries of sufficient caliber (>7 to 9 mm) to tolerate the passage of the graft as it is admitted into the infrarenal aorta. Features that are severe as relative contraindications to the procedure include short (<25 mm) and wide (>14 mm) common iliac arteries and the presence of mural thrombus in the aneurysmal sac. Funnel-shaped necks and excessive calcification are absolute contraindications to endovascular repair.

The exciting advances in this arena offer a less invasive approach to AAA management so that some patients considered unfit for open surgery may well be candidates for endoluminal repair. Results of endovascular intervention as compared to open repair are currently being assessed with prospective trials such as the ongoing Endovascular Arterial Reconstruction (EVAR) project. At this stage it would appear that endovascular repair offers mortality and morbidity rates similar to those of open surgery, but stenting has the advantage of a markedly reduced length of total in-hospital stay and diminished requirement for intensive care and high dependency support. The financial advantage of this, however, is offset by the major drawback of this approach, which is the cost of the stent graft itself.

Type of Endovascular Procedure

Three distinct endovascular prostheses are currently available for AAA repair. All the manufactured devices form the proximal seal in the infrarenal aortic segment, but differences exist in the location of their distal "landing site." The aorto-aortic straight graft resides entirely in the abdominal aorta but is only suitable in 5% of cases amenable to endovascular repair. Bifurcated stents can be used in 30% of patients, with the distal seals formed in the iliac vessels. The remainder (65%) of suitable aneurysms may be repaired with aorto-uniiliac stent graft devices. This latter method requires a combined surgical crossover procedure (usually femoro-femoral) for maintenance of contralateral lower limb blood supply following radiological embolization or surgical occlusion of the non-graft common iliac artery.

Perioperative Management

The patient should be assessed and prepared for endoluminal intervention as discussed earlier for open repair. Adequate appropriate radiological imaging should be obtained to enable calibration of both aneurysm and related vasculature for graft sizing. Informed consent should include the known specific complications associated with endovascular repair and also mention the possibility of conversion to open surgery if necessary. The operating room should be equipped with a C-arm or equivalent for intraoperative imaging, and adjunctive input is required from both the resident surgical and interventional radiology team.

After anesthesia induction, the patient is appropriately positioned, prepped, and draped. The procedure commences by surgical cutdown to the femoral artery to gain access to the arterial circulation. The device is admitted through the exposed artery and advanced proximally under radiological control until deployment of the appropriate site for aneurysm exclusion. Correct graft position and the absence of endoleak is confirmed by on-table angiography, and the groin is closed in a routine fashion unless a surgical crossover graft is to be performed. At the end of the procedure, the lower limbs should be assessed for evidence of graft thrombosis or embolism before transfer to the recovery area. The patient can be mobilized

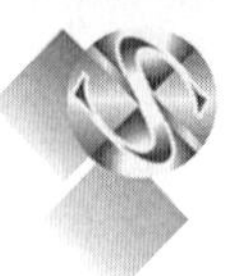

gently the day after surgery, and discharge can be expected at 5 to 7 days in uncomplicated cases with a satisfactory early postoperative CT scan. Follow-up guidelines currently advise 6-month CT and plain lumbar spine imaging in the first year and then annually thereafter.

Complications of Endovascular Abdominal Aortic Aneurysm Repair

Endovascular AAA repair unfortunately carries with it a distinct spectrum of specific complications in addition to "routine" causes of postoperative morbidity.

Iatrogenic Vessel Injury

The introduction of guidewires, large-bore catheters, and a stent graft poses the risk of arterial and proximal vessel injury such as rupture or dissection. Delayed manifestations of iatrogenic vessel damage may present later, with the development of a false aneurysm at the cannulation site, and requires prompt surgical repair.

Endoleak

Endoleak refers to the persistence of arterial flow of blood into the "excluded" aneurysm sac but outside the lumen of the deployed stent graft. It represents one or more of the following processes: incomplete sealing of the proximal or distal landing sites (type I); continued blood flow into the sac by collateral and lumbar vessels (type II); an incomplete seal at junctions of overlapping graft components or ruptured graft fabric (type III); or leakage of blood through a porous graft membrane (type IV). The incidence of endoleak is approximately 20% and may be further classified as immediate, early, or late. Without treatment, the aneurysm may continue to expand, thus carrying the risk of rupture, although most cases seal spontaneously with thrombosis. Bearing this in mind, the majority of vascular surgeons initially manage an endoleak with simple observation. If, after a prescribed time period, the endoleak persists or rapid aneurysm expansion is observed, further interventions such as endoluminal graft extension deployment, band ligation of the aortic aneurysmal neck, or even open repair may be indicated.

Embolization

Endoluminal stent graft deployment carries the risk of distal embolization of debris from the aneurysmal sac. This is particularly true in cases of extensive mural thrombosis, and therefore the benefits of endovascular repair should be questioned in these circumstances. Showering of microemboli may result in renal failure and leg ischemia requiring amputation.

Graft Migration, Dislocation, and Displacement

Long-term follow-up of endoluminal stenting has shown that the stent devices may migrate, resulting in endoleak, dislocating, and jeopardizing the seal and kink, with potential thrombosis. The advent of second-generation devices has attempted to address these problems with reinforcement of graft struts and the introduction of suprarenal uncovered fixation.

Postimplant Syndrome

Well described in the literature, postimplant syndrome refers to the presence of early back pain and fever without leukocytosis following endoluminal AAA repair. It lasts for up to 1 week after insertion. The condition is self-limiting and is managed conservatively.

Conversion to Open Repair

Failure of endovascular management of AAA may require conversion to open repair, occurring in 2% of cases. Indications for such measures include aortic rupture during a primary stenting procedure, persistent endoleak with failed secondary intervention, and graft infection.

Ruptured Abdominal Aortic Aneurysms

Ruptured aortic aneurysms are uniformly fatal without operative intervention, explaining the emphasis of AAA management of early detection and elective repair. Unfortunately, the vast improvements in outcome following elective AAA repair have not simultaneously been witnessed in the emergency situation, and operative mortality under these circumstances has remained static over the last 20 years at between 40% and 70%. Even this estimation can be considered conservative, as the figure does not take into account community prehospital deaths, and therefore an overall mortality following AAA rupture is probably in the region of 80% to 90%.

The exact process that triggers rupture of an AAA remains unknown. Several factors (discussed earlier) are known to suggest an increased likelihood of rupture and the most important of these is aneurysm size.

Clinical Presentation

A high index of suspicion is paramount in clinching the diagnosis. Any patient with a known AAA who presents with sudden severe abdominal or back pain has a ruptured aneurysm until proven otherwise. The difficulty arises in atypical presentations of patients with unknown aneurysmal disease leading to detrimental delays in surgical management. Ruptured AAA should feature in the differential diagnosis of any patient who presents with unexplained hypertension, severe abdominal pain, or cardiac arrest with no prior history of myocardial disease or trauma.

Clinical symptoms of rupture are varied, but classically comprise sudden back or abdominal pain with an episode of collapse, fainting, and maybe nausea. Examination reveals a pulsatile mass on abdominal palpation that may or may not be tender. The patient may be pale, irritable, clammy, tachycardic, and hypotensive. Maintenance of a normal blood pressure may indicate a contained rupture, affording the clinician time to confirm the diagnosis with appropriate imaging prior to surgery. This luxury is not offered in an uncontained ruptured AAA when the patient should be taken to the operating room for operative repair without delay.

Operative Repair of a Ruptured Abdominal Aortic Aneurysm

Perioperative management is aimed at stabilizing the precarious hemodynamic status of the patient. After an initial brief history and examination, venous access should be secured with at least two large-bore cannulae and blood samples withdrawn for biochemistry, hematology, and urgent crossmatch (at least 10 units) of packed red cells and blood products.

Arguments persist regarding the optimal goal of fluid resuscitation in cases of ruptured AAA. It has been suggested that overzealous fluid management runs the risk of a sudden increase in blood pressure and hence converting a contained leak into a frank rupture. Management strategies should aim to keep a systolic blood pressure of 90 mm Hg by infusion of intravenous fluids until operative repair can be performed. Patient response should be assessed with continuous hemodynamic monitoring and a urinary catheter inserted. Early involvement of both the surgical and anesthetic team is desirable in order to optimize patient status and minimize operative delay.

In some stable presentations of suspected AAA rupture, radiological imaging may be performed to confirm the diagnosis and delineate aneurysmal anatomy. The investigation of choice remains CT scanning. Ultrasound is of little benefit due to its inability to reliably distinguish a ruptured AAA.

Operative management for leaking AAA is by open repair by midline laparotomy. Although some centers have reported encouraging results, endovascular management currently plays little role in the management of ruptured AAA. Surgery should be expedient, performed by the most senior available member of the vascular team. Following incision, brisk but careful dissection should proceed with placement of the clamp in the infrarenal aorta, avoiding damage to the left renal vein. Temporary supraceliac clamping may be performed to initially control problematic bleeding and facilitate dissection for later re-siting in the infrarenal aortic segment. In extreme circumstances, the surgeon's fingers or an intra-aortic balloon may be used to gain proximal control. Intravenous antibiotics should be administered to limit graft infection, but unlike in elective cases, intravenous heparin is not routinely given. Once the aorta is cross-clamped, the operation is then performed as is described for elective AAA.

Outcome Following Repair of a Ruptured Abdominal Aortic Aneurysm

Significant postoperative morbidity following repair of ruptured AAA occurs in 50% to 70%

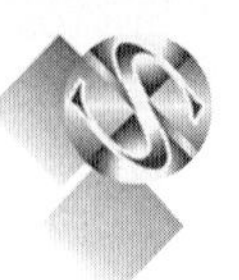

of cases (Heller et al., 2000). This figure represents both suboptimal patient preparation for major surgery and the sequelae of prolonged hypotension experience pending operative repair. Cardiorespiratory disorders and renal impairment are the most commonly encountered complications, closely followed by ischemic colitis. The latter condition carries a subsequent mortality of 25% and results from gut hypoperfusion secondary to aneurysm rupture. The clinician should anticipate its diagnosis.

Assuming operative survival, patients with a ruptured AAA enjoy a long-term prognosis as governed by their other comorbidities. Repair has not been shown to diminish the patient's quality of life postoperatively, and no different exists in outcome should the aneurysm have been repaired electively.

Inflammatory Abdominal Aortic Aneurysms

An important subdivision of infrarenal aortic aneurysmal disease is the inflammatory aortic aneurysm (Rasmussen and Hallett, 1997). Inflammatory AAAs were not classified per se until the early 1970s, and even today their nature in terms of being a distinct clinical and pathological entity is still disputed.

Definition of the inflammatory AAA depends on the presence of a triad of factors: a thickened aneurysmal wall, marked perianeurysmal/ retroperitoneal fibrosis, and dense adhesions involving adjacent abdominal viscera to the aneurysm. These aneurysms comprise 5% to 10% of all AAAs, and the typical patient is a male in his sixth decade. Females are rarely affected by the disease (male-to-female ratio of 20:1). Interestingly, the average age at diagnosis is about 10 years younger than those patients presenting with noninflammatory aortic aneurysms. Postulated risk factors that are specific for the development of inflammatory AAA include cigarette smoking and a genetic predisposition.

There is currently much debate regarding the etiology and pathogenesis of the inflammatory AAA. Until recently, it was generally upheld that these aneurysms were of a distinct exclusive nature and therefore to be considered different from their noninflammatory counterpart. This belief is now being challenged. An early hypothesis suggesting the periaortic fibrosis was secondary to retroperitoneal blood leakage from tiny perforations in a previously noninflammatory aneurysm has been rejected. Similarly, other theories of an initial prodromal atherosclerotic AAA developing into an aneurysm of inflammatory type remain unproven. The suggested mechanism for this transformation is by either lymphatic vessel compression by the expanding aneurysm resulting in stasis, edema and subsequent fibrosis, or as a direct consequence of an inflammatory reaction between blood in the aneurysmal sac and the aortic wall. Viral infection with herpes simplex or cytomegalovirus has also been proposed as a causal factor, with evidence of their presence in the aortic wall proven by DNA polymerase reactions.

A more convincing theory regarding inflammatory AAA development is that it is the result of a specific inflammatory process. This process is responsible for both inflammatory and noninflammatory AAAs, and thus we are not to consider the two pathologies as distinct pathological entities; rather, the former is an "inflammatory variant" of the latter. There seems to be good evidence for this theory. Initially, histological analysis revealed the presence of a chronic inflammatory infiltrate present in the walls of inflammatory and noninflammatory aortic aneurysms, with the only difference being an augmented level of inflammatory response in the putative inflammatory AAA. This finding was then supported by serial observations of a progressive inflammatory response from the initial atherosclerotic to the inflammatory AAA proven both under the microscope and radiologically. It is suggested that there is a primary inflammatory reaction to an antigen present in the aortic wall whereby there is gradual infiltration of B lymphocytes, T lymphocytes, and macrophages. Subsequent cytokine production from the infiltrate triggers a proteolytic cascade with increased turnover of MMPs, elastin, and collagen. With time the aortic wall begins to degrade, losing tensile strength, and the aneurysm begins to develop. It is proposed that this inflammatory response is accentuated further in smokers and those with a genetic predisposition, explaining an earlier presentation of aneurysmal disease.

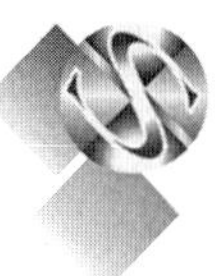

Clinical Features

The inflammatory AAA is typically symptomatic with only 20% cases being discovered incidentally. Classically, the presence of abdominal or back pain, weight loss, and an elevated ESR in patients with a known AAA confers a diagnosis of inflammatory aneurysm until proven otherwise. Clinical examination may reveal a pulsatile mass on abdominal palpation and generalized evidence of weight loss. Specific blood tests to be taken if an inflammatory AAA is suspected are an ESR, which will be raised in 70% cases signifying the acute phase response, and less reliably a white cell count. Serum electrolytes and creatinine should also be taken to look for evidence of obstructive uropathy and associated chronic renal failure (10% to 20% of patients).

Diagnosis

Despite symptomatology and available laboratory investigations, the inflammatory AAA still tends to be a diagnosis that is made at operation. Preoperative CT scanning can sensitively detect aneurysm wall thickening and perianeurysmal fibrosis but depends on the radiologist's awareness to make the diagnosis. Although ultrasound remains useful in routine AAA surveillance, it is less helpful than CT in distinguishing the inflammatory variant. If there is any suspicion of ureteric involvement by the retroperitoneal fibrosis, an intravenous pyelogram should be requested.

Management

Although inflammatory aneurysms are usually larger than their atherosclerotic counterpart, it is generally accepted that the risk of rupture is lower. Presumably this is due to the paradoxical strengthening of the periaortic tissue by fibrotic change. Some clinicians advocate administration of oral corticosteroids in an effort to attenuate the inflammatory aneurysmal response, but there is no evidence to support this. In fact there is a body of opinion that suggest steroid therapy may actually increase the risk of inflammatory AAA rupture by a reduction in the protective fibrosis. Ultimately, surgery remains the treatment of choice for inflammatory AAA.

Surgical Intervention for Inflammatory Aortic Aneurysms

At laparotomy the inflammatory AAA is easily recognized with its thickened aortic wall and shiny, smooth white appearance. There is periaortic and retroperitoneal change with adhesions invariably involving the duodenum and less commonly the inferior vena cava and left renal vein. Disease affecting the ureters occurs in 20% to 40% of cases, which may necessitate a team approach with both the vascular surgeon and urologist.

Aneurysm repair should proceed with as little dissection as possible. The propensity of these aneurysms to bleed compounded by the high risk of iatrogenic damage to neighboring structures poses potentially high surgical morbidity. Early inflammatory AAA surgery with futile attempts at periaortic adhesiolysis were complicated by needless duodenal enterotomies and inadvertent venous and ureteric injury, and this approach to repair has now been discarded. The method of surgical repair is otherwise as previously described for noninflammatory infrarenal AAAs, and operative mortality rates for elective inflammatory AAA repair should be comparable (3% to 4%). Ureterolysis at the time of AAA repair remains a controversial issue. Over half of inflammatory AAAs demonstrate ureteric involvement on preoperative CT scanning. We advise that such ureteric surgery be reserved for those exhibiting signs or symptoms of obstruction or proven incipient uropathy on preoperative investigation. Early consultation with the urology team is advisable in these circumstances.

Thoracoabdominal Aortic Aneurysms

Aneurysmal diseases affecting both the abdominal and thoracic aorta are known collectively as thoracoabdominal aortic aneurysms (TAAAs). In clinical practice these essentially refer to aneurysms arising above the celiac axis. Previously considered as quite a rare condition, recent advances in clinical diagnostic capability by methods such as angiography, CT, and MRI suggest that these aneurysms in fact account for up to 10% of the aortic aneurysm population. The management of these patients is complex and indeed may fall into the realm of both the vascular and cardiothoracic surgeon. It is therefore suggested that these aneurysms are best dealt with at a tertiary referral center with appropriate expertise and not routinely at the district general hospital.

Etiology

Atherosclerosis is the most commonly implicated factor in the development of TAAA disease. The classical fusiform aneurysm that results is typically seen in men over the age of 50 years, usually with evidence of arterial atherosclerotic pathology elsewhere. In fact, over half of TAAA presentations are subsequently discovered to have coexistent aneurysmal disease at an alternative site including the infrarenal aorta and femoral and popliteal arteries. Other causal factors to be excluded are thoracic dissection with secondary aneurysm formation, cystic medial necrosis (e.g., Marfan syndrome, Takayasu disease, trauma leading to false aneurysm), and infection. Previously the most common cause of this type of aneurysm, syphilitic aortitis leading to the classical Crawford type I (see later) saccular TAAA, has now thankfully declined and is rarely seen nowadays in non–Third World practice.

Clinical Features

Clinical presentation of TAAA can be categorized as asymptomatic, symptomatic but not ruptured, and ruptured.

Asymptomatic Thoracoabdominal Aortic Aneurysm

The vast majority of TAAAs are without symptoms. Unlike infrarenal and peripheral aneurysms, it is also improbable that routine clinical examination will yield the diagnosis. In these patients it is the review of the chest radiograph that initially arouses clinical suspicion of TAAA, for further investigations to confirm.

Symptomatic Nonruptured Thoracoabdominal Aortic Aneurysm

Symptomatic TAAAs usually result from local pressure effects, and this most commonly manifests as chest pain. The pain is central and radiates through to the upper back, depending on the neighboring anatomy (e.g., spinal nerves or vertebral column erosion). Irritation of the recurrent laryngeal nerve and bronchial structures may result in voice changes, stridor, and dyspnea. Gradual unexplained orthopnea, paroxysmal nocturnal dyspnea, and ankle swelling all indicate a failing myocardium, and this may be due to a compromised pulmonary circulation by TAAA compression. Occasionally, if the abdominal component of the TAAA is large enough, the clinician or even the patient may discover a pulsatile mass. Occult symptoms of distal embolization should always arouse suspicion of an ongoing proximal aneurysmal process, thus necessitating appropriate investigation for exclusion of TAAA.

Ruptured Thoracoabdominal Aortic Aneurysm

A TAAA rupture can be varied in its clinical presentation. There is usually a history of acute severe chest pain, and examination may reveal a hemodynamically unstable patient requiring vigorous resuscitation. The site of rupture and possible involvement of other thoracic structures govern other associated symptoms. Massive hematemesis may result if rupture occurs into the esophagus, whereas hemoptysis and dyspnea suggests the possibility of rupture into the tracheobronchial tree. Hemorrhage into the pleural cavity or retroperitoneal space can often result in a more delayed and profoundly hypovolemic presentation.

Diagnosis

Examination of a standard chest radiograph may reveal a widened mediastinum, loss of thoracic aorta outline, or a "mass" extending into the left hemithorax. Calcification in the wall of the aorta is seen in about one third of patients. In cases of TAAA rupture into the pleural space, evidence of a hemothorax should be seen. Confirmation of the diagnosis is achieved by spiral CT scanning, which usually gives all the required preoperative information regarding aneurysm size, visceral artery relation, and proximal extent of aneurysm. Magnetic resonance imaging techniques are equally

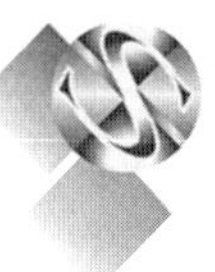

instructive, but their availability and cost limits their use. Unlike investigation of infrarenal aneurysms, ultrasound for TAAAs offers unreliable and poor quality results; hence, it plays no role in either radiographic diagnosis or surveillance. Angiography is indicated only if CT scanning does not give sufficient information regarding relationships to visceral (especially renal) arteries and for the evaluation of possible visceral artery stenoses.

Classification

Classification of thoracoabdominal aneurysms is into one of four types as described by Crawford:

Type I: Aneurysm involves the descending thoracic aorta as far as visceral artery branches

Type II: Aneurysm extends from the aortic arch, just distal to the left subclavian artery as far as the aortic bifurcation (involves visceral arteries)

Type III: Aneurysm commences in the midthoracic aorta and extends to the aortic bifurcation

Type IV: Aneurysm starts at or just below the diaphragm but above the renal arteries and extends as far as the aortic bifurcation

Of the four types, surgical repair is carried out most often on type IV.

Management of Thoracoabdominal Aortic Aneurysm

As in all surgery a balance must be struck between the high morbidity and mortality of operative repair, with a reported 5-year survival of 20% in nonoperative management. Aneurysmal size is important, and as general rule, asymptomatic aneurysms are not considered for intervention unless maximal diameter exceeds 6 cm. This threshold may be reduced in saccular pathology due to the increased propensity to rupture.

Extensive preoperative preparation is mandatory in order both to exclude patients with insufficient physiological reserve to survive operation and to allow adequate planning of proposed surgery. Required investigations are as outlined in the workup for AAA repair, with an emphasis on rigorous optimization of cardiorespiratory and renal status.

Open Repair of Thoracoabdominal Aortic Aneurysm

Following appropriate patient positioning, draping, and skin preparation, a left-sided thoracoabdominal incision is performed. In high aneurysms (types I and II) some surgeons advocate the use of extracorporeal circulation with atriofemoral or femorofemoral cardiopulmonary bypass to reduce the increased afterload and left ventricular strain induced by thoracic aorta cross-clamping. If this maneuver is not performed, the requirement for expedient surgery is further augmented. The thoracic and abdominal aorta are dissected out to enable proximal and distal control through nonaneurysmal aortic (and possibly iliac) crossclamping. Under normal circumstances heparin is not routinely given prior to clamp application to avoid unacceptable blood loss. An appropriately sized inlay prosthetic graft is introduced after opening the aneurysmal sac, and the proximal anastomosis is performed by continuous Prolene suture end-to-end with the thoracic aorta distal to the left subclavian artery. After confirmation of proximal anastomosis integrity, the visceral vessels (celiac axis, superior mesenteric, and renal arteries) are then reimplanted into the graft with sequential clamping in order to minimize organ ischemic time. Most high intercostal arteries are oversewn, but those in the region of T10 to L2 must be reimplanted for preservation of spinal cord blood supply. After verification of successful vessel anastomosis with evidence of perfusion, the distal anastomosis is formed at the level of the aortic bifurcation or iliac vessels. The aneurysm sac is closed over the graft and the patient closed in routine fashion. Postoperatively, the patient is transferred to the intensive care unit for close observation.

The nature of type I and type IV thoracoabdominal aneurysms may permit modifications to the outlined surgical technique in operative management. In certain low type IV aneurysms, a "rooftop" abdominal incision can be used for a total transabdominal access without the need for thoracotomy. The abdominal aorta is

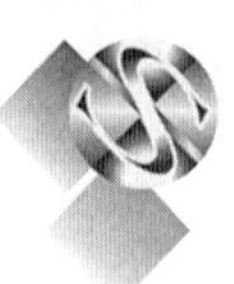

approached retroperitoneally with mobilization of the spleen, left kidney, and bowel to the contralateral side. A vascular clamp can then be applied to the suprarenal aorta to allow an oblique proximal anastomosis to be performed, incorporating a tongue of native aorta from which the celiac axis and superior mesenteric and renal arteries emerge. Once achieved, the clamp is reapplied infrarenally to allow organ perfusion following minimal ischemic time. Certain type I aneurysms may be approached with the need for thoracotomy only. In a similar manner to type IV repair, the distal anastomosis can be obliquely fashioned to incorporate a reversed tongue of native vessel from which the visceral arteries originate and so limit organ ischemic time.

Perioperative spinal fluid drainage is suggested as an adjunctive measure to lessen the risk of neurological complication. The technique aims to optimize spinal cord perfusion by enabling regulation of the increases in spinal fluid pressure that result from aortic cross-clamping. A fine-bore intrathecal catheter connected to a pressure transducer is introduced between the fourth and fifth lumbar vertebrae. If a potentially deleterious rise in spinal fluid pressure are observed, fluid drainage by a tap is performed to correct it. The catheter is removed once normal neurological function is confirmed in the early postoperative period.

Endovascular Repair of Thoracoabdominal Aortic Aneurysm

Endoluminal stent grafting may treat suitable descending thoracic aneurysms without visceral artery involvement. The principles of graft deployment were discussed earlier, with the exception that the aneurysmal neck is ideally situated at least 25 mm distal to the left subclavian artery. More proximal pathology may still be considered in the knowledge that compromised upper limb perfusion due to subclavian artery occlusion would require either operative reimplantation into the carotid artery or a carotid-subclavian bypass procedure.

Outcome of Thoracoabdominal Aortic Aneurysm Repair

As with AAA repair, cardiorespiratory morbidity remains the most frequently encountered complications postoperatively. Renal failure requiring replacement therapy with dialysis occurs in 10% and is more likely in those with preoperative renal dysfunction.

Postoperative paraplegia and paraparesis remain the most feared legacy of thoracoabdominal aneurysmal surgery. In spite of the outlined operative measures to reduce this risk, type I and II repairs are associated with a 15% to 20% chance of paraplegia compared to 5% to 10% occurring after types III and IV surgery. In general terms, higher thoracic aorta clamping equates to an increased risk of paraplegia, and this is supported by reported paraplegia rates of<1% for low type IV repairs performed by a total abdominal approach. Informed patient consent must include detailed discussion with respect to these risks prior to operative repair. If paraplegia does result from surgery, the clinician should make immediate referral to the local spinal rehabilitation team for early physiotherapy and patient support.

Mortality rates following TAAA repair are variable. Assuming appropriate case selection and sufficient surgical expertise, acceptable operative mortality rates of 10% to 15% for types I and II aneurysms and 5% to 8% for types III and IV are observed. Attempted repair of ruptured TAAA transmits inferior results, and postoperative death rates are reported as between 40% and 60%. If operative survival is accomplished, the patients' long-term prognosis is good and nearly two thirds of operated patients are alive at 5 years.

Peripheral Arterial Aneurysms

Aneurysmal disease affecting the nonaortic arterial vasculature may occur in isolation or more commonly as part of a generalized systemic arterial dilatation. It is for this reason that a thorough examination of all susceptible vessels should be performed after the initial assessment of the presenting peripheral aneurysm.

Popliteal Arterial Aneurysms

Popliteal aneurysms are the commonest nonaortic aneurysms, accounting for 70% of all diagnosed peripheral aneurysms (Dawson and van Bockel, 1997). Defined as an external diameter of one and a half to two times the normal proximal vessel, the true prevalence and incidence of the disease remains unknown. That said, it is estimated currently that approximately five patients present to a major vascular center on an annual basis with such lesions. Males in their sixth and seventh decades are most frequently affected, and the aneurysms are bilateral in around half of patients; 6% to 12% of presentations have a coexistent AAA.

The majority of popliteal aneurysms are associated primarily with atherosclerosis but other etiologies include trauma, infection, and popliteal artery entrapment syndrome. These should always be considered, especially in the younger patient. The aneurysms occur above the knee joint and are either fusiform or saccular in nature. The beaded fusiform popliteal aneurysms tend to be smaller (2- to 3-cm diameter) than the saccular variety with diameters reached of 4 to 6 cm.

Clinical Features

About one third of all popliteal aneurysms are asymptomatic; the diagnosis is made only after investigation of a lump in the popliteal fossa found on a routine clinical examination. The remaining two thirds are symptomatic and reflect the complications of these aneurysms: limb ischemia, rupture, or local pressure effects.

Limb ischemia remains the commonest presentation and is due to either aneurysmal sac thrombosis or distal embolization of intraaneurysmal clot. The emergence of ischemia (acute or chronic) is dependent on the presence of an established collateral circulation. In the more frequent case of acute thrombosis, such a circulation is usually poorly developed, and presentation is typically that of acute severe ischemia with threatened limb viability. Chronic thrombosis of popliteal aneurysms affords more time to the surgeon, resulting in one or more of symptoms of claudication, rest pain, blue-toe syndrome, or gangrene.

Local pressure effects of popliteal aneurysms may cause edema by compression of the adjacent popliteal vein and even local or referred pain by irritation of the neighboring sciatic nerve or its derivatives. Rupture of popliteal aneurysm is a rare presentation, necessitating immediate surgical attention in order to preserve the limb.

Diagnosis

The diagnosis of popliteal aneurysm should be suspected if an exaggerated pulsation is discovered on palpation behind the knee during clinical examination. A firm pulseless mass in the popliteal fossa may indicate a thrombosed aneurysm, especially if an aneurysm is found on examination of the contralateral limb. Further information regarding the lump should then be obtained by appropriate imaging.

Arterial duplex scanning is cheap, easily available, and therefore ideal for diagnosis confirmation, sizing, and subsequent popliteal aneurysm surveillance. Arteriography is of less use in the estimation of aneurysm size, but is paramount in the assessment of the regional vasculature for determination of planned surgical intervention. Computed tomograph and MRI can offer detailed assessment of the popliteal fossa contents and the nature of the intravascular thrombus content, but their expense and limited availability renders them of little use in the management of the routine popliteal aneurysm.

Management of Symptomatic Popliteal Aneurysms

Acute Ischemia and Rupture

Presentation of a pale, pulseless, cold, and paresthetic leg signifies an immediate threat to limb viability, and prompt intervention is needed to avert primary amputation. There are a variety of surgical procedures with adjuvant therapy (thrombolysis) for repair, depending on the aneurysm's size, embolic potential, and the status of proximal and distal vessels.

Ideally, a preoperative angiogram should be obtained and the patient taken for arterial reconstruction without delay. The aim of surgery is limb preservation and popliteal aneurysm exclusion. After adequate exposure by either the medial or the posterior approach (see later), the aneurysm is excluded by means of ligation and bypass grafting, inlay grafting, or resection with primary anastomosis. There should be a low threshold for performing an additional fasciotomy as indicated by the individual clinical picture.

Bypass grafting after proximal and distal aneurysm ligation remains well established and

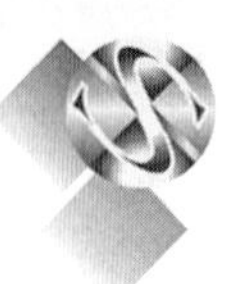

is the usual technique employed. The conduit may be prosthetic graft or preferably autogenous saphenous vein if available. Improved distal run-off can be achieved by the intraoperative use of balloon-tipped embolectomy catheters, and enhanced perfusion following surgery should be confirmed by an on-table angiogram. The commoner complications of this surgery include graft thrombosis, infection, and deep vein thrombosis. Resection of popliteal aneurysms is indicated only in the larger, saccular type that involves a short segment of popliteal artery, so the resultant end-to-end anastomosis can be performed without tension. Great care must be taken in resection to avoid damage to the adjacent popliteal vein, and for this reason some surgeons avoid this method of aneurysm repair.

Thrombolysis has an important role to play in the management of acute symptomatic popliteal aneurysmal disease. In thrombosed aneurysms with acute ischemia, a percutaneous transfemoral arterial catheter can be inserted and lodged in the aneurysmal thrombus. Infusion of thrombolytic agent [recombinant tissue-type plasminogen activator (rtPA), streptokinase, or urokinase] is commenced at an appropriate dose, and check angiograms are performed at suitable intervals (every 4 to 6 hours) to confirm the clinical observations of improved blood supply. Angiographic demonstration of adequate run-off is an indication to stop thrombolytic infusion and proceed to bypass grafting. Long periods of thrombolysis carry the risks of bleeding and embolization of released intraaneurysmal thrombus. Strict observation for excessive hemorrhage and worsening foot ischemia must be adhered to during treatment, and they mandate cessation of the infusion if they occur. In advanced ischemia with loss of sensation and muscle power, attempts at surgical revascularization should not be delayed, and thrombolysis should be restricted to intraoperative use in an effort to clear tibial and peroneal vessel run-off.

Chronic Ischemia

Symptoms of chronic ischemia in popliteal aneurysmal disease may be due to thrombosis or distal embolization. A conservative nonoperative approach may be considered in the case of thrombosed popliteal aneurysm, as an acute deterioration is unlikely due to the established collateral circulation. Distal embolization, on the other hand, involves a persistent blood flow through the aneurysm (unlike thrombosis), putting the patient at risk of further embolic episodes and worsening limb ischemia unless the aneurysm is surgically excluded.

Management of Asymptomatic Popliteal Aneurysms

Discovery of these aneurysms is usually on examination following diagnosis of aneurysmal disease elsewhere such as the abdominal aorta or contralateral popliteal artery. Subsequent treatment remains a controversial issue with as yet no clear guidelines for surgical intervention. The recent trend of aggressive repair in the majority of asymptomatic popliteal aneurysms is currently under review in an effort to balance the inherent surgical morbidity of repair and the fact that for many patients their popliteal aneurysm will be associated with no long-term adversity. Review of the literature suggests that following factors favor elective surgery: aneurysm size >2 cm, the presence of mural thrombus (potential embolic source), autogenous conduit availability, absent ankle pulses (indicating possible "silent" embolization), and a long life expectancy. Classical popliteal aneurysm exclusion and bypass as described earlier is the operation of choice in this situation. Endovascular procedures have been described in the treatment of popliteal aneurysms but the long-term patency rates and outcomes are at present unknown.

Surgical Approach in Popliteal Artery Aneurysms

Access to the popliteal artery in aneurysmal surgery is achieved by either the medial or posterior approach.

In the medial approach the knee is partially flexed and the skin incision follows the course of the long saphenous vein, taking care to preserve the vein for later harvest. The adductor muscles are retracted, allowing entry to the popliteal space with decent exposure and better access to the superficial femoral and tibial arteries than with the posterior approach. A further advantage of this method is that the incision may be easily extended without the need for patient repositioning.

The posterior approach requires the patient to be prone, and the incision is made between the heads of the gastrocnemii extending proximally. Excellent exposure of the popliteal artery is achieved, but access to more proximal or distal vessels proves more problematic. Furthermore, unless the short saphenous vein is to be used for bypass, this approach compels a second incision for vein harvest.

Femoral Arterial Aneurysms

Femoral arterial aneurysms can be divided simply into true or false aneurysms. Due to its ease of accessibility and the trend for more invasive medical investigation and treatment (e.g., cardiac catheterization, intra-aortic balloon pumps), iatrogenic injury of the femoral artery leading to false aneurysm is a relatively common occurrence. This chapter discusses only true femoral aneurysms, and false aneurysms are considered in detail elsewhere.

Although rare, true femoral aneurysms are the second commonest peripheral aneurysm after those affecting the popliteal artery. They occur in between 2% and 3% of patients with aortic aneurysms and tend to be a disease of elderly men (male-to-female ratio of 30:1). The condition is frequently bilateral and similar to popliteal aneurysms; a coexistent generalized aneurysmal process may be manifest in other anatomical sites such as the aortoiliac or popliteal arteries. Multiple factors are implicated in their development including atherosclerosis, turbulent blood flow (at proximal major vessel bifurcations and infrainguinally), and repeated hip flexion. Other etiologies to exclude are infection, inflammation (e.g., systemic lupus erythematosus, Takayasu's disease), trauma, and connective tissue disorders (e.g., Marfan syndrome).

Classification

True femoral aneurysms are distinguished by the Cutler and Darling classification:

Type 1: aneurysm involves common femoral artery (CFA) only, not the bifurcation

Type 2: aneurysmal disease of the bifurcation, the commencement of the profunda femoris (PFA), or the superficial femoral artery (SFA)

Clinical Features

Femoral aneurysms may be symptomatic or asymptomatic. The latter group is usually discovered incidentally on clinical examination of a patient with an aneurysm elsewhere or suffering symptoms of chronic limb ischemia. Presentation of a symptomatic femoral aneurysm can include a pulsatile groin mass (which may or may not be painful), leg swelling (in large aneurysms due to femoral vein compression and deep vein thrombosis), or features associated with chronic ischemia attributable to aneurysm thrombosis/embolization.

Diagnosis

Once clinical suspicion has been aroused, the diagnosis should be confirmed with a duplex scan. If surgery is being considered (e.g., in CFA thrombosis or embolization), preoperative angiography is desirable for further information regarding the proximal and distal vessels.

Management of Femoral Aneurysms

Symptomatic femoral aneurysms are themselves an indication for surgical intervention. As with popliteal disease, the management of the asymptomatic case is less clear. It is generally accepted, however, that if aneurysms are >4 cm or aortoiliac disease is present (with indicated surgery), then operative repair is warranted.

Surgical Repair of Femoral Aneurysms

The skin incision extends from a point approximately 4 cm proximal to the inguinal ligament, following the course of the artery (and thus aneurysm) to a point just distal to the CFA bifurcation. Once proximal and distal control is achieved, heparin and intravenous antibiotics are administered so that aneurysmal repair can be performed. In Type 1 aneurysms, the CFA-restricted disease, may be addressed by aneurysm resection and insertion of an interposition graft [polytetrafluoroethylene (PTFE)/Dacron]. Repair of type 2 aneurysms is by graft (autogenous saphenous vein or prosthetic) interposition with an end-to-end technique between the nonaneurysmal CFA and the larger of the bifurcated vessels (SFA or PFA). The smaller vessel is then reimplanted into the side of the graft directly, or by the use of a second graft. Patency rates following repair are good, 80% to 85% at 5 years with a low operative mortality and morbidity.

Iliac Artery Aneurysms

Isolated iliac aneurysms are rare with a reported incidence of only 1% to 2% of all aortoiliac aneurysmal disease. The aneurysms tend to be large (4 to 8 cm), with annual expansion rates comparable to that of AAAs. Males over the age of 70 years are most frequently affected, with the atherosclerotic process implicated in the vast majority of cases. Other reported etiologies include infection (TB, syphilis), trauma (pelvic fractures and iatrogenic during surgery), inflammation, and pregnancy.

Clinical Features

Iliac aneurysmal disease may be asymptomatic or symptomatic. Human pelvic anatomy accounts for the fact that even very large iliac aneurysms may remain "silent" until an incidental diagnosis. Any symptoms experienced are typically due to local effects on neighboring structures including the ureter, small bowel, iliac vein, and femoral or sciatic nerve.

Abdominal examination may reveal the diagnosis but is usually normal. Palpation of a pulsatile mass on rectal or vaginal examination should alert the clinician to the possibility of iliac aneurysmal disease.

Diagnosis

Duplex ultrasound scanning is cheap, readily available, and thus the preliminary investigation of choice in diagnosis confirmation. Conventional angiography is extremely informative, but due to contrast load and radiation exposure its use is restricted to preoperative instruction. The cost and availability of spiral CT and magnetic resonance angiography negates their use routinely, but the quality of information obtained remains impressive.

Management of Iliac Aneurysms

Management strategies are outlined depending on whether the common iliac (CIA) or internal iliac (IIA) artery is involved.

Common Iliac Aneurysms

Small CIA aneurysms (<3 cm) do not require surgery and can be managed conservatively. If the maximal aneurysm diameter lies between 3 and 4 cm, patients should be kept under ultrasound surveillance (every 6 months) and operation offered if expansion to >4 cm. Isolated CIA aneurysms may be repaired by means of an interposition graft and oversewing of the IIA origin. Alternatively, the CIA aneurysm can be ligated (proximally and distally) with execution of an iliofemoral or femorofemoral crossover graft.

Internal Iliac Aneurysms

Unilateral IIA aneurysms can be addressed by either radiological or operative techniques. Coil embolization of the IIA successfully excludes the aneurysm from the circulation with minimal long-term sequelae. Surgical intervention requires simple proximal and distal aneurysm ligation for treatment in these cases. Bilateral IIA aneurysms pose an interesting problem as bilateral aneurysm ligation or embolization is not a viable option to preserve adequate colorectal and perineal blood supply. In this scenario an attempt at surgical revascularization should be made. The bypass graft runs from the nonaneurysmal CIA to the distal IIA with proximal aneurysm ligation. Extensive hemorrhage can often be encountered in this difficult procedure for which the surgeon should be prepared.

Visceral Artery Aneurysms

Aneurysmal disease involving the visceral arteries is uncommon but an important cause of vascular admission. As imaging techniques continue to improve, there will no doubt be a corresponding increase in the diagnostic yield of these aneurysms, so it is hoped that management strategies can be applied to the elective rather than the emergency presentation.

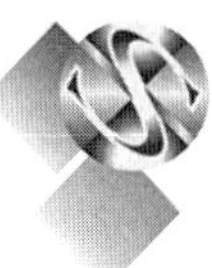

Splenic Artery Aneurysms

The splenic artery is the most common visceral artery to be affected by aneurysmal disease, accounting for 60% of all visceral aneurysms. They are the second most common abdominal aneurysm after the aorta, with an estimated population incidence of 1%. Vessel dilatation is usually minimal (<2 cm) and about one fifth of these aneurysms are multiple. Contrary to aneurysmal disease elsewhere, it is multiparous women who are classically affected. The etiology of splenic artery aneurysm is unknown, but theories include the vascular sequelae of multiple pregnancies, altered flow dynamics in portal hypertension, and multifactorial vessel wall degradation.

Eighty percent of splenic artery aneurysms are asymptomatic. The remaining proportion may present with a nonspecific pain in the left hypochondrium or epigastrium that can radiate to the left flank or be referred to the left shoulder by diaphragmatic irritation. As aneurysmal progression continues, the symptoms worsen and are further aggravated by excessive movement. Abdominal examination is usually normal, although splenomegaly is detected in 20% of patients. Rupture occurs in 5% to 10% of splenic artery aneurysms, and in these cases the patient presents with severe upper abdominal pain, hypotension (volume loss), and frank peritonism. Nearly all ruptures occur during pregnancy, and associated mortality rates are high (75% mother, 95% fetus).

Diagnosis of splenic artery aneurysms is usually incidental on imaging modalities such as plain abdominal radiographs (calcification), angiogram, spiral CT, or MRI scanning. Alternatively, these lesions may be discovered during laparotomy for other pathology. Management planning in splenic aneurysms tends to be dependent on whether symptoms exist. As a general rule, the majority of asymptomatic aneurysms may be treated conservatively, but in those experiencing symptoms, surgical intervention is indicated at an early stage. Operative procedure is governed by the anatomical location of disease within the splenic artery. Proximal aneurysms (in the first third of the splenic artery) are treated by either ligation or excision and grafting after an approach through the lesser sac. Ligation is indicated in aneurysms affecting the middle third of the artery, whereas either splenectomy or aneurysmal excision (for splenic conservation) is advocated for distal disease. Coil embolization performed by a member of the resident interventional radiology team may be successfully used to treat appropriate splenic aneurysms in high-risk patients.

Hepatic Artery Aneurysms

Aneurysmal disease involving the hepatic artery accounts for approximately one fifth of visceral aneurysms. They occur more often in the male population with an average age at presentation of 40 years, somewhat lower than is observed in other aneurysmal processes. Site of aneurysm formation is either intrahepatic (25%) or extrahepatic (75%), the latter aneurysms being usually solitary affecting the common hepatic artery (60%). Isolated involvement of the right and left hepatic arteries is less frequent, but if present, a predilection for the right hepatic artery is seen (seven times more common). The cause of extrahepatic aneurysm is normally atherosclerosis, but factors such as infection, trauma, and cystic medial degeneration must be considered. Conversely, intrahepatic disease tends to be false aneurysms resulting from trauma.

Nonruptured hepatic aneurysms are usually asymptomatic but may present with discomfort in the right hypochondrium or epigastrium. As its size increases, the pain radiates into the back. Sudden development of acute abdominal pain, hypotension, and peritonism indicates rupture of the aneurysm, occurring in 20% of cases. Unless the aneurysm has indeed ruptured, clinical examination is invariably normal, although detection of a pulsatile mass and bruits have been reported.

Prerupture clinical diagnosis of hepatic aneurysm is problematic. Elevated serum amylase, bilirubin, and white cell counts may be observed, but more often than not diagnosis depends on ultrasound and CT findings. Once suspected, the investigation of choice for hepatic aneurysm is selective celiac and superior mesenteric angiography.

Due to high rates of rupture-related mortality of approximately 40%, proven hepatic aneurysms merit aggressive management. The exact surgical procedure is again guided by anatomical location of aneurysms: for extra-

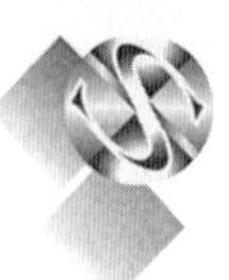

hepatic aneurysms proximal to the gastroduodenal artery, simple aneurysm ligation should be performed (hepatic blood supply maintained by gastroduodenal and right gastric arteries); if the aneurysm location is distal to the commencement of the gastroduodenal artery, then an excision and graft procedure should be attempted. Intrahepatic aneurysm repair is more difficult. Both embolization and limited liver resections have been performed, but not all aneurysms are suitable for coil deployment, and operative mortality in these cases remains high.

Renal Artery Aneurysms

Renal artery aneurysms are about as common as hepatic aneurysms, accounting for one fifth of all visceral aneurysms. The true incidence of these aneurysms lies between 0.3% and 1.3%, with less than 10% of those affected exhibiting symptoms. They occur in both sexes, with women of childbearing age considered to be of highest rupture risk. Etiologies of renal artery aneurysms are varied, but the majority (80% to 85%) are caused by the degradation of the internal elastic lamina at the renal arteriolar divisions leading initially to microaneurysm formation that then progresses into frank aneurysmal disease. Other factors to consider in aneurysm development include previous renal trauma and generalized arteritis. As already mentioned, the vast majority of these aneurysms are clinically silent, but if present, symptoms include flank pain on the affected side, hematuria, and systemic hypertension. Clinical examination may reveal a bruit on auscultation. Rupture is manifest by acute localized pain and hypovolemia due to either retroperitoneal hemorrhage or rupture into the neighboring renal vein, resulting in a high-output arteriovenous fistula.

Diagnosis is usually made at laparotomy for a different abdominal pathology or incidentally on radiographic imaging such as CT scanning, angiography, or MRI. Management of asymptomatic, low-risk renal artery aneurysms should be nonoperative, as the procedure carries a significant (5%) risk of nephrectomy. On the other hand, "high risk" asymptomatic populations (defined as women of fertile age) and symptomatic patients should proceed to aneurysm repair irrespective of aneurysmal size. Operative procedures include excision with direct end-to-end arterial anastomosis, graft interposition (prosthetic or autogenous vein), and nephrectomy. Suitable aneurysms may be treated with embolization, but these techniques carry a significant risk of parenchymal damage.

Superior Mesenteric Artery Aneurysms

These aneurysms are rare, representing approximately 8% of all visceral aneurysms. Both sexes are equally affected, with infection implicated as the causal factor in two thirds of cases. Other etiologies include atherosclerosis and trauma. Age at presentation is variable, mycotic aneurysms being more common before 50 years of age, whereas atherosclerotic aneurysms usually present later (over 60 years of age). Superior mesenteric artery aneurysm management tends to be aggressive, as there is a high rate of rupture whatever the size of the aneurysm. Surgery should attempt to ligate the aneurysm without reconstruction or excision due to the high risk of damaging adjacent structures. Again, embolization may be considered, but it carries the potentially fatal complication of intestinal ischemia.

Celiac Artery Aneurysms

Celiac aneurysms are even less common than those affecting the superior mesenteric artery, representing 3% to 4% of all visceral aneurysms. There is an equal sex distribution, and most are due to atherosclerosis and medial degeneration. The majority are without symptoms, but if present they include epigastric pain, nausea, and vomiting. A bruit may be heard on clinical examination. Diagnosis is confirmed by CT scanning or abdominal ultrasound, and subsequent management involves surgical excision (for small aneurysms) or reconstruction.

Gastroduodenal, Pancreaticoduodenal, and Pancreatic Artery Aneurysms

Aneurysms of these arteries are extremely rare, collectively accounting for 3% of visceral aneurysms. The patient is usually a man in his sixth decade with a prior history of pancreatitis. Symptoms, if present, are of epigastric pain radiating through to the back, and angiography

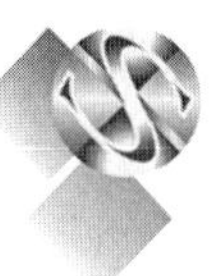

or CT scanning reveals the diagnosis. Rupture-related death rates are high (about 50%); therefore, a low threshold should exist for surgical repair. Operation is by aneurysm ligation, or in suitable cases coil embolization may be appropriate.

Jejunal, Ileal, and Colic Artery Aneurysms

Together these aneurysms constitute 2% to 3% of all visceral aneurysms. Sex distribution appears to be equal, with an average age at presentation of 75 years. These aneurysms tend to be small, isolated, and asymptomatic until rupture. Diagnosis is invariably made at subsequent laparotomy, where repair is by either aneurysm ligation or excision. Concomitant limited bowel resection may have to be performed if the vascular repair threatens an inadequate intestinal blood supply.

Axillary and Subclavian Artery Aneurysms

Aneurysmal disease affecting the upper extremity is rare but remains of importance due to the severity of possible sequelae associated with the disease. Ideal management, therefore, aims at early diagnosis and repair in order to minimize this potential morbidity. Pathology in this region is divided anatomically into one of three types, each with a distinct etiology.

Subclavian Artery Aneurysms

Subclavian aneurysms (SCAs) are arbitrarily classified as proximal or distal in reference to the location of diseased arterial segment. Proximal aneurysms are totally confined to the parent artery and are usually caused by degenerative disease, trauma, or infection. They occur more commonly in men and over the age of 60 years. In contrast, distal subclavian aneurysms tend to occur in the younger female population.

Clinical features associated with SCA can be considered as local or distant. The patient may complain of a painless pulsatile mass in the lower neck, whereas acute aneurysm expansion or rupture causes pain experienced in the chest, neck, or shoulder. Local symptoms due to compression are common and include neuropathic pain (which may be referred) due to brachial

plexus irritation, an ipsilateral Horner syndrome from sympathetic chain compression, hoarseness due to recurrent laryngeal nerve pressure, stridor due to partial extrinsic tracheal obstruction, and upper limb edema caused by venous outflow obstruction. Pulmonary erosion by the aneurysm explains any hemoptysis, whereas distant manifestations of the condition can include acute or chronic limb ischemia from thromboembolism and Raynaud syndrome. Examination may reveal a supraclavicular pulsatile mass with an audible bruit. An assessment of full upper limb neurovascular status is mandatory, which classically reveals normal pulses in the evidential face of prior microembolism and altered neurology in the corresponding segment of brachial plexus or sympathetic chain.

Duplex or CT scanning confirms the diagnosis of SCA, but angiography is also required to plan appropriate intervention. Proximal SCA management is by resection with end-to-end anastomosis for (small aneurysms) or by surgical resection with interposition arterial graft. Proximal vascular control can be difficult, and occasionally sternotomy (right SCA) or extended thoracotomy (left SCA) is required. Surgical correction of the distal SCA adheres to the same principles as for proximal pathology, with the advantage that adequate exposure is achieved by simple supraclavicular incision.

Axillosubclavian Artery Aneurysms

These aneurysms involve the junction between the terminal subclavian and proximal axillary arteries at the border of the first rib. They are invariably poststenotic aneurysms from a thoracic outlet syndrome caused by either a cervical rib or fibrous band. The disease is more common in younger females, probably because it is this population that has the highest incidence of cervical rib.

Symptoms are similar to those outlined for isolated subclavian aneurysms, but it is worth noting that there is an increased frequency of embolic phenomena. Investigation of axillosubclavian disease is initially by duplex ultrasonography, but arteriography is advised for all cases to be considered for surgery. Exact management depends on both aneurysmal size and the presence of distal thromboembolic complications. Large (defined as more than twice the arterial

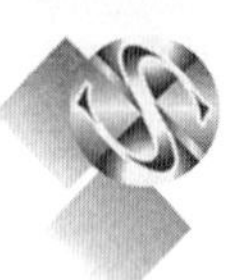

diameter) or symptomatic aneurysms require arterial repair by means of excision and graft interposition with synchronous removal of the antecedent cause (e.g., excision of cervical rib or division of fibrous band). Small, asymptomatic aneurysms may well recede once the thoracic outlet syndrome has been surgically corrected so that arterial reconstruction is often not required.

Axillary Artery Aneurysms

Isolated axillary artery aneurysms are very rare but typically affect young males as a consequence of trauma. Repeated blunt trauma to the axillary artery, classically due to long-term crutch-use, may result in aneurysm development and the subsequent complicating symptoms of acute or chronic upper limb ischemia. Penetrating trauma tends to result in false aneurysm formation. A rich collateral blood supply in this region may lead to delayed and atypical presentations, so a high index of suspicion is needed to make the diagnosis.

Investigation is by duplex ultrasound followed by arteriography, and appropriate surgery is aneurysm resection and arterial reconstruction by interposition autogenous vein graft (saphenous vein). Prosthetic grafts have been successfully used but are associated with inferior long-term patency rates. Recently, successful management with axillary endovascular stent grafts has been reported, but the long-term results of this intervention are presently unknown.

Carotid Artery Aneurysms

Extracranial carotid aneurysmal disease requiring vascular surgical expertise is extremely rare.

True carotid aneurysms are located either in the carotid bifurcation, internal carotid system or external carotid, in decreasing frequency of that order. Etiological factors are varied, but the most common include atherosclerosis, trauma, previous carotid surgery (e.g., endarterectomy), and carotid artery dissection. Historically, infection used to be the major culprit causing disease, but widespread antibiotic availability has rendered this mechanism responsible in only a minority of cases.

The patient may present with an awareness of a pulsatile mass in the neck that may or may not be painful. Other symptoms are attributed to local compression and include dysphagia as a result of pharyngeal proximity, deafness or facial pain due to cranial nerve compression, and hoarseness caused by vagus nerve impingement. Distal central nervous neurological symptoms such as stroke, amaurosis fugax, or transient ischemic attack (TIA) indicate thromboembolic complications from the carotid aneurysm and are in fact the most common presenting feature of the disease. Large aneurysms have also been implicated in posture-related transient neurology as a result of limitation and even occlusion of blood flow through the neighboring internal carotid artery. Ruptured carotid aneurysms are fortunately rare but are usually fatal if they occur.

It is interesting that despite the paucity of the disease, carotid aneurysms remain overdiagnosed. True aneurysms must be distinguished from the much commoner reality of tortuous or coiled carotid vessels, and other diagnoses such as cervical lymphadenopathy, carotid body tumors, and branchial cysts. In the majority of cases history and clinical examination alone should be sufficient to expose the bona fide aneurysm, but confirmation can be obtained with duplex or CT scanning. If intervention is being contemplated, an angiogram must also be obtained.

The aim of management is ultimately prevention of the neurological complications associated with carotid aneurysmal disease. Current opinion regarding preferred treatment is divided between surgical and endovascular methods. In the former, the aneurysm is resected, arterial reconstruction is performed, and cerebral blood flow is maintained during carotid clamping with an operative shunt. The adequacy of this maneuver is assessed by some surgeons with the use of intraoperative transcranial Doppler or electroencephalography in order to confirm distal perfusion. Surgery is notoriously perilous in proximal internal carotid disease and in larger aneurysms where "distal" control can be difficult to secure. The most feared complication of carotid aneurysm surgery is disabling stroke, occurring in 6% to 10% of cases, which may result from cerebral hypoperfusion or intraoperative dislodgment of debris from the vessel wall. Another specific risk of surgery is cranial nerve palsy, resulting from local tissue handling or careless dissection. The condition affects 20% of patients and is usually temporary, but must nonetheless be mentioned to the patient preoperatively while obtaining informed consent.

Endovascular approaches to carotid aneurysm management may soon render surgery as second-line treatment for extracranial carotid aneurysmal disease. Graft stenting and coil embolization of such lesions is reported to be as effective as surgical repair, without the need for operation. These techniques may be especially appropriate in large aneurysms, revisional surgery, or the case of high carotid aneurysm close to the base of skull so that access is problematic. The risk of neurological complications following the procedures remains, but these cerebrovascular events appear less common in this approach to treatment. Still in its infancy, these initial encouraging results may be tempered as we await the longer term results of endoluminal intervention.

Controversial Issues

- Should there be a national screening program for the detection of AAA?
- Are all elective AAA repairs best performed at tertiary referral centers?
- Is open repair preferable to endovascular therapy in elective AAA repair?
- What is the optimal management of type I and type III endoleaks?
- Does routine uterolysis have a role in the management of the inflammatory AAA?
- Do all high (Crawford types I and II) thoracoabdominal aneurysm repairs mandate the use of cardiopulmonary bypass and spinal fluid drainage?
- What is the best treatment for the asymptomatic popliteal aneurysm?
- When should carotid aneurysms be repaired with endovascular methods?

References

Dawson I, Sie RB, van Bockel JH. (1997) Br J Surg 84: 293–9.

Hallin A, Bergqvist D, Holmberg L. (2001) Eur J Vasc Endovasc Surg 22:197–204.

Heller JA, Weinberg A, Arons R, et al. (2000) J Vasc Surg 32:1091–100.

Rasmussen TE, Hallett JW Jr. (1997) Ann Surg 225:155–64.

Wassef M, Baxter BT, Chisholm RL, et al. (2001) J Vasc Surg 34:730–8.

Wilmink AB, Quick CR. (1998) Br J Surg 85:155–62.

Woodburn KR, May J, White GH. (1998) Br J Surg 85: 435–43.

18

Renovascular Hypertension and Ischemic Nephropathy

Sherry D. Scovell

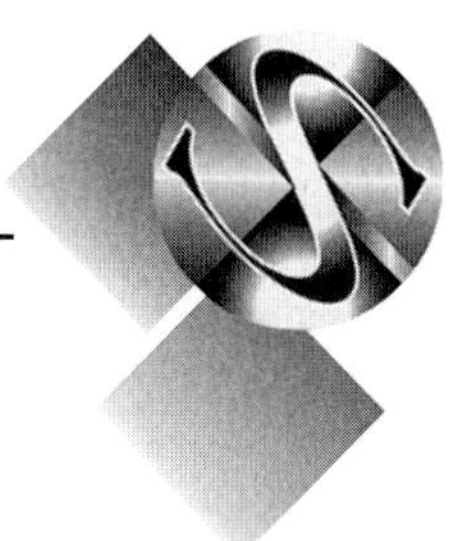

Renovascular hypertension is a relatively uncommon cause of hypertension and is only seen in 5% to 10% of the hypertensive population. However, this translates to at least 600,000 people in the United States alone when considering that nearly 60 million people in the United States have some degree of hypertension. Renal artery stenosis (RAS) often produces an unclear clinical picture. Patients may be asymptomatic. However, they may also present with severe, uncontrolled hypertension referred to as renovascular hypertension or with evidence of renal insufficiency, otherwise known as ischemic nephropathy. This chapter focuses on the clinical characteristics that may be helpful in identifying those patients who may be at risk for RAS, how to accurately diagnose RAS, and how to correlate RAS with the symptoms of uncontrolled hypertension or ischemic nephropathy. It also outlines the options available for treatment, including medical management, endovascular correction of RAS via angioplasty with or without stenting, and open surgical revascularization.

Characteristics

With renovascular disease being responsible for only 5% to 10% of the hypertensive population, it would be helpful to define certain clinical characteristics that are prevalent in this population to aid in screening patients. Typically, renovascular hypertension produces severe diastolic hypertension, which is defined as diastolic blood pressure greater than 115 mm Hg. In a blood pressure screening program 137 patients with new-onset hypertension were diagnosed in a shopping center. Further workup consisted of angiography followed by renal vein renin measurements and split renal function tests in patients with evidence of critical renal artery stenosis. None of the 102 patients with a diastolic blood pressure between 90 and 115 mm Hg had evidence of renovascular hypertension. However, nine of the 35 patients (26%) with a diastolic blood pressure of 115 mm Hg or higher did have evidence of renovascular hypertension. With respect to race, none of the African-American patients had renovascular hypertension, whereas nine of the 22 (41%) Caucasian patients did have renovascular hypertension.

Renovascular hypertension has also been described as having a bimodal age distribution, with patients at the two extremes of age carrying the highest incidence of having renovascular disease responsible for their hypertension. It is typically seen in children younger than 5 years old and in patients over 60 years of age.

Based on observations such as these, additional characteristics thought to be associated with renovascular hypertension were postulated to include recent onset of hypertension, young age, lack of family history of hypertension, and the presence of an abdominal bruit. The most comprehensive study used to compare these characteristics in hypertensive patients both

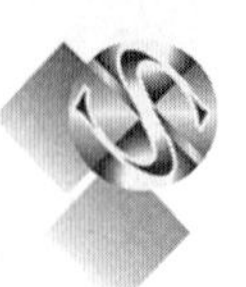

with and without RAS was the Cooperative Study of Renovascular Hypertension (Simon, 1972). One of the ultimate conclusions of this study was that neither the above four criteria nor any other clinical criteria could accurately predict the presence of renovascular hypertension. Indeed, the majority of patients with renovascular hypertension do not present with what were once thought to be the "classic" characteristics delineated above. As a result of these studies, it is necessary to maintain a high index of suspicion in patients whose hypertension is difficult to control with medical management and to rely on screening examinations in patients with severe diastolic hypertension.

Etiology

The etiology of RAS is primarily atherosclerotic in approximately 90% of patients. The second most common etiology is fibromuscular dysplasia (FMD). Other less common causes of RAS include aortic dissection, vasculitis, emboli, radiation, and extrinsic compression from masses or tumors.

Atherosclerotic renal artery stenosis is seen predominantly in males. The majority of these lesions are believed to be ostial encroachment of an aortic plaque on the orifice of the renal artery or arteries. As a result, 50% of the time these lesions are bilateral. As well, these lesions are typically eccentric and irregular luminal stenoses. It is well known that atherosclerotic disease is progressive and the renal artery in not an exception. RAS will be progressive in 30% to 70% of cases. Approximately 11% of the time, patients with a greater than 60% stenosis of the renal artery will progress to total occlusion within a 2-year period (Zierler, 1994).

The stenoses caused by FMD are primarily nonostial and often extend into the branches of the renal arteries. Fibromuscular dysplasia may be divided into three types: medial fibrodysplasia, perimedial dysplasia, and intimal fibroplasia.

Medial fibrodysplasia is the most common type, accounting for 85% of all FMD lesions. Women are predominantly affected, usually between 25 and 45 years of age. In 55% of patients, the disease is bilateral. If it is unilateral, it is more likely to affect the right renal artery when compared to the left renal artery. The angiographic appearance is that of a string of beads. There are two distinct types of medial fibrodysplasia—diffuse and peripheral.

Perimedial dysplasia is seen in only about 10% of patients with FMD. This subtype is again seen most often in women in the fourth or fifth decades of life. This type may be more progressive when compared to medial fibrodysplasia.

Finally, intimal fibroplasia is seen in 5% of patients with FMD. These lesions are long, irregular, tubular regions of stenosis. They tend to progress more rapidly than those caused by medial fibrodysplasia.

Pathophysiology

Any comprehensive review of renovascular hypertension must cite Goldblatt's (1934) classic experiments. He described both the two-kidney, one-clip model of unilateral RAS in the setting of a normal contralateral kidney, as well as the one-kidney, one-clip model that represents unilateral RAS in a patient with only one kidney.

In the two-kidney, one-clip model, one renal artery is clamped while the other one is left open. In this model, there is decreased renal blood flow seen by the ipsilateral juxtaglomerular apparatus. This leads to increased secretion of renin by the clipped kidney. Through the renin-angiotensin-aldosterone system, there is mild sodium retention as a result of increased aldosterone and increased blood pressure secondary to angiotensin II–related vasoconstriction. The contralateral kidney then suppresses its release of renin to compensate. When an angiotensin-converting enzyme (ACE) inhibitor is administered to a patient in the two-kidney, one-clip model acutely, there is a dramatic reduction in blood pressure. This demonstrates that the elevation in blood pressure is primarily angiotensin II–dependent.

In the one-kidney, one-clip model of renovascular disease, a clip is applied to the renal artery supplying a single kidney. In this case, there is an initial elevation in renin. This initial rise in the renin leads to activation of the renin-angiotensin-aldosterone system, and there is peripheral vasoconstriction as well as an increase in sodium and water retention. Blood pressure rises as a result of both of these mechanisms. This model is both an angiotensin-dependent system as well as a volume-driven

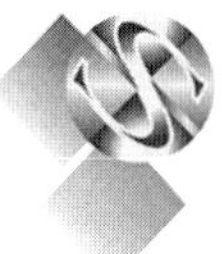

system and produces a more persistent form of hypertension.

Diagnostic Evaluation

The patients who are well served by renal revascularization are those with severe RAS in the setting of either uncontrolled hypertension or ischemic nephropathy. Patients without an association between the anatomical stenosis and these symptoms are not well served by correction of the RAS. Therefore, it is necessary to establish a correlation between the anatomical RAS and the uncontrolled hypertension or ischemic nephropathy to determine who will benefit from an attempt at revascularization. This is done primarily through the combination of both anatomical screening tests as well as studies that document associated physiological consequences. Anatomical tests are those that delineate RAS and document associated hemodynamic data. Physiological tests attempt to establish an association between the anatomical stenosis and the alterations in the renin-angiotensin-aldosterone axis.

Anatomical Tests

Duplex Ultrasound

Duplex examination of the kidneys and the renal arteries is an extremely useful screening modality as it is a noninvasive examination. The only preparation necessary is an overnight fast, and it is not necessary to discontinue antihypertensive medications for reliable results. Renal artery duplex examination is able to identify hemodynamically significant renal artery lesions. It offers information on renal length as well as on the renal artery blood flow. The resistive index (RI) indicates the degree of renal artery resistance and should be calculated. It is defined as the peak systolic shift minus the minimum diastolic shift over the peak systolic shift. A normal RI is less than 0.70. The RI may be predictive of outcome with respect to renal revascularization (Radermacher et al., 2001). However, caution should be taken in the interpretation of RI as it may also be increased in patients with intrinsic renal disease, decreased cardiac output, or perinephric fluid collections.

The degree of RAS is typically calculated based on the renal-to-aortic ratio (RAR) as well as the peak systolic velocities in the renal artery. The RAR is the ratio of the peak systolic velocity of the renal artery to the aortic peak systolic velocity. If the RAR is less than 3.5 with a peak systolic velocity of greater than 180 cm/sec, there is a less than 60% stenosis. If the RAR is greater than 3.5 and the peak systolic velocity is greater than 180 cm/sec, this is diagnostic of a greater than 60% stenosis. If there is no detectable renal artery signal with a kidney length of less than 9 cm, the renal artery is considered occluded.

Although this is an excellent screening test to detect the presence of renal artery stenosis, duplex examination is unable to accurately predict the clinical response of either the hypertension or renal insufficiency following correction of the RAS. It is also unable to accurately identify all accessory branches of the renal artery and their contribution to the clinical picture. This is, however, an appropriate noninvasive screening test to evaluate for RAS and is useful for following the patient with serial examinations after intervention.

Angiography/Digital Subtraction Angiography

The gold standard for the identification of RAS still remains angiography, although it is an invasive test and not an optimal screening tool. It serves to define the presence, severity, and location of intraluminal anatomical defects in the renal artery. It facilitates a full evaluation of the abdominal aorta as well as the renal artery orifices and the accessory branches of the renal artery. Multiple accessory renal arteries exist in up to 25% of patients and are well defined with angiography. It is able to define a nephrogram. It is still controversial whether angiography should be utilized as a screening test for renovascular disease. It is likely best used as an adjunct when duplex examination is unable to visualize the renal arteries, or smaller accessory branches are suspected of contributing to severe renovascular hypertension.

Technically, the renal arteries usually arise posterolaterally from the aorta and require oblique views for adequate visualization of their orifices. Peak systolic pressure gradients across the lesion of >20 mm Hg or mean gradients of

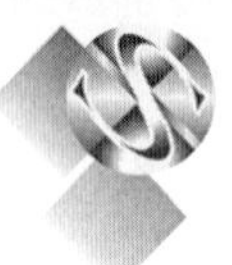

10 mm Hg have been used as objective criteria to define a significant reduction in blood flow.

It has been well documented that angiography may exacerbate renal failure in patients with baseline renal insufficiency. Nonionic, low-osmolar contrast material is recommended for the evaluation of the renal arteries and is associated with a lower incidence of contrast-induced nephropathy (Barrett and Carlisle, 1993). In patients with an elevated creatinine, CO_2 or gadolinium may be substituted without an increase in contrast-induced nephropathy. As well, preintervention hydration is critical as is acetylcysteine in select patient groups.

The calculation of RAS is determined by comparison of the narrowest segment of the renal artery to the normal diameter of the renal artery either proximal to the stenosis or distal to any region of poststenotic dilatation. Poststenotic dilatation is common in many cases of long-standing arterial stenosis.

Patient Selection

Renal artery stenosis alone, in the absence of symptoms, does not mandate repair. The coexistence of RAS and hypertension does not establish a causal relationship. For this reason, it is essential to determine the functional significance of the anatomical stenosis.

Patients with RAS and symptoms attributable to that stenosis are considered for treatment and correction of the anatomical lesion. Symptoms of hypertension, renal insufficiency, or pulmonary edema in the setting of a greater than 60% RAS serve as criteria for repair. Clinical criteria for revascularization have been defined recently in the Guidelines for Reporting on Renal Artery Revascularization in Clinical Trials (Rundback, 2002). Based on these guidelines, hypertension was classified as either accelerated with sudden worsening in the setting of previous control, refractory hypertension resistant to medical management with three or more anti-hypertensive medications including a diuretic, or malignant hypertension with evidence of severe end-organ damage as a result. The presence of hypertension in the setting of a unilaterally shrunken kidney was also used as an indication for intervention. With respect to renal insufficiency, the clinical criteria for intervention were defined as unexplained worsening of renal function or a decrease in renal function

with the addition of an ACE inhibitor, as well as renal dysfunction not attributable to another obvious etiology. Finally, recurrent episodes of "flash" pulmonary edema not able to be explained on the basis of severe left ventricular dysfunction in the setting of RAS was also considered an indication for revascularization. The value of prophylactic renal artery revascularization in asymptomatic patients is unproven at this point, and that is why physiological tests are significant in these patients.

Physiological Tests

When a unilateral RAS is defined by anatomical studies, the functional significance must be determined. In the past, many different tests were attempted in order to define this correlation including intravenous urography, nuclear medicine studies, conventional angiography, computed tomography, and magnetic resonance imaging. More recently, this is accomplished through the use of renal vein renin assays or by isotope renography. The value of these tests is not as great in patients with severe bilateral renal disease or RAS in a solitary kidney when compared to unilateral renal disease and a functioning contralateral kidney.

Physiologically, there is a functional increase in plasma levels of renin from the affected kidney, which is characteristic in the setting of RAS. Originally, systemic levels of renin were obtained in an attempt to establish a diagnosis. However, utilizing this method, the rate of false-negative and false-positive results were high, 43% and 34%, respectively, in patients with confirmed renovascular hypertension. As well, roughly 20% of patients with essential hypertension had an elevated plasma renin level. The value of selective renal vein sampling of renin, although an invasive procedure, has been found to be more sensitive and specific. This test compares the renin levels between the ipsilateral and contralateral kidneys. If the renal vein/renin ratio is greater than 1.5, there is lateralization of renin secretion. This, as well, seems to be predictive of improvement following renal revascularization. However, the failure to demonstrate lateralization does not reliably predict failure of revascularization procedures. In addition, there are unfortunately strict prerequisite guidelines required prior to performance of this test. Antihypertensive medications must be held for up to

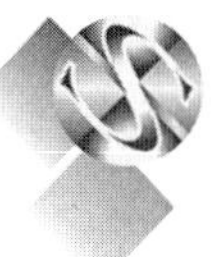

3 weeks prior to the test, which is not without clinical consequences.

For these reasons, other physiological tests became more favorable. Initially, isotope renography was developed as a screening procedure for renovascular hypertension. The theory was that the underperfused kidney would have delayed uptake and excretion of solute when compared to the normal, well-perfused contralateral kidney. Various nucleotides were utilized; however, this test still yielded a high rate of false-negative results. More recently, the results of this functional test have improved through the use of the ACE inhibitor captopril. Angiotensin II is elevated in patients with RAS, and this elevation leads to selective vasoconstriction of the efferent arterioles in an attempt to maintain glomerular filtration. The use of captopril blocks angiotensin II production, and thus filtration drops precipitously. The finding of a decrease in the uptake and excretion of the tracer is more pronounced in patients after captopril in the setting of clinically significant RAS. Through the use of captopril, this study has most recently demonstrated a 92% sensitivity and a 94% specificity.

Therapeutic Options

The options for the treatment of symptomatic RAS include medical management utilizing multiple antihypertensive medications, the endovascular approach including angioplasty with or without the placement of a stent, or open surgical management.

Medical Management of Symptomatic Renal Artery Stenosis

The medical management of symptomatic RAS is accomplished using a variety of antihypertensive medications in an attempt to control the hypertension. Control of the hypertension in itself is critical, as uncontrolled hypertension is a major risk factor for myocardial infarction, cerebrovascular accident, and chronic renal insufficiency. Thus, the goals of medical management of symptomatic RAS are to reduce the blood pressure, to control cardiovascular risk factors, and ultimately to prevent end-organ damage from sustained hypertension.

However, the natural history of uncorrected RAS is not benign. It has previously been documented that 11% of patients with a greater than 60% stenosis of the renal artery progress to occlusion within a 2-year period. As well, over 40% of patients with a critical stenosis of the renal artery will have a decrease in glomerular filtration by greater than 25% with progressive deterioration in renal function being common in this group of patients.

As a result of these findings, there have been numerous studies designed to evaluate medical management for symptomatic RAS compared to both open surgical repair as well as endovascular management.

Hunt and Strong (1973) orchestrated a comparative analysis examining drug therapy compared to operative therapy to treat symptomatic RAS; 114 patients were in the medical treatment arm and 100 patients were in the surgical treatment arm. The follow-up was over the course of 7 to 14 years. Overall, 84% of patients were alive in the surgical group compared to 66% alive in the group treated medically. Of those alive in the surgical group, 93% were cured or significantly improved, whereas of those patients in the medical treatment group, 21% subsequently required surgical intervention for uncontrolled hypertension. Another seven patients from that group continued to have uncontrolled hypertension but were not taken to surgery. In addition, death was twice as common in the medically treated group. These differences were statistically significant ($p < .01$) for both atherosclerotic and FMD lesions. This study demonstrated that in patients with renovascular hypertension, there is a need to treat symptomatic lesions surgically. Indeed, in this series, surgical intervention offered better symptomatic relief of hypertension, which translated to a lower incidence of end-organ damage.

Webster and colleagues (1998) performed the first prospective randomized trial comparing medical management with renal artery angioplasty in 55 patients. All patients were hypertensive and showed evidence of ≥50% RAS on angiography. They found that only patients with bilateral RAS demonstrated a significant decrease in blood pressure with angioplasty. There was no significant improvement in renal excretory function. Otherwise, there was no statistical difference between the two groups. This study suggested that there might be a significant benefit to be derived from the endovascular management of symptomatic RAS over medical management of these patients, which ultimately led to the validation of this therapeutic option.

Based on the results of the above studies as well as other smaller studies, it became clear that intervention, either endovascular or open surgical, should play a significant role in the treatment of symptomatic RAS.

Endovascular Repair of Renal Artery Stenosis

In addition to open surgical repair for symptomatic RAS, renal artery angioplasty with or without stenting offers a less invasive method to correct the anatomical stenosis. Although still a matter of great debate, it is clear that angioplasty with or without stenting may offer at least short-term improvement in blood pressure and, in certain circumstances, renal function. Although this option is especially appealing for patients, it is certainly necessary to further evaluate and better define what the role of endovascular management of symptomatic RAS should be through a multi-institutional randomized, prospective trial.

There is much debate regarding the need to place a stent in the renal artery compared to angioplasty alone. Typically, renal artery angioplasty alone is utilized for fibrodysplastic lesions and lesions that do not involve the origin of the renal artery. However, as mentioned previously, RAS that is atherosclerotic in etiology is often an extension of aortic plaque. For this reason, angioplasty alone is not as durable. It has been demonstrated that atherosclerotic lesions of the renal artery seem to have lower rates of re-stenosis following angioplasty and placement of a stent for this reason. In addition, it is clear that if there is a residual stenosis following initial angioplasty or evidence of dissection, a stent should be placed at that time.

There has been some concern that renal artery angioplasty and stenting may make operative intervention difficult or impossible secondary to postangioplasty periarterial fibrosis. This is especially true for transaortic renal endarterectomy. In the case of a previously placed renal stent placement, renal artery bypass grafting to a site on the renal artery distal to the stent may be the best option.

However, in certain cases, endarterectomy may still be feasible (Pak, 2002).

Although it is widely practiced at most institutions, renal artery angioplasty and stenting is a topic that is still the subject of modest debate. There are only a few prospective randomized controlled trials that compare medical therapy, endovascular management, and open surgical repair of symptomatic RAS.

Weibull and associates (1993) prospectively and randomly assigned 58 patients with symptomatic RAS to either renal angioplasty or surgical renal revascularization. Percutaneous transluminal angioplasty (PTA) was initially technically successful 83% of the time, whereas surgical management was successful 97% of the time. The primary patency rate after 2 years was 75% in the PTA group compared to 96% in the surgical group. Secondary patency was 90% versus 97%, respectively, in the PTA and surgical patients. Hypertension was improved in 90% after PTA and 86% following open surgical renal revascularization, and improvement in renal function was seen in 83% and 72%, respectively. The authors concluded that PTA is a reasonable option when compared to surgical revascularization. Indeed, the primary patency was lower in the endovascular group, but the secondary patency was comparable. Patients treated with angioplasty of RAS clearly require close surveillance and often subsequent procedures to maintain patency.

Martin and colleagues (2003), as well, have demonstrated a 30% incidence of re-stenosis following initially technically successful renal artery angioplasty. This high incidence of re-stenosis with respect to renal artery ostial lesions is likely due to the fact that these lesions represent extension of an aortic plaque. The idea of placing stents in the renal arteries as a method of preventing re-stenosis was introduced by Palmaz in 1976, initially in animal models and subsequently in humans. Currently, the indications for the placement of a stent in a renal artery following renal artery angioplasty include substantial elastic recoil, resistance of the plaque, or dissection.

Bush and colleagues (2001) retrospectively examined the results of renal artery stenting in 73 consecutive patients over a 7-year period. In this study, the majority of stents were placed for residual stenosis following angioplasty or dissection. The technical success rate was

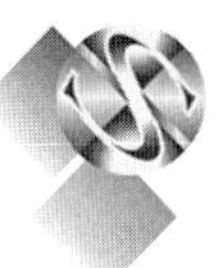

89%, with one patient requiring thrombolytic therapy for intrastent thrombus. The complication rate was 9.1% with renal artery thrombosis, extravasation, and hematoma. In this study, the authors noted a significant decrease in both systolic and diastolic blood pressures ($p < .001$) as well as a decrease in the number of medications required to treat the hypertension ($p < .01$). Over the course of an average of 20 months' follow-up, serum creatinine levels decreased by more than 20% in 22% of patients. It remained unchanged in 48% of patients and deteriorated in 25% of patients. Of the 25% of patients who had an increase in serum creatinine, 12% eventually required hemodialysis. Five of these patients had a preoperative creatinine level over 4.0 mg/dL. Over the course of approximately 11 months' follow-up, 10 patients had evidence of re-stenosis in a total of 14 renal arteries. Overall, this retrospective study established the safety of endovascular management with respect to these lesions as an alternative to open surgical repair.

Attempts to validate the endovascular management of symptomatic RAS seem to be beneficial, at least in the short term. This method of treatment, although less invasive than open surgical repair, appears not to be as durable over the long term. This group of patients needs close post–angioplasty and stent surveillance to detect re-stenosis and subsequent intervention to have results that are comparable to open surgical repair. However, this still remains an option that is feasible for the treatment of these lesions and attractive for the patients. It is hoped that through the use of a well-constructed trial, more data will be available to formulate more solid conclusions on angioplasty and stenting of symptomatic renal artery stenosis.

Open Surgical Renal Revascularization

Open surgical repair or reconstruction of symptomatic renal artery lesions still remains the gold standard in treatment. Options for direct open surgical repair include aortorenal bypass, reimplantation of the renal artery, and thromboendarterectomy. Indirect renal revascularization may be accomplished via splenorenal or hepatorenal artery bypass. This option is especially useful because aortic cross-clamping may be avoided. The conduits available for use include autologous vein grafts, synthetic polytetrafluoroethylene (PTFE) and Dacron prosthetic grafts, and autologous hypogastric artery. Nephrectomy, as well, may be considered in patients with unreconstructable renal disease with a nonfunctioning ipsilateral kidney.

The operative approach may be through a midline xiphoid to pubis incision, a supraumbilical transverse incision, an extended flank incision, or a subcostal incision. The midline approach is useful for atherosclerotic lesions as well as lesions combined with aortic procedures, whereas the subcostal or flank incisions are efficacious for fibrodysplastic lesions or splanchnorenal bypass. When combined with mesenteric artery bypass grafting, the extended flank incision may be useful. Thromboendarterectomy may be easily accomplished via a retroperitoneal trapdoor approach.

With respect to exposure of the distal renal artery, the left renal artery lies posterior to the left renal vein. The vein must be sufficiently mobilized with division of the gonadal and adrenal veins. The renal vein may be retracted either cephalad or caudad to expose the renal artery. There is also a lumbar vein that enters the posterior aspect of the renal vein that may be easily avulsed if not carefully identified and ligated. Distal exposure of the renal artery is essential to clearly identify the extent of the atheroma, and the renal artery should be dissected free distal to the atherosclerotic plaque. Silastic loops may be used for distal arterial control, as they are less traumatic compared to metal clamps.

The aortic anastomosis is typically performed utilizing an aortotomy that is two to three times the diameter of the conduit. The anastomosis is usually placed on the anterolateral aspect of the aorta. It is essential to prevent the graft from kinking. For right-sided revascularizations, the aortorenal graft is typically placed in a retrocaval position, although this must be individualized. With respect to left-sided revascularizations, the graft is usually placed beneath the left renal vein.

Subsequently, the renal anastomosis is completed. This is typically anastomosed in an end-to-end fashion with spatulation of both the graft and renal artery. Spatulated anastomoses are ovoid and less prone to the development of

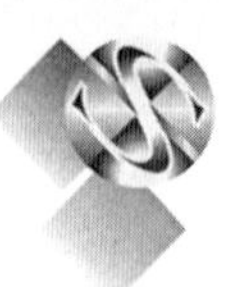
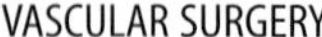

strictures. Intraoperative evaluation of blood flow is typically accomplished using a directional Doppler device. Intraoperative angiography is usually unnecessary; however, many surgeons advocate baseline angiography prior to discharge to establish a baseline and to confirm the adequacy of repair.

Hansen and colleagues (1992) retrospectively reviewed the data on 200 patients who underwent open surgical renal revascularization over a 54-month period. There was a mortality rate of 2.5% and only a 1.4% primary failure rate at 30 days. In this series, the hypertension was cured in 21% of patients and improved in another 70%. Of the patients with ischemic nephropathy, 49% demonstrated an improvement in glomerular filtration; 36% of these patients remained stable and only 15% worsened. This study clearly demonstrates that open surgical renal revascularization is a safe option that is successful in treating the underlying clinical manifestations of the RAS in the majority of patients.

Recently, Cherr and associates retrospectively reviewed the clinical outcome of 500 consecutive patients with renovascular hypertension. The perioperative mortality was 4.6% at 30 days. The hypertension was cured in 12%, improved in 73%, and unchanged in only 15%. With respect to ischemic nephropathy, 43% had an improvement in renal function, 47% were unchanged, and 10% became worse. Interestingly, of the 43% of patients who demonstrated an improvement in renal function, 28 patients were removed from dialysis dependence. These data confirm the findings of Hansen and associates and once again demonstrate that open surgical repair of severe, flow-limiting, symptomatic RAS is efficacious in improving hypertension and ischemic nephropathy in the majority of patients. It adds the point, however, that if there was a blood pressure cure or an improvement in renal function, there was an association with dialysis-free survival. This has a significant impact on patient lifestyle as well as on health care dollars.

At this time, there is significant controversy regarding the optimal treatment in patients with symptomatic RAS. It is important that a multicenter, prospective, randomized clinical trial be organized in an effort to further define the best possible treatment options for these patients.

Conclusions

Renovascular hypertension is an uncommon cause of hypertension in the general population. However, it may cause considerable morbidity with respect to end-organ damage from uncontrolled hypertension as well as progression of ischemic nephropathy. It appears as if duplex ultrasound is at least a reasonable screening tool in patients suspected of having hypertension that is renal in origin. However, there clearly needs to be correlation between the anatomical stenosis and the physiological effect. For this purpose, there is not a clearly optimal test, although captopril renography seems to offer the best results at this time.

Once diagnosed and found to be functionally significant, there are several options for the treatment of RAS, including medical management, endovascular angioplasty with or without stent placement, or open surgical revascularization. From the data that are available, it is clear that there is a patient population that does benefit from revascularization, either endovascular or surgical. Surgical revascularization is more durable, and long-term success has been previously demonstrated. Angioplasty with or without stent placement is indeed less durable over the long-term; however, with close surveillance and secondary intervention, it may offer results comparable with open surgical repair.

Although there have been a multitude of attempts to define which patients with symptomatic RAS would benefit from renal revascularization, both surgical and endovascular, there is still no clear consensus at the present time. Recently, the American Heart Association released the guidelines for the reporting of renal artery revascularization in clinical trials. This document serves to clearly outline criteria and definitions for randomized, controlled clinical trials, which are needed to further dictate the optimal management of symptomatic RAS. At this time, it is clear that certain patients do benefit from restoration of blood flow to the kidney, but a multicenter, prospective, randomized, controlled study will be better able to define which patients benefit from surgical repair compared to endovascular management and which patients, if any, should merely be treated medically.

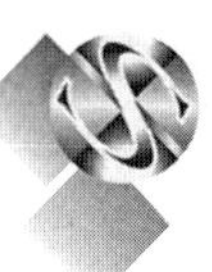

References

Barrett BJ, Carlisle EJ. (1993) Radiology 188:171–8.

Bush RL, Najibi S, MacDonald MJ, et al. (2001) J Vasc Surg 33:1041–9.

Goldblatt H. (1934) J Exp Med 59:347.

Hunt JC, Strong CG. (1973) Am J Cardiol 32:562–74.

Martin LG, Rundback JH, Sacks D, et al. (2003) J Vasc Interv Radiol 14:5297–310.

Pak LK, Kerlan RK, Mully TW, Messina LM. (2002) J Vasc Surg 35:808–10.

Radermacher J, Chavan A, Bleck J, et al. (2001) N Engl J Med 344:410–17.

Rundback JH, Sacks D, Kent KC, et al. (2002) J Vasc Intervent Radiol 13:959–74.

Simon N, Franklin SS, Bleifer KH, Maxwell MH. (1972) JAMA 220:1209–18.

Webster J, Marshall F, Abdalla M, et al. (1998) J Hum Hypertens 12:329–35.

Weibull H, Bergqvist D, Bergentz SE, Jonsson K, Hulthen L, Manhem P. (1993) J Vasc Surg 18:841–50; discussion 850–2.

Zierler RE, Bergelin RO, Isaacson JA, Strandness DE Jr. (1994) J Vasc Surg 19:250–7; discussion 257–8.

19

Visceral Ischemic Syndromes

George Geroulakos, Peter A. Robless, and
William L. Smead

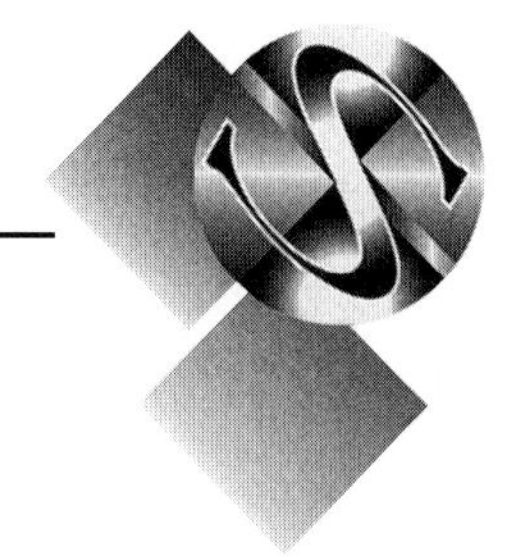

The disorders of the visceral circulation are infrequent mainly because of the very extensive and efficient collateral system connecting the celiac, superior mesenteric, and inferior mesenteric arteries. However, there is a lot of interest in the optimal management of these conditions, because of their catastrophic outcomes that are usually associated with a high morbidity and mortality. Over the last two decades there has been a greater awareness of these conditions, which was followed by the introduction of new diagnostic and therapeutic techniques such as duplex ultrasound, computed tomography (CT), magnetic resonance angiography (MRA), and angioplasty/stenting.

Visceral ischemic syndromes can be classified as acute or chronic. Acute ischemic syndromes are the result of embolic or thrombotic occlusion of a visceral branch of the infradiaphragmatic aorta. In addition, it could be the result of mesenteric venous thrombosis. Chronic visceral ischemia is usually caused by stenotic or occlusive atherosclerotic lesions involving two or more visceral vessels.

Acute Mesenteric Ischemia

Acute mesenteric ischemia (AMI) is a life-threatening condition seen in 1 per 1000 hospital admissions with mortality rates ranging between 60% and 100% despite advances in operative technique and perioperative management (Bradbury et al., 1995). Early diagnosis and aggressive management are essential. However, the relative rarity of this condition, along with the nonspecific physical findings makes early diagnosis difficult and is often delayed. Furthermore, patients with AMI are often elderly, malnourished, and have significant comorbidity that increases the risk of major surgical intervention.

The most common causes of AMI are superior mesenteric artery embolization (50%) or thrombosis (25%), nonocclusive mesenteric ischemia (20%), and acute mesenteric venous thrombosis (5%). Rarer causes include vasculitis, fibromuscular dysplasia, dissection, trauma, and mesenteric aneurysm rupture or thrombosis.

Pathophysiology

Two thirds of mesenteric blood flow supplies the gut mucosa. Splanchnic autoregulation fails when perfusion pressure falls below 40 mm Hg, and prolonged gut ischemia results in anaerobic metabolism. The extent of injury is related to the duration and the anatomical extent of mesenteric ischemia. At the cellular level, adenosine triphosphate (ATP) is depleted with a buildup of catabolic products and lactate. Mucosal and vascular permeability increases and tissue injury occurs. Hemorrhagic necrosis follows with mucosal sloughing, bowel wall edema, and intestinal hemorrhage (Table 19.1). The bowel wall becomes permeable to gut bacteria once the mucosa is shed. Peritonitis results

Table 19.1. Pathophysiology of mesenteric ischemia

Mucosa—villous sloughing
Increased capillary permeability—Edema
Submucosal hemorrhage
Transmural necrosis

from transudation of microflora across the intestinal wall. Septicemia develops as the organisms enter the portal circulation. Massive fluid shifts into the bowel wall and peritoneum follow, resulting in hemoconcentration, oliguria, and hypotension. Serum levels of lactate dehydrogenase (LDH), serum glutamic oxaloacetic transaminase (SGOT), and creatine kinase (CK) become markedly elevated with the death of intestinal cells.

Ischemia reperfusion injury due to free radical production through the xanthine oxidase pathway may result from subsequent reperfusion of the acutely ischemic gut. There is a high mortality rate from the ensuing multiorgan dysfunction syndrome.

Acute Mesenteric Embolism

The main presenting symptom is usually the sudden onset of severe central abdominal pain. The severity of the pain is usually out of proportion to the physical findings. This may be accompanied by vomiting or diarrhea.

Mesenteric emboli can originate from the heart or the supradiaphragmatic aorta and most frequently occur in patients with cardiac arrythmias, valvular disease, or following myocardial infarction. If the embolus disintegrates and travels distally, the resulting ischemia may be patchy, typically affecting the duodenum, proximal jejunum, and colon. The majority of emboli lodge in the superior mesenteric artery (SMA) distal to the origin of the middle colic artery, often sparing the proximal jejunum and ascending/transverse colon. Owing to the lack of adequate collaterals, this may lead to reactive vasoconstriction, thereby reducing existing collateral blood flow and increasing the ischemic injury.

Mesenteric Artery Thrombosis

Thrombosis of the SMA or celiac axis occurs as a result of underlying mesenteric atherosclerotic stenosis progressing to occlusion. This usually occurs at the origin of the vessel. Other causes include systemic vasculitic and prothrombotic syndromes. Less common causes include aortic and visceral artery aneurysms or dissection. Some patients may describe prodromal symptoms compatible with chronic mesenteric ischemia. These patients often have coexisting multilevel atherosclerotic disease. Unlike acute mesenteric embolism, the onset of pain is often gradual, with nonspecific central abdominal pain. The extent of infarction usually involves the duodenum to the transverse colon and is typically more extensive than that seen with acute embolism.

Nonocclusive Mesenteric Ischemia

Nonocclusive mesenteric ischemia (NOMI) develops in patients with low-cardiac-output states, especially in the presence of digoxin or vasoconstrictors. Secondary mesenteric vasoconstriction results in segmental vasospasm of the secondary and tertiary branches of the SMA. It is not caused by underlying atherosclerosis or venous obstruction. Causes of low-flow states include cardiac failure, shock, and hypovolemia. The use of vasoconstricting agents that affect the splanchnic circulation such as digoxin, cathecholamines, angiotensin II, vasopressin, beta-blockers, and cocaine has been associated with NOMI.

Diagnosis

Acute mesenteric ischemia presents classically with acute onset of abdominal pain out of proportion to the physical findings. Central abdominal pain occurs as a result of mid-gut ischemia and spasm. Gastrointestinal emptying, with emesis and bloody diarrhea may occur. Laboratory findings including leukocytosis, acidosis, hyperkalemia, raised hematocrit, LDH, SGOT, and CK occur later. However, no single laboratory investigation or combination of tests has proved to be sensitive or specific enough to enable the early diagnosis of AMI.

Early recognition of AMI is crucial, as bowel necrosis develops in many patients by the time of surgery and investigations should not produce unnecessary delays in revascularization.

Plain abdominal x-rays may show nonspecific findings of intestinal dilatation, gasless abdo-

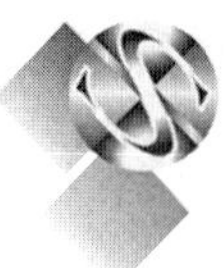

men, or other signs of ileus. Occasionally mural "thumb printing" is caused by submucosal edema or hemorrhage. Pneumoperitoneum or portal vein pneumatosis may be seen in advanced cases with transmural infarction. Ultrasonography in patients with AMI may reveal a thickening of the bowel wall, signs of ileus with distended bowel loops, intraperitoneal fluid, or air in the portal vein. Ultrasonography is also helpful in excluding other causes of an acute abdomen.

Ultrasound and plain x-rays are not very specific in diagnosing AMI and other imaging modalities such as CT, MRA, and contrast angiography play a major role in the diagnosis. Computed tomography angiography is sensitive for the diagnosis of mesenteric occlusion or bowel ischemia. Computed tomography scanning also facilitates the identification of nonvascular causes of acute abdominal pain. Computed tomography angiography with three-dimensional reconstruction may facilitate identification of vascular anatomy and pathology with good enough detail for diagnosis and operative planning (Fock et al., 1994).

Differentiation of the three forms of mesenteric arterial occlusion can be done with aortography and it facilitates planning of treatment. Selective mesenteric angiography remains the most reliable and definitive diagnositic tool for AMI. Endovascular interventions or catheter-directed vasodilator therapy can be started immediately after angiography (Park et al., 2002).

Thrombotic occlusion of the SMA produces a sudden cut-off at the vessel origin or within 1 to 2 cm of the SMA trunk. Extensive collaterals in the distal SMA indicate a chronic occlusion. Mesenteric arterial emboli produce a sharp, rounded filling defect with a typical meniscus sign on angiography. Vasospasm may be present with mesenteric thrombosis or embolism. Angiographic criteria for NOMI include a diffuse narrowing of the SMA and its branches, alternating areas of narrowing and dilatation of the SMA branches (string of sausages sign), spasm of the peripheral vascular arcades, impaired filling of the intramural vessels, and a sluggish flow with reflux of contrast during selective SMA injection. Increased vessel diameter following papaverine infusion and the absence of atherosclerotic disease on angiography supports the diagnosis of AMI.

Treatment

Regardless of the etiology of the AMI, the goals of surgical treatment are to reestablish good pulsatile flow to the SMA, to restore adequate blood flow to the ischemic but viable gut, and to resect the necrotic bowel. Adequate volume resuscitation and correction of acid base and electrolyte imbalance must also be undertaken. Cardiac output has to be optimized, and any arrhythmias treated. Broad-spectrum antibiotics are given if signs of peritonitis are present.

The single factor in improving the results of surgical treatment of acute mesenteric insufficiency has been the addition of transcatheter intraarterial vasodilator infusion perioperatively (Boley et al., 1981).

The decision to undertake second-look laparotomy is made at the time of the initial laparotomy. It allows the reassessment of bowel viability and to decide if further bowel resection is required. Bowel viability can be assessed by physical examination, handheld Doppler scan examination, and intravenous injection of fluorescein (Ballard et al., 1993).

Acute Mesenteric Artery Embolism

Surgical revascularization in the presence of an embolism is performed with balloon embolectomy usually with patch angioplasty of the SMA. Patients with chronic proximal occlusion or stenosis undergo revascularization with bypass grafting. Autogenous vein is the graft material of choice if resection of necrotic bowel is necessary. Resection of the infarcted bowel is performed following revascularization.

Acute Mesenteric Artery Thrombosis

The thrombotic process occurs in a severely atherosclerotic proximal SMA. Therefore, these patients require placement of a bypass graft to the SMA distal to the occlusive segment. Antegrade or retrograde bypass may be performed depending on anatomical considerations or according to surgeon preference.

Thrombolytic therapy is a potential consideration in patients with acute thrombosis and no clinical signs of peritonitis. Successful lysis returns the mesenteric circulation to its chronic, stable state. Subsequent operative revascularization or balloon angioplasty of the stenotic vessel can be undertaken electively. However, this does not allow inspection for bowel viability following reperfusion and may delay operative revascularization if thrombolysis is unsuccessful. Thrombolysis in AMI therefore should be reserved for selected patients (Park et al., 2002).

Nonocclusive Mesenteric Ischemia

The treatment of NOMI is primarily nonsurgical. A metabolic cause of the problem should be identified and corrected. The SMA is selectively catheterized, and vasodilating agents such as papaverine (or tolazoline hydrochloride) are administered. Resection of nonviable bowel may be required (Park et al., 2002).

Chronic Visceral Ischemia

Clinical Presentation

The most common pattern of symptoms is chronic abdominal pain that is associated with involuntary weight loss. The pain is usually epigastric, dull, or colic. The patient experiences the pain 15 to 30 minutes after eating, and it lasts for 1 to 3 hours before disappearing. The pain becomes so severe that soon the patient develops fear of food and limits the oral intake. This results in a pronounced weight loss. Absence of weight loss may put in doubt the diagnosis of chronic visceral ischemia. Other gastrointestinal complaints may include diarrhea, nausea or vomiting, and constipation. The most typical feature of the clinical presentation is that the symptoms are atypical. We and others have shown that the majority of the patients affected are women in their sixth decade of life. The reasons for this sex predilection remain undetermined. On examination, the patient looks emaciated, mimicking a patient with advanced malignant disease. These is often an epigasric bruit present.

Untreated patients with symptoms of chronic visceral ischemia are at an increased risk of death from complications of acute visceral ischemia. In a large series of patients presenting with acute mesenteric ischemia over a period of 10 years, 43% had prior chronic symptoms.

Investigations

Gastrointestinal contrast studies, endoscopy, and computed tomography are not essential to the diagnosis but are important in eliminating other sources of abdominal discomfort. Microulceration of the gastric mucosa and atypical colonic mucosa ulceration are uncommon endoscopic findings.

Duplex ultrasound examination of the celiac and the superior mesenteric artery origin can be successfully obtained in 80% to 95% of the cases, and in these it is a reliable screening test for chronic visceral ischemia. To obtain optimal visualization of the celiac and superior mesenteric arteries, patients should be on a clear liquid diet on the day before the examination and should refrain from oral intake for 6 hours before the study. Lateral views of biplane aortography remains the primary diagnostic modality in demonstrating visceral occlusive lesions compatible with the diagnosis. In a typical patient there is involvement of two or all three visceral arteries. Aortography also reveals the meandering mesenteric artery (arch of Riolan or arch of Treves), a large collateral tortuous vessel of uniform caliber residing in the left upper quadrant of the abdomen. It connects the middle colic artery with the patent trunk of the inferior mesenteric artery.

Treatment

Angioplasty

Mesenteric percutaneous transluminal angioplasty (PTA) is a valuable treatment option in patients with chronic visceral ischemia who are considered high operative risk. The initial technical success rate is good, with the majority of patients having symptomatic improvement and continuous relief of symptoms at short-term follow-up. However, long-term patency results are unknown. Allen et al. (1996) presented a series of 19 patients treated by PTA. The only technical failure resulted in mesenteric artery dissection, thrombosis, bowel infarction, and a fatal outcome. Complete symptomatic relief was attained in 15 patients. Recurrent symptoms developed in three patients (20%) at a mean interval of 28 months. Percutaneous transluminal angioplasty may also be used for the management of recurrent symptoms following the

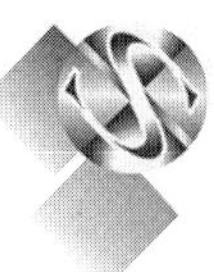

development of a stenosis in the aortomesenteric bypass.

Surgery

A variety of techniques have been developed to correct atherosclerotic obstruction of the major visceral branches of the thoracic aorta. Techniques of revascularization include transection of the mesenteric artery and reimplantation on the aorta, bypass grafting, and thromboendarterectomy. There is no consensus regarding the best surgical approach for the treatment of chronic visceral ischemia. Bypass grafting is the most common type of visceral revascularization performed today. It provides immediate restoration of flow and may originate from several different locations that include the suprarenal aorta (antegrade reconstruction) or the infrarenal aorta and the common iliac arteries (retrograde reconstruction). The distal thoracic aorta is usually free of atherosclerosis and is an excellent origin of a short bypass placed in the direction of normal flow. This design eliminates the possibility of kinking and thrombosis by compression or traction from the overlying mesentery, which may be observed with retrograde grafts. The distal thoracic aorta may be approached from the abdomen or via a thoracoabdominal incision. The retrograde bypass has the advantage that its origin is in a more familiar territory, but it is more commonly affected by atherosclerotic or aneurysmal disease. Park et al. (2002), in a large series of 98 reconstructions for chronic visceral ischemia, reported a 5-year symptom-free survival of 92%. The rate of recurrence was unaffected by the number of vessels revascularized or the orientation of the bypass. In contrast, others have reported that revascularization of as many visceral vessels as possible is important in reducing the risk of recurrent intestinal ischemic symptoms (Rheudasil et al., 1988). Thus the number of vessels that need to be revascularized remains a controversial issue.

Thromboendarterectomy has been used by a small number of groups with excellent results. The aorta is approached via medial visceral rotation. For the majority of ostial stenoses, a "trapdoor" arteriotomy is made around the celiac and superior mesenteric arteries as they emerge from the aortic wall. A retrograde endarterectomy facilitates direct removal of the aortic plaques. Duplex scanning should be routinely used at the end of the procedure to document the technical result at the distal end point of the endarterectomy in the mesenteric/celiac artery. A comparison of antegrade bypass (n =004 26) and transaortic endarterectomy (n = 48) showed the same incidence of perioperative mortality and 5-year recurrence-free survival for both groups (Cunningham et al., 1991).

Mesenteric Venous Thrombosis

Mesenteric venous thrombosis is a rare but potentially lethal form of intestinal ischemia that accounts for 5% to 15% of all cases of mesenteric vascular events. Improved survival depends on early recognition and appropriate treatment of this entity.

Etiology

Low-flow states in the mesenteric venous circulation that may be produced by liver cirrhosis, portal hypertension, and congestive heart failure could lead to mesenteric venous thrombosis. Intraabdominal infections from organs that drain to the mesenteric venous system such as appendicitis, diverticulitis, pelvic abscess, and pancreatitis can be associated with mesenteric venous thrombosis. Other conditions that may predispose to mesenteric venous thrombosis include hypercoagulable states associated with malignancy, oral contraceptives, and recent operations, particularly splenectomy followed by thrombocytosis. Thrombophilia is common in this group of patients. In a series of 31 patients, 13 (42%) were diagnosed to have a hypercoagulable state. Twelve patients were found to have protein C, protein S, or antithrombin III deficiency. A single patient had activated protein C resistance. Six patients had prior thrombotic episodes, including deep venous thrombosis (n = 5) or arterial thrombosis (n = 1). Four patients had a history of cancer, and five patients had previously undergone a splenectomy (mean platelet count 487,000) (Morasch et al., 2001).

Clinical Presentation

The most common presenting symptom is abdominal pain. The pain is constant, colicky, and poorly localized. Often the complaints of abdominal pain are out of proportion to the clinical findings. Other symptoms include vomiting, diarrhea, and constipation. In a series of patients with mesenteric venous thrombosis, upper and lower gastrointestinal bleeding occurred in 10% and 19% of the patients, respectively. Physical findings in patients who had gradual onset of abdominal symptoms may reveal low-grade pyrexia, abdominal distention, increased bowel sounds, and generalized abdominal tenderness. When the pain is localized, it may be located in either the upper or lower quadrants of the abdomen.

Peritoneal signs such as guarding and rebound are present when infarction of the bowel has occurred.

Investigations

Plain abdominal films are abnormal but not specific in the majority of the patients. Edematous and dilated small bowel loops are the most common finding.

Contrast-enhanced CT scanning is the most sensitive tool in detecting acute mesenteric venous thrombosis. The presence of a mesenteric venous filling defect is diagnostic of this condition. Other CT findings include free fluid; an enlarged, dilated superior mesenteric vein; mesenteric edema or stranding; bowel wall thickening or edema; and dilated small bowel loops. Selective mesenteric angiography may show intense spasm of the arterial branches supplying the involved part of the bowel, prolonged opacification of the thickened bowel wall, contrast extravasation into the lumen of the bowel, visualization of the venous thrombus, or nonvisualization of the venous phase. Currently, angiography is not recommended as the initial investigation.

Treatment

Patients with mesenteric venous thrombosis and no signs of peritonitis are treated with fluid resuscitation, prophylactic antibiotic therapy, and intravenous heparin. Close clinical and hemodynamic monitoring is indicated, preferably in an intensive care unit. If peritoneal signs are present, a laparotomy should be performed and the infarcted bowel should be resected. An ileostomy should be considered if there is extension of the macroscopic involvement at the resection margins. The macroscopic features of the affected part of the bowel are striking, and consist of a dark red coloration and thickening of the bowel. It is often difficult to distinguish viable from nonviable bowel. In a recent series 82% of patients who underwent bowel resection (about 100 cm length) did not have transmural necrosis. Bowel viability assessment by direct inspection may be improved by Doppler ultrasound techniques or fluorescein examination under a Wood's lamp. Several case reports have been published indicating that thrombolysis may be a useful treatment option for patients with no signs of peritonitis. Antegrade transarterial thrombolysis via the superior mesenteric artery has been effective in a small number of cases in lysing the thrombus and providing good symptomatic relief (Antoch, 2001). Postoperatively, patients should be anticoagulated to prevent recurrent episodes of thrombosis. The duration of anticoagulation is determined by the expected duration of the predisposing factors.

References

Allen RC, Martin GH, Rees CR, et al. (1996) J Vasc Surg 24:415–21; discussion 421–3.

Antoch G, Taleb N, Hansen D, Stock W. (2001) Vasc Endovasc Surg 20:471–2.

Ballard JL, Stone WM, Hallett JW, Pairolero PC, Cherry KJ. (1993) Am Surg 59:309–11.

Boley SJ, Feinstein FR, Sammartano R, Brandt LJ, Sprayregen S. (1981) Surg Gynecol 153:561–9.

Bradbury AW, Brittenden J, McBride K, Ruckley CV. (1995) Br J Surg 82:1446–59.

Cunningham CG, Reilly LM, Rapp JH, Schneider PA, Stoney RJ. (1991) Ann Surg 214:276–87; discussion 287–8.

Fock CM, Kullnig P, Ranner G, Beaufort-Spontin F, Schmidt F. (1994) Eur J Radiol 18:12–14.

Morasch MD, Ebaugh JL, Chiou AC, Matsumura JS, Pearce WH, Yao JS. (2001) J Vasc Surg 34:680–4.

Park WM, Gloviczki P, Cherry KJ Jr, et al. (2002) J Vasc Surg 35:445–52.

Rheudasil JM, Stewart MT, Schellack JV, Smith RB 3rd, Salam AA, Perdue GD. (1988) J Vasc Surg 8:495–500.

20

Endovascular Approaches and Techniques

Steven M. Thomas, Kong T. Tan, and Mark F. Fillinger

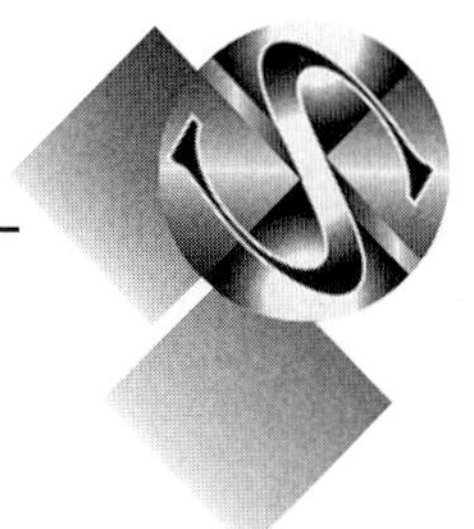

This last chapter describes the equipment commonly used during endovascular procedures; some of the commonly used endovascular techniques, beginning with arterial access technique; and the endovascular interventions for arterial occlusive disease and aneurysmal disease. Embolotherapy is also discussed.

Equipment for Access, Angiography, and Vascular Intervention

Needles

In general terms, there are two types of needles available for obtaining vascular access: one-part and two-part. The one-part needle has a sharp cutting bevel, whereas the two-part needle has a sharp inner stylet with a blunt outer needle. The two-part needle is preferred by many for vascular access at the femoral artery, because it reduces the risk of vascular damage at the access point, either due to movement of the needle tip or passage of the guidewire into the subintimal plane (see Access Technique, below). The most commonly used needle calibers are 18 and 19 Stubs needle gauge (18 being the larger and equivalent to about 1.25 mm in outer diameter). For most purposes the 19-gauge needle suffices, though it does not accommodate an 0.038-inch-diameter guidewire if required. A newer variant of the one-part needle designed to reduce arterial injury is the 20- or 22-gauge needle typically used as part of a "micropuncture" set. The micropuncture technique uses a 0.014- or 0.018-inch guidewire and standard Seldinger technique to introduce a short 4-French sheath, which is then used to place the typical 0.035-inch guidewire.

Wires

Guidewires are integral to successful catheterization; they support the catheter and allow the catheter to be steered to its intended location. Guidewires come in many diameters and lengths, and degrees of stiffness, slipperiness, and steerability. All wires have a softer, more flexible, curved, or "floppy" leading end to minimize damage to the vessel as it is advanced, though the length of the flexible segment may vary. This is because a long flexible segment may be useful if a vessel is extremely tortuous, or a very short flexible segment may be needed to allow maximum support for an advancing catheter or sheath.

Diameter

Most standard guidewires are 0.035 inch in diameter, though some very stiff wires are 0.038 inch in diameter. It is important to ensure that the wire used is compatible with the lumen diameter of the catheter to be placed over it. If small-caliber catheters are used, small-diameter wires such as 0.014 or 0.018 inch are required.

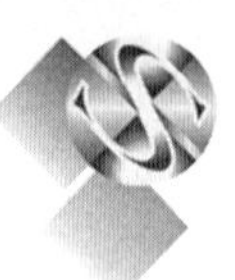

However, many of these wires do not have the same stiffness as larger diameter wires, and hence may kink or result in poor tracking of the catheter. If a kink is produced, it is usually very difficult to pass a catheter over the wire, and a new wire is required. The hydrophilic Terumo (Terumo, Leuven, Belgium) guidewire has a nitinol core and is difficult to kink.

Length

The usual length of guidewire required is about 150 cm, and this is adequate for most diagnostic imaging. However, in some circumstances longer wires are required, usually ranging from 200 to 300 cm. This is particularly the case in a peripheral location, where the catheter has to be changed, or a guiding catheter, angioplasty balloon, or stent has to be introduced. When using monorail balloon catheters or stents for intervention, this is usually less of a problem compared to systems that are fully over the wire. This is because in a monorail system the wire passes through the wire guide for only about 30 cm from the tip of the catheter or device, rather than through the whole length of the catheter or device as occurs in a fully over-the-wire system. Aortic stent-graft interventions also tend to require long (260 cm) guidewires due to the length of the delivery system for most aortic stent grafts. However, systems tend to be manufacturer-specific, as some newer aortic stent-graft systems require only 180-cm guidewires.

Stiffness

The degree of guidewire stiffness varies considerably (Table 20.1). It is generally easier to track a catheter or device over a stiffer guidewire; however, a very stiff guidewire may be more difficult to manipulate into a vessel origin or through a diseased vessel. Exchanging wires is often necessary for different parts of a procedure, but a stiff wire should always be placed through a catheter that has been positioned using a more conventional wire to prevent damage to the vessel during advancement of the stiff wire.

Slipperiness

Some wires (e.g., Terumo Glidewire or Cook Nimble guidewire), have a hydrophilic coating that, once lubricated, becomes very slippery and

Table 20.1. Variation in guidewire stiffness

Floppy
Bentson
Movable core
Standard J or straight
Hydrophilic
More supportive
Heavy duty J or straight
Stiff hydrophilic
Wholey
Stiff
Amplatz super stiff
Amplatz extra stiff
TAD
Flexfinder
Very stiff
Meier
Lunderquist

nearly frictionless. They are very useful for negotiating tortuous vessels and crossing stenoses and occlusions. They can be difficult to handle because when slippery, the wire may slip back through the operators hands during catheter exchanges, and if allowed to become dry, can stick to the operator's gloves and are then easily pulled out inadvertently. These problems can be minimized by keeping hydrophilic wires moist, handling the wires with a damp gauze to allow slightly more friction than a glove, using a "torque device" when manipulating the wire, and using caution when moving the wire in or out of the patient.

Steerability

A completely straight wire and a J wire have little or no inherent steerability. A straight wire, to which a curve has been introduced, can be directed using the curve, and this is enhanced if a directional catheter is also used. Many wires have tips that can be deformed into a curve or even into a J if required. Some hydrophilic wires have a preformed curve or angle, and if the core is made of nitinol (an elastic nickel-titanium alloy with "memory"), this cannot be changed. This gives more torque control and makes the wire very steerable.

Catheters

There are a plethora of catheters available, to be placed over the guidewire to facilitate arteriog-

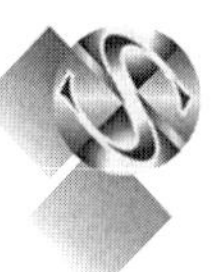

raphy, selective entry to branch vessels, device delivery, and so on. The size of catheter is denoted using the French (F) system, which describes the outer circumference (external diameter of 3F = 1 mm external diameter). Smaller caliber catheters have the advantage that the access puncture site can be kept small, although the turning ability or torque control is often compromised. For nonselective angiograms this is not usually a problem, and 3F or 4F catheters can be used, but if a selective catheterization is required, then larger caliber catheters may be required.

It must be remembered that catheters are thrombogenic to some extent, and should always be regularly flushed with heparinized saline while in the patient. In the case of guide catheters, this is often best achieved using a bag of heparinized saline (using a pressure bag) connected via a side arm.

Most catheters are reasonably radiopaque, though hydrophilic-coated "glide catheters" and smaller caliber catheters can be relatively radiolucent. Some catheters have radiopaque material added to them toward the tip, or a radiopaque band at the tip to enhance visibility.

Catheter Types

Most catheters can be divided into two main groups: nonselective and selective.

Nonselective Catheters

These are used to inject large volumes of contrast at high rates into large vessels. They have multiple side-holes to allow high injection rates and reduce the risk of subintimal injection by the end-hole jet of contrast. The most commonly used nonselective catheter is the pigtail catheter, the workhorse of diagnostic angiography. If the vessel is too small to accommodate the pigtail loop, a straight multi–side-hole catheter can usually be used instead.

Selective Catheters

These are shaped catheters that have directional properties that aid selective catheterization of side branch vessels. Some, such as the Multipurpose, Cobra, Berenstein, and Sidewinder catheters, can be used for a variety of selective examinations, whereas others such as the inter-

nal mammary or renal double-curve catheters are designed to aid catheterization of particular vessels. In practice, most angiographers prefer to have a range of catheters available and sometimes many may be used to achieve a difficult selective arterial position. Probably the six most commonly used selective catheters are Berenstein (or similar Kumpe), Cobra, Sidewinder, Headhunter, Sos Omni, and Multipurpose. Catheters such as the Sidewinder and Cobra come in a range of sizes designated 1 to 3 dependent on the degree of catheter curve or loop. These are useful for varying the degree of angulation at the catheter tip, and the ease of manipulation as the diameter and tortuosity varies substantially in large vessels. When using a Sidewinder catheter in the aorta, if the loop is too large, the catheter tip will be held away from the aortic wall and will not engage branch vessels. This may be modified by introducing a guidewire into the apex of the catheter curve, but this often means that a smaller Sidewinder or a Sos Omni catheter should be used instead.

Most of these catheters can be used as soon as the wire is removed from them, and will engage side branches if advanced or retracted. The Sidewinder and smaller Sos-Omni catheters need to be re-formed so that the reverse curve of the catheter can be used to engage side branch vessels. The Sos Omni, being of a smaller curve than the Sidewinder catheters, can usually be re-formed in the aorta. The Sidewinder catheter usually has to be re-formed using a variety of techniques. The simplest and safest is to place a guidewire over the iliac bifurcation using a pigtail catheter and re-form the sidewinder in the lower aorta. If this is not possible, it can usually be easily reformed in the aortic arch by twisting and advancing the unformed catheter. Once formed, the catheter is pulled back to engage the origins of arterial side branches.

When choosing a catheter, it is important first to select the appropriate gantry angle to view the origin of the vessel and its "true" degree of angulation relative to the parent vessel. The angle of origin of the vessel being catheterized often dictates which catheter is most likely to successfully engage the arterial origin, so, for example, vessels that are angled back toward the site of access are often best approached with a Sidewinder or similar catheter. There are also catheters that have hydrophilic coatings, and these are often very useful for tracking a catheter to peripheral locations, particularly for embolization.

Microcatheters

These are coaxial catheters that are only 2F to 3F in diameter that will pass through the 0.035- or 0.038-inch lumen of the selective catheters mentioned above. They were originally developed for cerebral catheterization and intervention, but can be useful for superselective catheterization of visceral or peripheral vascular beds, particularly for embolization procedures.

Sheaths

Sheaths are used to establish a secure pathway from the skin to the arterial lumen. This allows catheters and devices, such as balloons and stents, to be exchanged in an atraumatic manner. The sheath is a plastic tube with a hemostatic valve and an attached side arm to allow flushing. The size designation of the sheath refers to the size of catheter that will pass through it (i.e., the internal diameter). Hence, a 7F sheath allows the passage of a 7F catheter or device. As a result the external diameter of any sheath is approximately 1F larger than its designated size for smaller sheath sizes, and 2F to 3F larger when the sheath size is in the 12F to 25F range. The thickness of the sheath is also somewhat dependent on its length and intended application, generally thicker for longer sheaths intended to pass stents or stent grafts through tortuous arteries. If the puncture is at a steep angle or in obese patients, the smaller sheaths may kink, particularly with an antegrade puncture. There are reinforced sheaths that are resistant to kinking, but they have an external diameter 1F to 2F greater than standard sheaths.

Most sheaths are short, but longer sheaths and guiding catheters can be useful during interventional procedures to provide stability to aid selective catheterization and delivery of balloons or stents. Guiding catheters are larger than standard catheters, often 6F to 7F, because they are designed to work with a standard catheter within. Because they are catheters, it is important to remember that their size is designated by the external diameter, unlike a sheath, despite similarities in appearance. Guiding catheters come in a variety of lengths and shapes to aid introduction into the vessel ostium, allowing conventional catheters to be introduced through them for more distal catheterization. Guiding catheters can perform a similar role to sheaths, but they do not usually have an integral hemostatic valve, and their internal lumen is smaller. Thus, in some cases a guiding catheter may be placed within a short sheath with a hemostatic valve, or used in combination with a Y adapter and a Tuohy-Borst valve for hemostasis.

Commonly Used Medications

When performing vascular interventions, a number of medications are frequently required. Examples in a number of broad groups are provided, but this is not a comprehensive description. Practioners should be familiar with local guidelines for medication use, and if in doubt should consult standard sources to check dosages and interactions.

Local Anesthetics

Local anesthetic is used for nearly all diagnostic and interventional procedures. The most commonly used agent is lignocaine hydrochloride (lidocaine in the United States). It has a low incidence of side effects when used as a local anesthetic, but a total dose of 200 mg (20 mL of 1% solution) should not be exceeded, as overdosage may lead to central nervous and cardiovascular system toxicity. Alternative agents are prilocaine hydrochloride or bupivacaine hydrochloride, which are longer acting and may be useful in certain circumstances. Depending on the agent, some adjustments may be advised for renal impairment, primarily related to metabolites that are renally excreted, or hepatic impairment. For any of these agents, direct intraarterial or intravenous injection should be avoided, due to risk of seizure and other potential immediate systemic effects.

Heparin

Heparin is added to saline flushes and used routinely in higher doses during interventional procedures. In both cases it helps prevent pericatheter or vessel thrombosis during the pro-

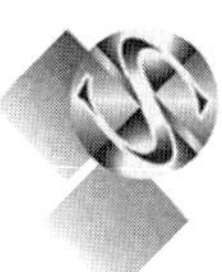

cedure. For flushes, it is used in a dose of about 5000 IU per liter of normal saline. For interventional procedures, doses of between 3000 and 5000 IU are given depending on the size of the patient and the proposed length of the procedure. For aortic stent-graft procedures, the sheaths may be totally occlusive, and systemic heparinization is commonly used. Systemic heparinization is also common in carotid stent procedures, due to the risk of emboli and to prevent thrombosis related to distal protection devices. As the half-life of heparin is 45 to 60 minutes, further doses should be considered if a procedure is prolonged. During longer cases or for systemic heparinization, dosing may be based on the activated clotting time (ACT), with target levels in the 250 to 300 s range depending on the procedure, the degree of vascular occlusion by devices, and the thromboembolic risk.

Vasodilators

Vasodilators are used for prophylaxis or treatment of vascular spasm, and during intraarterial pressure measurements, to augment distal flow and give a better assessment of the significance of a pressure drop across a lesion. Commonly used intraarterial agents are glyceryl trinitrate (GTN, 100 μg) (nitroglycerin in the U.S., 50 to 100 μg) and papaverine (30 mg). Of course, vasodilators may produce significant hypotension, so attention should be paid to patient hydration status and coexisting cardiac disease. Vasodilators should not be used in patients with significant aortic stenosis, as they may produce severe hypotension in this circumstance. Nifedipine (10 mg) can be given orally prior to a procedure if significant spasm is likely, such as embolization of the testicular vein.

Atropine/Glycopyrronium Bromide

These agents are given routinely during carotid stenting to reduce the risk of bradycardia and hypotension during balloon inflation in the carotid bulb. Glycopyrronium bromide (600 μg) is preferred in patients with a history of cardiac disease because it has a better side effect profile (U.S. equivalent is glycopyrrolate, adult dosage 100 μg IV repeated every 2 to 3 minutes as necessary with a reasonable upper limit of 600 μg).

Sedation/Analgesia

Sedation is rarely required for vascular procedures, short of aortic stent grafts. Patients with limb ischemia should have their pain adequately controlled prior to investigation, as patients in severe pain can rarely lie still for prolonged periods. If sedation is required, small doses of short-acting benzodiazepines such as midazolam (2 to 10 mg IV) are preferred, with the aim being to relax, not anesthetize, an agitated patient. If anesthesia is produced, an anesthetist must be in control of it, but if oversedation does occur, the effects of the benzodiazepine can be reversed (temporarily) with flumazenil (200 μg over 15 s and then 100 μg every 60 s up to a total dose of 1 mg). If analgesia does become necessary, opiates such as morphine or pethidine (25 to 100 mg) can be given IV, or an appropriate oral opiate can be given, though the onset of action may be considerably delayed. In all cases with analgesia and sedation, IV administration is preferred, as IM absorption is unpredictable and cumulative effects can result in sudden overdosage.

Antibiotics

When and which antibiotics are used varies according to local policy. Common indications are when prosthetic graft material is likely to be punctured during a procedure, when prosthetic material is to be placed (especially aortic stent-grafts), or for some embolization procedures.

Antiplatelet Agents

All patients with peripheral vascular disease should be advised to take antiplatelet agents, predominantly for their cardioprotective effect. Dosages of aspirin likely need be no higher than 75 mg daily, although the precise optimal dosage has not been definitively determined. If the patient is intolerant of aspirin then dipyridamole (25 to 50 mg) or clopidogrel (75 mg) are alternative agents. In our practice, patients are given clopidogrel 75 mg at least 3 days prior to and for 30 days following carotid stent insertion. If the patient has not taken a dose prior to the day of the procedure, a loading dose of 300 mg is given on the day of procedure. In the U.S., most centers use both aspirin and clopidogrel for carotid stents.

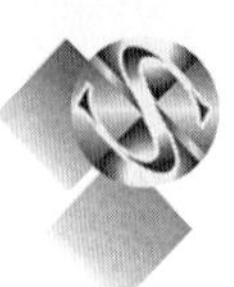

Drugs for Treating Contrast Reactions

It is imperative to be aware of the risk of a severe contrast reaction and its treatment. The drugs to do this should be readily available on the resuscitation trolley in the angiography suite. All centers should have a protocol for treatment of severe contrast reactions. This should be prominently displayed and usually involves the use of some or all of the following: chlorpheniramine (10 to 20 mg IV); adrenaline or epinephrine (0.5 mL of 1:1000 solution subcutaneous or 0.1 mL of 1:10,000 solution IV), usually given if there is severe anaphylactic shock; hydrocortisone (200 mg IV), though its effects are not immediate; cimetidine (300 mg IV), may be useful as a second-line drug following adrenaline; atropine (500 μg to 1 mg IV) can be used for severe bradyarrhythmia.

Devices for Vascular Intervention

Various devices may be required to perform vascular interventional procedures, such as balloon catheters and stents for treating arterial occlusive disease, or coils for embolization. The specifics of these devices are described during discussion on their use elsewhere in this chapter.

Closure Devices

Arterial puncture site closure devices aim to eliminate or reduce the need for manual compression of the puncture site, reduce the time to patient mobilization, and reduce the risk of significant bleeding, especially when using larger sheath sizes. For most centers it is the increased throughput of patients and the ability to perform intervention as a day case that justifies their use.

There are a number of devices available, divided into two main groups: "stitchers" and "pluggers." The Closer (Perclose, CA) device is the original "stitcher." It percutaneously places a suture through the artery at the puncture site, and the patient can be fully mobilized immediately. It can be used for closure of up to a 10F sheath size. Another suture-based device, Prostar XL (Perclose), has been used successfully for closure of 24F femoral artery access. One of the authors has personally used these devices with good success for totally percutaneous endovascular aortic aneurysm repair, both abdominal and thoracic. The primary issues are vessel size and calcification, which can affect the ability of the device to capture the sutures properly. Obesity and prior surgery or dense scar can also affect these devices. The vessel can be immediately reaccessed if necessary and other than the suture, there is no other residual material to cause problems if surgery is required at the access site. There are a number of plugging devices, such as the Angioseal (St. Jude Medical, St. Paul, MN), the Duett (Vascular Solutions Inc., Minneapolis, MN), and the Vasoseal (Datascope Corp., Montvale, NJ). The authors are also quite familiar with the angioseal. This is quick and simple to use and comes as a 6F or 8F device. An absorbable shoe remains inside the artery and a collagen plug is deployed over the puncture site outside the artery. The device now uses a knot mechanism to hold the collagen plug in position, and the patient can mobilize in 2 to 4 hours. The primary issues with this device are vessel size and the size of the arterial access device used for the procedure.

Access Technique

Before any diagnostic or interventional procedure can begin, vascular access has to be established. The basic technique remains the same as that described by Seldinger:

- Vessel puncture
- Guidewire introduction
- Placement of the catheter over the guidewire

Vessel Puncture

For the purposes of this chapter, only arterial access is discussed; venous access is discussed in Chapter 13. In general, which vessel to puncture is dictated by the site of disease to be inves-

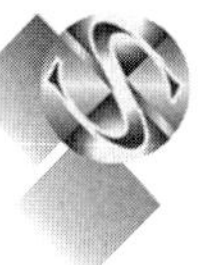

Table 20.2. Arterial access sites

Access site	Main indications
Ipsilateral common femoral artery (CFA)	All accessible stenotic/occlusive lesion
Contralateral CFA	Occluded ipsilateral CFA Lesion to be treated close to ipsilateral groin Scarred groin
Low superficial femoral artery (SFA)	Percutaneous transluminal angioplasty (PTA) of ipsilateral CFA (rare), SFA origin or proximal graft anastomosis but contralateral femoral puncture not possible
Profunda femoris (PF) artery	PTA of PF origin PTA of CFA (rare) if SFA occluded and contralateral approach not possible
Direct graft puncture	Arteriography in patients with graft crossing both groins Intervention at graft anastomoses Occluded graft, to allow accelerated thrombolysis
Popliteal artery	PTA of occlusions involving the origin of the superficial femoral artery Failure of guidewire passage antegrade, often due to steep, large collaterals at the proximal site of an occlusion
Brachial artery	Bilateral aortoiliac occlusions PTA of a supraaortic branch occlusion or stenosis Severe aortoiliac disease and vascular tortuosity
Axillary artery (brachial approach preferred)	As above
Radial artery	Arteriography as above; limited intervention possible

tigated or treated, and the strength of the arterial pulses at various sites. The commonly used arterial puncture sites are shown in Table 20.2.

For most purposes, the common femoral artery is used, as it is a relatively easy artery to puncture, the artery is readily compressed over the femoral head, and most vascular beds are easily within reach. The vessel is punctured at the point of maximal pulsation, not by means of external anatomical landmarks. At this point the vessel is over the femoral head. The site is first cleaned and draped, and local anesthetic inserted. A two-part needle is preferred for most access as this avoids the risk of damaging the vessel if the tip of the needle has to be repositioned. There is also a reduced risk of the wire passing into a subintimal position. This can occur because the long bevel of a one-part needle may imply the needle tip is in the center of the lumen of the vessel, when it is only partially through the wall of the artery. The needle is guided at about 45 degrees to the skin surface toward the pulse, and the vessel is speared. The central stylet is then removed and the needle gently withdrawn until the tip is felt to flick into the lumen of the artery, and this should be accompanied by the free pulsatile backflow of arterial blood.

Bony landmarks for the femoral artery on fluoroscopy can also be used, namely the medial aspect of the femoral head, but direct palpation is preferable. If there are difficulties gaining access or if the pulse is weak or absent, then generally the best approach is to use ultrasound to directly visualize the arterial target. This is particularly useful for antegrade femoral artery punctures, as it often avoids the need to use fluoroscopy to guide a wire into the superficial femoral artery (SFA) for distal intervention, and hence reduces the risk of irradiating the hands of the operator. In cases of difficult access, a micropuncture set is commonly used to reduce the risk of arterial injury, and in most of these sets the guidewire is specifically designed with an echogenic tip to aid visualization of the small 0.018-inch wire. Once arterial access is obtained with a short 4F introducer, an exchange is made for a larger guidewire and 5F sheath.

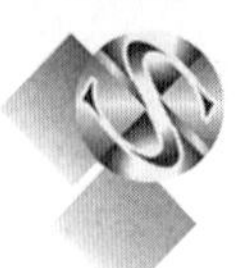

Guidewire Introduction

Once the needle is in position, a guidewire is introduced through it. For most purposes a standard 3-mm J wire is used to secure access and to allow initial introduction of catheters and sheaths. The wire should pass smoothly and easily into the artery. If any resistance is felt, fluoroscopy should be used to ensure the wire is following an appropriate course and is running freely. If the wire does not pass beyond a certain point, then a limited angiogram may be required to identify the problem, but this requires that at least some wire is within the arterial lumen to allow the introduction of a sheath or dilator. If the wire does not pass out of the needle, then there is probably an arterial plaque at the puncture site. The needle tip can often be repositioned without losing an intraarterial position, but sometimes re-puncture is necessary, perhaps using ultrasound to guide the optimal site for puncture.

Catheter Placement

Once the wire has been advanced into a suitable position, a catheter or sheath can be introduced over it. The wire is held under slight tension as the catheter is introduced, as this helps to avoid the wire kinking in the soft tissues and makes tracking the catheter easier. Once the catheter has been advanced into position, the guidewire can be removed, the catheter flushed, and the intraluminal position verified with a test injection of contrast.

If the site of insertion has dense scar from a prior procedure, then insertion of even a small sheath or dilator may be difficult. If this is the case, then it is often prudent to use a stiffer guidewire initially or to change to one through a 4F dilator and then place a sheath for use during the rest of the procedure. Current micropuncture sets also have stiff versions for these cases. Although not needed frequently, these stiffer versions can be quite helpful.

Endovascular Techniques for Arterial Occlusive Disease

The mainstay of vascular intervention for arterial occlusive disease remains balloon angioplasty, though arterial stenting also has an important role to play. Some techniques, such as laser treatments, have come and gone. Atherectomy has a limited role for occlusive disease, predominantly for graft or stent re stenosis, and stent grafts are being evaluated for occlusive disease to see if the expense can be justified over simple angioplasty or stenting.

Angioplasty

The technique of balloon angioplasty is used extensively to treat arterial stenoses and occlusions, and the principles and equipment are largely the same regardless of where they are applied. The basic principle is to place a guidewire through an arterial narrowing and over this to position an appropriately sized angioplasty balloon. The balloon is then inflated to high pressure, disrupting the stenotic arterial plaque. The luminal area, therefore, is increased and blood flow improved.

As with all vascular intervention, planning is important and consideration should be given to the following:

Access site: Access should usually be as near to the site to be treated as possible. This optimizes tactile control of wires and catheters, minimizes a tortuous approach to a lesion, and may help avoid an awkward approach to a vessel origin. For distal lower limb intervention, this usually means an antegrade femoral artery puncture.

Crossing the lesion: The guidewire has to lie in an intraluminal position above and below the site to be treated (even in cases of subintimal angioplasty). For simple stenoses, the lesion is crossed intraluminally, often using a directional catheter, such as a Cobra and a curved wire, with or without a hydrophilic coating. Particularly when treating occlusions, the wire may pass (intentionally or otherwise) into the subintimal space within the diseased section. The wire usually buckles on itself when this happens, and if a hydrophilic wire is then used, a loop is formed with it. The wire must then reenter in an intraluminal position in the more normal distal vessel before balloon dilatation is performed. This often occurs by advancing the wire loop in the subintimal space, with reentry occurring where a collateral arises

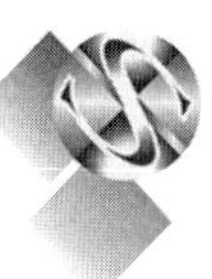

or at a vessel bifurcation—the basis of subintimal angioplasty. A Berenstein or other directional catheter can also be used to direct the wire back into the true lumen, and as with other steps in subintimal angioplasty, this should be performed with caution to avoid vessel perforation. New intravascular ultrasound catheters with wire guides and over-the-wire "spreading" devices have recently been produced to help cross-total occlusions, but are typically needed only in difficult cases.

Dilatation of the lesion: Angioplasty balloons fall into two main groups—compliant and noncompliant. Noncompliant balloons inflate to only one size, regardless of pressure, up to their burst rating. Compliant balloons vary in size, dependent on the pressure/volume of fluid within them. Most interventionists prefer noncompliant balloons because they often can be inflated to higher pressure and the risk of oversizing of the balloon for the vessel is smaller. The size of balloon chosen is dependent on the size of the adjacent normal vessel, though most operators use an approximate guide based on experience and scale the size up or down for individual patients (e.g., petite elderly women have small, fragile vessels). Inflation of the balloon can be performed by hand or using an inflation device. The latter has the advantage of a pressure gauge, allowing more control of the pressure and less likelihood of exceeding the maximum balloon inflation pressure. Inflation is performed with a contrast/saline mix and the balloon should fully inflate with no "waist." Some operators inflate for a short period, others for 2 to 3 minutes, and some initially at high pressure, reducing to a prolonged low-pressure inflation. The basis for this is to reduce the risk of distal embolization and significant dissection. However, the evidence that these strategies achieve these aims is lacking.

Following angioplasty a completion angiogram should be performed to assess the appearance of the treated segment and the "runoff."

Of primary importance is exclusion of vessel rupture with contrast extravasation, particularly in the iliac arteries. If there is arterial rupture, reinsertion of the balloon and inflation under low pressure proximal to the site of rupture should stop or minimize further bleeding. This may suffice for a small hole. It is prudent to inform a vascular surgeon of the problem. An angiogram should be performed after a trial of low-pressure balloon inflation. If extravasation continues, then the balloon should be immediately reinflated, and, if available, an appropriately sized stent graft inserted. If this is not possible, then surgical repair of the arterial tear is required.

If there is no injury and the treated segment remains significantly stenosed, then it may be that the balloon was undersized, in which case increasing the balloon size is often all that is required. In the iliac arteries, a pullback pressure can be performed through the lesion to assess if there is a significant pressure gradient at the site treated. This is usually taken to be a peak systolic pressure drop of 10 mm Hg across the lesion following administration of a distal vasodilator, such as GTN or papaverine. At other sites, for example, in the SFA, pressures are often not useful, as the catheter has to cross the treated segment for a pressure reading to be obtained distally, and this may in itself produce a pressure drop if the lumen is small. A normal distal pressure, however, is reassuring that the stenosis has been treated adequately. If there is still a significant pressure drop in the iliac arteries after apparently adequate balloon inflation, then secondary stenting is warranted. If elastic recoil seems to be occurring on balloon deflation, again, stenting should be considered, depending on the site of the lesion.

Often following angioplasty, a local dissection is visualized; however, most of these will remodel and do not require further treatment. If there is evidence of flow limitation, then there is a risk the segment will acutely occlude, and further investigation/treatment is warranted. Again a pressure measurement can be performed. For further treatment a long low-pressure inflation may tack back the dissection, but if this is unsuccessful, stenting may be required.

Imaging the runoff vessels ensures that there has been no distal embolization. If this has occurred and the embolus is in an important vessel or producing poor flow/limb ischemia, then thrombo-aspiration should be performed

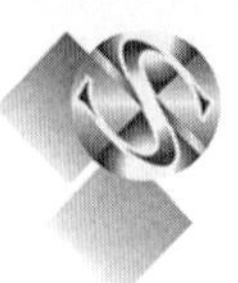

using an appropriate-size catheter for the occluded vessel and a sheath with a removable hemostatic valve.

Stenting

Intravascular stenting places a metallic scaffold inside the vessel to hold open the lumen. Stents were developed as an adjunct to balloon angioplasty in recognition that angioplasty alone was occasionally unsuccessful. In this circumstance, the role of stenting is secondary to the primary treatment of angioplasty and is used to salvage a failed angioplasty. However, there are occasions when stenting is the initial treatment, so-called primary stenting. Examples include the treatment of ostial lesions, such as ostial renal artery stenosis (Fig. 20.1); most iliac occlusions; and carotid stenosis. The basis for stenting is to reduce problems caused by elastic recoil or distal embolization. Stents are generally avoided below the inguinal ligament, as there is no evidence they are superior to balloon angioplasty alone in this location. In these lower flow vessels, stents may result in early thrombosis and thus are reserved for bailout situations after angioplasty.

There are a huge number of types of stents available for intravascular use, and choice of stent is usually at the discretion of the practitioner. The common types of stent are described here, with some examples given of those with which the authors are most familiar.

Types of Stent

Stents fall into two main groups: balloon-mounted or self-expanding. Balloon-mounted stents are usually made of stainless steel and are positioned on an angioplasty balloon for expansion and deployment. There is usually little shortening with expansion, and balloon-mounted stents are particularly useful where positioning of the stent is critical, enhanced by their radiopacity. Larger balloon-mounted stents, for example, unmounted Palmaz stents, shorten considerably when expanded on a large-diameter balloon, making their placement more difficult. As these stents are quite inflexible, they may be difficult to position through tortuous vessels. Their rigidity, however, gives them good radial strength, but if deformed once placed, for example, in superficial locations, or near joints, they will remain deformed and may themselves cause vascular obstruction. Most of these stents now come premounted on an angioplasty balloon ready for deployment, for example, Bridge stent (Medtonic AVE, Santa Rosa, CA), Genesis, or premounted Palmaz (Cordis, Miami Lakes, FL). Others have to be manually crimped to an appropriate balloon prior to use, for example, SAXX (C.R.

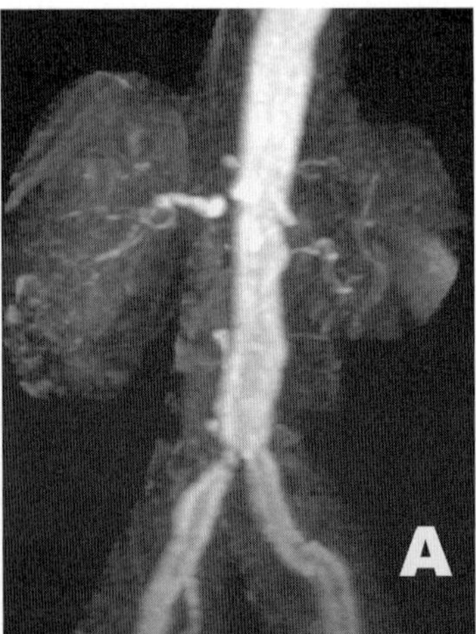

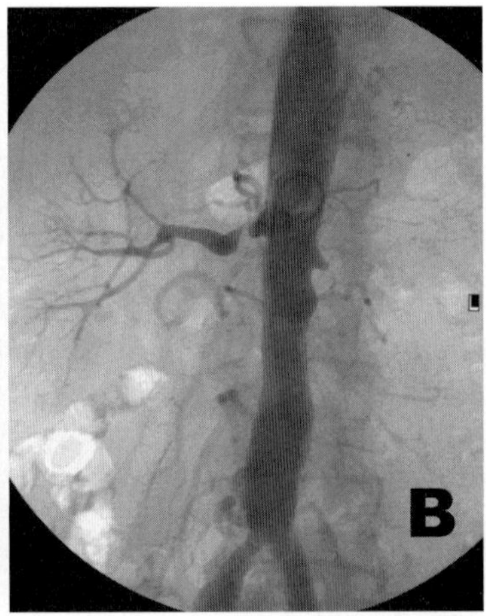

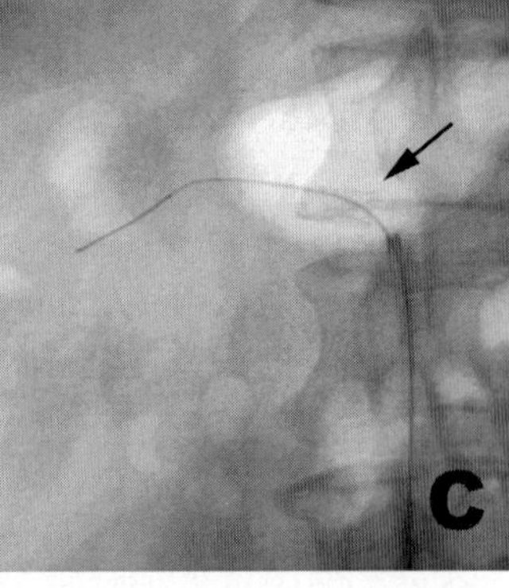

Figure 20.1. Renal artery stenting. Gadolinium-enhanced magnetic resonance imaging (A) showing a tight stenosis in the solitary kidney, confirmed by catheter angiography (B) and successfully stented with a balloon-mounted stent (C). Note the left renal artery is occluded (arrow).

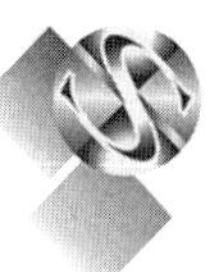

Bard, Murry Hill, NJ, USA) and the unmounted Palmaz (Cordis). The premounted stents are less prone to dislodgment from the balloon. This can occur as the stent is passed through the sheath and into its position for use, or during balloon inflation if a "dumbbell" is not formed around the stent as the balloon is initially inflated, in which case the stent may be squeezed off the deploying balloon. The latter problem is caused by movement of the stent from the center of the balloon or poor initial positioning so that one end of the balloon inflates first. Care is therefore required when using these stents, and if the stent has moved on the angioplasty balloon prior to deployment, it should not be used.

Self-expanding stents all have an inherent ability to expand to a predetermined length and/or diameter. They are compressed onto the delivery catheter and are typically constrained by a covering sheath. As this sheath is withdrawn, the stent expands and is deployed. Being self-expanding, the stent continues to exert an expansile force on the vessel wall once deployed, and will show some flexibility and recovery to their expanded shape if compressed or kinked. Stents such as the Wallstent (Boston Scientific, Boston, MA) are made of surgical grade stainless steel and rely on their design to be self-expanding. Newer stents tend to be made from nitinol, for example, the Memotherm Luminex (C.R. Bard), or the SMART stent (Cordis). Nitinol is a highly elastic nickel-titanium alloy that displays the property of thermal memory, returning to its preformed shape when released in the body. The "memory" properties of nitinol can be made to be more or less sensitive to temperature, which can be an advantage in certain situations.

The Wallstent shortens considerably as it expands, with its final length governed by the diameter achieved in the vessel. This can make accurate placement difficult. It is very flexible, but has a relatively low expansile force once in place. Nitinol stents show considerably less shortening during expansion, and though nitinol is poorly radiopaque, many stents now have gold or platinum markers on their proximal and distal struts to aid accurate placement.

All stents come in a range of diameters and lengths to suit their use in different-sized vessels and different lesion lengths. Placement of a stent usually requires a larger sheath to allow entry of the stent into the vascular system, though many self-expanding and balloon-mounted stents can now be introduced through 5F to 6F sheaths.

The basic principles of stenting are analogous to those of angioplasty, in the approach to the lesion and use of guidewires and catheters to cross the lesion. If there are difficulties tracking the stent to the lesion, a stiffer guidewire may be required than for balloon angioplasty alone. The size and length of stent are selected for the size of vessel and the length of the lesion. For self-expanding stents the diameter of the stent is usually oversized by 1 to 2 mm, compared to the vessel diameter. Use of fluoroscopic roadmapping techniques help ensure that the stent is appropriately positioned, both prior to and during deployment, but this may require the use of a guiding catheter or catheter positioned from another access site to perform angiography. Many self-expanding stents, as they deploy, move away from the operator. Gentle back traction on the delivery system and continuous screening during deployment should be used to maintain the position of the stent markers. Following deployment of self-expanding stents, balloon dilatation can be used to ensure adequate expansion and apposition to the vessel wall. In some circumstances, for example, small external iliac arteries, ballooning to the desired vessel diameter may not be possible because the patient may experience pain, and there is a risk of arterial rupture. In these circumstances it is prudent to use a self-expanding stent, and in most cases the stent will expand adequately over the next few days with no adverse outcome. As with angioplasty, check angiography with runoff views should be performed.

Atherectomy

As with many new interventions, there was initially much enthusiasm for atherectomy. However, the lack of evidence that the technique was superior to simple balloon treatment for atheromatous disease has meant there is now limited use for this technique. Pending data from newer devices and techniques, the role of atherectomy is mainly limited to removal of neointimal hyperplasia from graft anastomoses or from within stents. Such lesions tend to be elastic and resist balloon angioplasty alone. Stenting is often counterproductive as it may exacerbate the hyperplastic process (at least pending data using new drug-eluting stents in

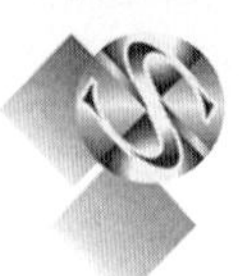

this role). However, the obstructing material can often be removed percutaneously using atherectomy devices.

Stent Grafting

Stent grafts are predominately used in the domain of aneurysmal disease. They have been advocated as an alternative to angioplasty and/or stenting for occlusive disease, often as a form of endovascular bypass procedure. As yet the technique has not shown superior effectiveness compared to angioplasty or conventional stenting in the iliac arteries, and studies on their use for long occlusions elsewhere are ongoing.

Thrombolysis/Thrombectomy

Thrombolysis may be considered if there is acute critical limb ischemia due to thrombosis. Thrombolytic agents have the potential to break down the clot, restore perfusion, and reveal the underlying abnormality that led to thrombosis in the first instance. The thrombolytic agents with which there is most experience for peripheral use for limb ischemia are recombinant tissue-type plasminogen activator (rtPA), streptokinase, and urokinase. Urokinase was withdrawn for some time, but has recently been returned to commercial availability.

Thrombolysis is indicated only if there is critical limb ischemia, and only then if the limb is salvageable, there is sufficient time for lysis to be instigated, and there are no contraindications to giving lytic agents. Its use is usually limited to the following clinical situations:

- Graft thromboses
- Native vessel thromboses
- Thrombosed popliteal aneurysm with occluded runoff

In general terms the fresher the thrombus, the more likely the thrombolysis is to be successful. Many clinicians do not consider thrombolysis if the thrombus is more than 2 weeks old, based partly on the STILE trial data that suggested that surgery is associated with a better outcome for more chronic ischemia (Weaver et al. 1996).

When considering thrombolysis, access should be as close as possible to the thrombosed segment. This may mean performing a preliminary ultrasound to identify the upper extent of clot if a distal graft or the SFA is thrombosed, to ensure ipsilateral access is possible. This allows easy access to the thrombus and aids adjunctive procedures such as angioplasty or thromboaspiration if necessary. Use of a single arterial wall puncture technique is preferred, and once access is achieved the guidewire traversal test should be performed. If the wire does not pass through the thrombus, the success rate for thrombolysis is reduced, as the thrombus is likely to be organized. A catheter and/or infusion-type wire should be placed through the thrombus and lytic agents delivered into the thrombus. If the catheter is positioned above the thrombosed segment, lytic agents are usually carried away by collaterals and the only lytic effect will be systemic. A number of infusion techniques are available; the most commonly used is bolus lacing of the thrombus (e.g., 5 mg of rtPA or 100,000 to 250,000 units of urokinase) followed by a low-dose (e.g., 0.5 mg/h of rtPA, or 10,000 units/h urokinase) infusion of lytic agent with the catheter embedded in the proximal extent of the thrombosed segment. There is no evidence that a high-dose technique (e.g., 5 mg/h of rtPA) or pulse spray techniques improve outcomes. However, it may be necessary to use these techniques if the degree of ischemia does not allow time for a low-dose approach, because although they are labor intensive, they do achieve lysis more quickly.

The catheter and sheath should be secured using a suture to minimize the risk of displacement. Loss of the sheath at the groin may result in hemorrhage, and if the catheter is pulled back, the effectiveness of the lytic infusion will be lost. Patients undergoing lysis are in danger of a number of complications, predominantly those of hemorrhage and the effects of reperfusion injury, and should be monitored in a high-dependency area. Analgesia should be given IV and the amount required reviewed regularly, as reperfusion injury may also cause pain. The effect of the lytic regime is checked angiographically after an appropriate period, and if necessary the catheter position changed and lysis continued. If there has been no effect after a reasonable period, then lysis is deemed to have failed and alternative surgical strategies may be considered. Complications may lead to the procedure being abandoned. If the thrombus

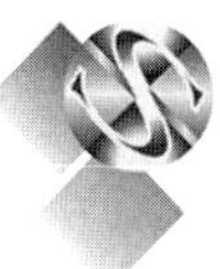

clears, partially or completely, then adjunctive endovascular or surgical treatment may still be necessary.

There is usually an underlying cause for graft or vessel thrombosis, and to maintain patency these should be treated immediately after they are revealed, usually with angioplasty and/or stenting. If clot clearance is only partial, it may be appropriate to attempt percutaneous thrombectomy. This can be simple aspiration of clot using a large-caliber catheter through a removable hemostatic valve, or using specialized mechanical thrombectomy devices such as the Amplatz Thrombectomy Device (Microvena, White Bear Lake, MN) or the Hydrolyser (Cordis). Mechanical thrombectomy devices macerate the thrombus, with the residue either aspirated or small enough to pass through the capillary circulation. Surgical intervention may be required even if lysis is apparently successful, for example, fasciotomy for reperfusion effects, though more commonly it is needed if lysis is only partially successful, with treatments such as graft revision or surgical thrombectomy.

Endovascular Techniques for Aneurysmal Disease

The aim of stent grafting is to line the aneurysm and adjacent normal arterial segments with graft material, therefore excluding the aneurysmal segment. There are now many commercially produced devices, manufactured using a variety of stent and graft materials, usually as a fully supported device with a metal frame covered by graft material.

Much of the focus in recent years has been on the use of stent grafts to treat abdominal aortic aneurysms (AAAs). In these circumstances, special modular bifurcated devices are the most frequently used to exclude the aneurysmal infrarenal aorta and allow flow into both iliac arteries. As with any stent graft procedure, it is necessary to have a segment of normal-caliber vessel above and below the aneurysm to anchor the device and produce exclusion of the sac from pressure (and preferably flow as well). Initially, only about 5% of infrarenal AAAs could be treated with this technique, but this expanded to 25% to 30% of infrarenal AAAs with the advent of bifurcated and aorto-uniiliac

grafts. At the present time, 50% or more of infrarenal AAAs fulfill the necessary criteria to allow stent grafting depending on device availability and the criteria applied for iliac access and sealing. Common reasons for unsuitability are an inadequate aortic "neck" below the renal arteries; poor access, with small-caliber or tortuous iliac arteries; and extensive iliac aneurysmal disease. To some extent, problems with iliac access can be dealt with by using iliac or iliac–femoral conduits, but this diminishes some of the advantages with regard to morbidity and recovery time. Extensive iliac aneurysmal disease can also be handled by coiling or covering the internal iliac arteries, but this is not without some risk of added morbidity compared to standard endovascular repair. Although undoubtedly a feasible technique with good short-term outcomes, concerns about the long-term results, especially the durability of the devices, mean that patients require lifelong surveillance, and in the United Kingdom the technique is offered only as part of an ongoing study. Lifelong surveillance and participation in organized data collection or a clinical trial are also recommended in the U.S., but commercial use of stent grafts for endovascular aneurysm repair has been accepted in most parts of the country following Food and Drug Administration (FDA) approval of the first devices in 1999.

Although most commonly applied to infrarenal AAAs, stent grafts can be used for a number of other applications: to exclude an aneurysmal section of a single vessel such as the iliac artery or the thoracic aorta; to treat vessel rupture, including partial aortic transection following deceleration injury, or iatrogenic rupture from balloon angioplasty; and to treat the acute ischemic complications of thoracic aortic dissection. In the case of thoracic aortic dissection, this is achieved by stent grafting the true lumen covering the entry tear, which usually lies just beyond the origin of the left subclavian artery. As a result there is a shift of blood flow from the false to the true lumen and a resolution of many of the ischemic complications that frequently occur due to compression of the true lumen by a high-pressure false lumen. Although coverage of the entry tear achieves the acute objectives, stable long-term fixation of the device should be in the normal aorta proximal and distal to the dissection to prevent erosion of the device

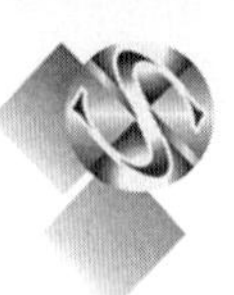

through the weakened segment of the aortic wall. Treatment of acute dissections requires a thorough understanding of the physiology related to flow in the false lumen, and may require adjunctive techniques such as balloon fenestration of the dissection distally or stenting of branch vessels.

The endovascular techniques used during stent grafting are essentially those of stenting generally. Devices are sized in terms of length and diameters to ensure adequate anchorage and to produce a seal proximally and distally and to cover the aneurysmal section of vessel, according to manufacturer guidelines. Appropriate selection of patient anatomy, device type, device diameter, and length are all crucial to the success of the procedure (Broeders et al., 1997; Fillinger, 1999; Wyers et al., 2003). Being large, most stent graft devices have to be introduced through an arterial cutdown at the groin, although recently the successful use of arterial closure devices for total percutaneous repair have been described. Also, as the devices are often bulky and fairly rigid, very stiff guidewires, such as the Amplatz Superstiff, Lunderquist (Cook Inc., Bloomington, IN) or Meier (Boston Scientific, Boston, MA), are used to facilitate tracking of the device into position for deployment (Fillinger, 1999; Wyers et al., 2003). Accurate deployment is vital to ensure that renal or internal iliac arteries are not inadvertently covered by the graft material, and this usually requires adjusting the gantry angle for the aortic neck angle. Deployment for most systems involves the unsheathing of the device, but deployment mechanisms may include self-expansion (e.g., Medtronic AneuRx or Talent), a release mechanism for a self-expanding device (e.g., Gore Excluder), a combination of these (e.g., Cook Zenith), or balloon expansion after retraction of the sheath (e.g., Edwards Lifepath). Most devices require adjunctive or optional balloon inflation to seat the device within the vessel. In part this is because hooks or some other attachment device may be present to help anchor the proximal or distal stents. For modular devices, the different parts are deployed separately, reducing the size of the individual delivery systems.

At completion, angiography is performed to ensure that there is no evidence of leak into the aneurysm sac. The key for completion angiography is to confirm the absence of type I (attachment site) or type III (stent-graft junction) endoleaks, which are the most dangerous and should be treated prior to leaving the endovascular suite if at all possible. Type IV "graft porosity" endoleaks should seal spontaneously in 24 hours, and type II [lumbar artery or inferior mesenteric artery (IMA) branch] endoleaks usually seal spontaneously as well, over a period of weeks to months. Care should be taken not to assume that the endoleak is a more benign variety, but to confirm the source prior to removing guidewires and catheters. Confirmation may require maneuvers such as retrograde injection near the distal end point, injection within the graft at the location of a modular junction, or other techniques.

Following endovascular aneurysm repair (EVAR) it is essential that adequate imaging surveillance be performed, as set out in Chapter 4. This should enable late complications to be detected with a view to appropriate treatments, as necessary, whether by endovascular or conventional surgical means.

Embolotherapy

Embolization techniques involve the deliberate blocking of blood vessels. This may be necessary to stop arterial hemorrhage, to exclude an aneurysm or pseudoaneurysm, to occlude a branch vessel that may contribute to an "endoleak" as part of endovascular aneurysm repair, or to treat vascular tumors and arteriovenous malformations. It is beyond the scope of this chapter to describe the use of embolization in detail for all these indications, but some general principles and techniques are described.

In all cases of embolization there are four main considerations:

- What is the anatomy?
- What needs embolizing?
- What embolic material should be used?
- Maintain patient safety.

Usually noninvasive testing or the clinical scenario will indicate the likely answers to the above considerations. However, an understanding and knowledge of the vascular anatomy is vital. This can usually be helped by high-quality angiography, which should be performed before embolization begins, during embolization as flow dynamics may change, and at completion.

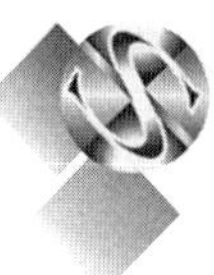

Once the anatomy becomes clear, then the target for embolization should also become clear. It may be a whole vascular bed or a single inflow vessel. The type of embolic material is dictated by the embolization site and whether permanent or temporary occlusion is required. During embolization procedures, a separate trolley should be used for the preparation of the embolization material. In addition, to avoid accidental injection of the material, all contaminated syringes, contrast, and saline should be discarded and replaced.

Before starting, consideration should be given to the approach to the embolization site. The shortest, straightest route is usually the best. Preliminary angiography may reveal the need for equipment, such as guiding catheters or microcatheters. Single end-hole catheters should always be used, and a guide catheter may be used to help ensure that a stable catheter position is achieved. When embolizing, always consider the effects of collaterals, as they may carry embolic material away from their target and damage normal tissues, in which case the catheter position needs to be closer to the target. When embolizing a vessel that is not an end artery, it is important to "close the back door" to prevent potential back-filling once the entry vessel is occluded. If this is not done, then a lesion will not have been effectively treated, and as the "front door" has been closed, further access for embolization will be impossible.

The main embolic agents to choose from are the following:

Particles: for example, Gelfoam, polyvinyl alcohol (PVA) microspheres

Mechanical devices: for example, coils and balloons

Liquids: for example, sclerosants, glues

When particles are injected they flow into distal vessels, occluding the vessels according to the age of the particles used. Correct selection of the size of the particles is important; small particles may pass through a lesion, causing undesirable embolization, whereas large particles may not successfully occlude the vascular bed. Gelfoam is a temporary embolic material, most commonly used by cutting up a sheet of Gelfoam into pledgets about 1 mm × 1 mm, that when mixed with contrast can be injected through a conventional catheter. PVA is a permanent embolic agent that comes in a range of

sizes from 150 to 1000 μm in diameter. When injecting particles, it is important to ensure that full stasis is not obtained before all embolic material in the catheter has been injected; otherwise further injection will produce significant reflux. Flush the embolic material mixed with contrast from the catheter with saline, and then it is safe to perform angiography.

Coils are permanent embolic agents that act as a focus for thrombosis within the vessel. They are metallic, but covered by thrombogenic threads. They are best used to occlude a single vessel or number of discrete feeding vessels to isolate a vessel or area of the circulation. Coils come in a variety of sizes. The wire diameter varies from 0.014 to 0.038 inch and is important to consider, as a large gauge will not pass down a small-lumen catheter, such as a microcatheter. Coil length also varies, with shorter coils being most easily managed. The formed coil diameter dictates the size the coil will form in the vessel and should be appropriate for the location being embolized: too small and the coil may migrate; too large and it may not form well in the vessel. Always check the stability of the catheter position prior to deploying the first coil. This is done by advancing the pusher wire to the end of the catheter and ensuring the catheter tip does not recoil or advance. The appropriate wire is stiff enough to push the coil but not so stiff as to dislodge the catheter. A Wholey wire has a straight flexible tip with a prominent radiopaque mark on the tip to distinguish it from the coil being pushed. If this wire is too stiff, a Bentson or other more flexible wire might be preferable. The coil is introduced into the catheter by pressing the coil introducer into the catheter hub and using the appropriate pusher wire to push the coil into the catheter, then out the distal end of the catheter, deploying the coil in the appropriate place.

Liquid agents are permanent agents and the most potent. They have the potential to rapidly produce hemodynamic changes resulting in inadvertent embolization and can be difficult to control in this respect. As such, their use should be limited to those with the most experience. Absolute alcohol causes immediate thrombosis as it enters a vessel. It is the ultimate permanent embolic agent and produces so much pain that patients usually require general anesthesia. Its principal use is for vascular malformations. Glues, such as cyanoacrylate, solidify on contact with ionic substances in blood, and are injected

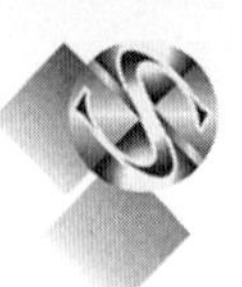

with lipiodol and dextrose solutions to ensure they do not solidify in the catheter. Once again, it is an unforgiving material but can be useful and does not produce the severe pain likely with other liquid agents. In general, liquid agents are best mixed with a contrast agent if they are not already radiodense, so the amount of injection and extent of delivery can be detected under continuous fluoroscopic guidance.

References

Broeders IA, Blankensteijn JD, Olree M, Mali W, Eikelboom BC. (1997) J Endovasc Surg 4:252–61.
Fillinger MF. (1999) Surg Clin North Am 79:451–75.
Weaver FA, Comerota AJ, Youngblood M, Froehlich J, Hosking JD, Papanicolaou G. (1996) J Vasc Surg 24: 513–21.
Wyers MC, Fillinger MF, Schermerhorn ML, et al. (2003) J Vasc Surg 38:730–8.

Index

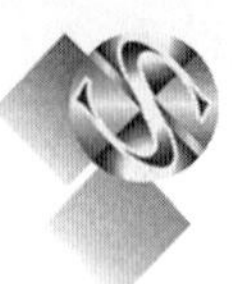

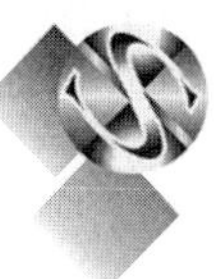

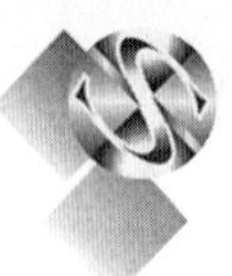

C

Calcitonin gene-related peptide, 74, 78–79
Calcium channel blockers, as Raynaud's
    phenomenon treatment, 76, 77–78
Calf muscle, venous blood pumping function of,
    106–107
Capillaroscopy, 76
Capillary refill test, 13
CAPRIE (Clopidogrel *versus* Aspirin in Patients at
    Risk of Ischemic Events) study, 56, 167
Captopril, 225
Carbon dioxide, as vascular contrast media, 27–28
Cardiac failure, high-output, 145
Cardiovascular disease, as mortality cause, 1
Carotid arteries
    aneurysms of, 218–219
        false, 158
        true, 158, 159
    dissection of, 127, 129, 158–159, 163
    external, in carotid endarterectomy, 171
    internal
        in carotid endarterectomy, 171, 172–173
        elongation and kinking of, 158
        fibromuscular dysplasia of, 158
        occlusive disease of, vertebral artery occlusive
            disease-associated, 189
        thrombosis of, as stroke cause, 156
    proximal common, occlusive disease of, 187–188
    stenosis of, 22, 182
    tortuous, 33, 158
    traumatic injuries to, 127, 160
Carotid artery disease, 155–180
    clinical presentation of, 161–163
    epidemiology of, 155
    investigation of, 164–166
    management of, 166–175
        medical, 166–168
        surgical, 169–175
    pathology of, 157–160
    postoperative management of, 175–179
    prognosis of, 164
    radiological investigations of, 32, 33
Carotid body tumors (CBTs), 32, 160
Carotid bypass, 175
Carotid-subclavian bypass, 187
Carotid surgery, anesthesia in, 69–70
Catheterization
    central venous, 141, 142
    epidural, 66
    equipment for, 237–240
    as vascular injury cause, 126
Catheters, 238–240
    central venous, 141, 142, 143–144, 146–147
    complications related to, 140, 146–147
    for embolotherapy, 251
    flushing of, 101, 147, 239, 240–241
    placement of, 244
    types of, 239–240

CAVATAS study, 180
Cavography, 109
Celiac artery
    aneurysms of, 216
    duplex ultrasound examination of, 234
Cerebral perfusion pressure (CPP), 69
Cervical plexus block, 69, 70
Cervical rib, 76, 185, 187, 217
Charles operation, for lymphedema, 122
Chest, vascular injuries to, 128
Chewing tobacco, as Buerger's disease cause, 86
Cholesterol, hepatic production of, 3
Churg, Jakob, 84
Churg-Strauss syndrome, 84–85
Chylomicrons, 3, 4
Cilostazol (Pletal), 61–62, 95
Claudication
    as amputation cause, 95
    chronic limb ischemia-related, 10
    cystic adventitial disease-related, 88
    exercise testing evaluation of, 20
    innominate artery occlusive disease-related, 181
    intermittent, 60
        drug therapy for, 61–62
        dyslipidemia-related, 58
        effect of smoking cessation on, 2
        exercise programs for, 60
        lower limb ischemia-related, 53, 91, 92–93, 95,
            98
        medical management of, 54
        natural history of, 53
        risk factors for, 55, 58
    of the jaw, 163
    neurogenic, differentiated from vascular
        claudication, 92–93
    thoracic outlet syndrome-related, 186
    upper-limb, 11
    venous, 108
Clinical status, 150–151
Clopidogrel, 56, 166, 167, 241
Clopidogrel *versus* Aspirin in Patients at Risk of
    Ischemic Events (CAPRIE) study, 56
Closure devices, arterial, 25, 26, 242
Clotting disorders. *See* Coagulation disorders
Coagulation cascade, 42
Coagulation disorders
    acquired, 46–47
    complications related to, 139–140
    inherited, 42–46
Cogan's syndrome, 81–82
Coils, embolic, 251
Colic artery, aneurysms of, 217
Colonic ischemia, postoperative, 202, 206
Colonoscopy, 202
Colorectal cancer, mortality rate in, 54
Common femoral artery, orthopedic surgery-related
    injuries to, 126
Compartment pressures, measurement of, 103

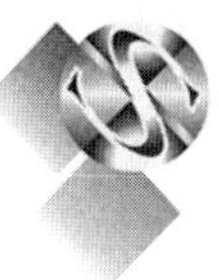

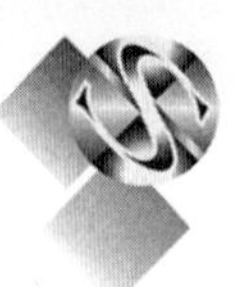

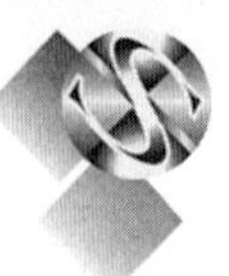

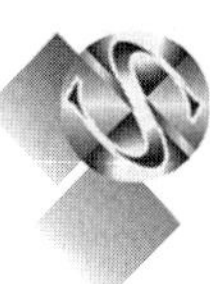

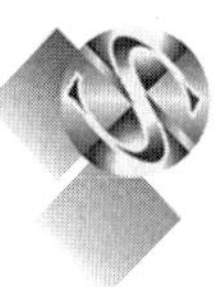

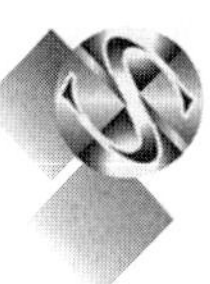

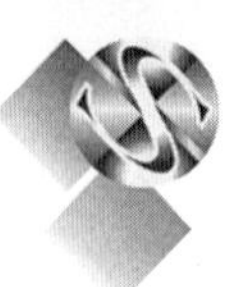